GENERAL PRACTICE PSYCHIATRY

EDITED BY
GRANT BLASHKI
FIONA JUDD
LEON PITERMAN

The McGraw·Hill Companies

Sydney New York San Francisco Auckland
Bangkok Bogotá Caracas Hong Kong
Kuala Lumpur Lisbon London Madrid
Mexico City Milan New Delhi San Juan
Seoul Singapore Taipei Toronto

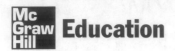

First published 2007

National Library of Australia Cataloguing-in-Publication data:
General practice psychiatry.
Bibliography.
Includes index.
ISBN 0 074 71351 5.
1. Mental illness. 2. Family medicine – Australia.
3. Psychiatry – Australia. I. Blashki, Grant, 1967– .
II. Judd, Fiona K. III. Piterman, Leon, 1947– .
616.89075

Published in Australia by
McGraw-Hill Australia Pty Ltd
Level 2, 82 Waterloo Road, North Ryde NSW 2113
Publisher: Nicole Meehan
Production Editor: Catherine Day
Editor: Sarah Baker
Permissions Editor: Jared Dunn
Proofreader: Kerry Brown
Indexer: Max McMaster
Internal design: Jennifer Pace Walter
Cover design: Jan Schmoeger, Designpoint
Cover image: Photolibrary
Illustrator: Alan Laver, Shelly Communications
Typeset in Berkeley by Jennifer Pace Walter
Printed on 80 gsm woodfree by RR Donnelley, China

FOREWORD

Increasingly, policymakers worldwide are recognising that general practitioners (GPs) and a growing number of other primary care professionals (PCPs) are not only the first port of call for most people experiencing mental illness in the community but also the main providers of care for those experiencing non-psychotic illnesses and significant providers of care for those with psychotic illness. Primary care is also the best setting in which to assess and understand the varied presentations of mental illnesses in the community, which often comprise a mixture of psychological symptoms, physical symptoms, physical comorbidities and substance abuse. Australia is at the forefront of raising public awareness of these issues as well as supporting and training GPs through a range of initiatives, such as the highly successful *beyondblue* campaign and the Better Outcomes in Mental Health Care program, with which the authors of this book have been involved.

Through their successful Masters of General Practice Psychiatry and numerous short courses, the editors Grant Blashki, Leon Piterman and Fiona Judd have a long track record of delivering GP-friendly mental health training to GPs. To my knowledge, this is the first general practice psychiatry book where each chapter has been co-developed by GPs in collaboration with mental health experts who have substantial experience working with and training GPs. In this way the GP perspective is strongly emphasised. In addition to this impressive collaborative process, the format of each chapter reflects a commonsense GP approach to mental illness: most chapters start with a case history, followed by a summary of the key points and practical advice on assessment and management. This mirrors the best of liaison consultation methods for face-to-face supervision and learning.

Having long been concerned about the wellbeing of GPs, who spend a huge part of their day listening to their patients' problems without any systematic support or supervision, I am very pleased to see a special chapter dedicated to GP self-care. The editors recognise that GPs are not immune to stress and mental illness, and are often reluctant to seek proper care for themselves. I have not seen this topic covered in such a book before.

General Practice Psychiatry covers common psychiatric conditions, providing a clinical approach for different age groups and cultural groups as well as specific advice on both medico-legal issues and the proper use of psychometric tools. The latter chapter would be of use to English GPs, who are now rewarded for using self-report patient scales to assess baseline severity of depression.

Although *General Practice Psychiatry* is designed primarily for an Australian readership (comprising GPs, medical students who are seeking a community approach to psychiatry, and specialists working at the primary care interface), I think it could be of use to other primary care professionals as well as GPs and PCPs in other countries.

I wholeheartedly recommend this text and fully expect it to become a recognised key text in primary care psychiatry.

André Tylee
Professor of Primary Care Mental Health
Institute of Psychiatry
Kings College
London, United Kingdom

CONTENTS

PREFACE

Worldwide, the impact of mental illnesses on individuals, their families and communities is enormous. The scale of the problem means that any attempt to improve the situation through public health measures will involve the primary health sector and necessarily involve general practitioners (GPs).

At the same time it is not simply a matter of imparting specialist psychiatric skills to GPs. The clinical setting of general practice has unique attributes that impact significantly on the provision of mental health care—the longstanding relationships with patients and their families, the intense time pressures and the multiple health care roles GPs are expected to fulfil.

We have endeavoured to provide a practical perspective to psychiatric care in general practice by involving GPs at all levels of the book's development. Each chapter has had input from a GP and specialist mental health care providers who work closely with GPs as consultants or who have provided training to GPs. This is an example of the interdisciplinary collaboration that we believe is necessary for effective primary mental health care.

The overall approach of the book and the structure of individual chapters reflect a GP-centred perspective. Chapters include case studies and key points that are designed so that readers can quickly overview the main points of a subject. Context is critical in providing mental health care and the first section of the book explores cultural, legal and consumer and carer issues. We recognise that GPs are not immune from mental illness and are pleased to present a chapter dedicated to GP self-care.

Whilst the book can be read from start to finish, we expect that most readers will select areas of relevance to their clinical work, based on specific conditions or particular age groups. For those involved in teaching, the case studies in each chapter can provide a basis for discussion.

Creating this book has been a team effort. We express our sincere appreciation to all the contributors for sharing their expertise. Thank you to Ms Sue Whyte and Dr Lisa Ciechomski for their assistance throughout the editing process. We also express our appreciation to McGraw-Hill for its support and in particular to Ms Catherine Day, who worked tirelessly to bring the book to completion.

At this time we are seeing unprecedented reforms of our mental health care system and clearly GPs will continue to have an important role to play. We hope that this book will be of assistance to GPs, medical students and specialists who work at the interface between primary and specialist mental health care, and that it will ultimately lead to better care for all those who experience mental illness.

Sincerely
Grant Blashki, Fiona Judd and Leon Piterman

ABOUT THE EDITORS

Grant Blashki (MD, MBBS, FRACGP) is a practising GP, a Fellow of the Royal Australian College of General Practitioners and a Senior Lecturer at Monash University (honorary), University of Melbourne and Kings College London (honorary). He has a strong commitment to improving mental health care in primary care settings and has written over 40 peer reviewed publications as well as undertaken numerous research projects relating to this field. For over a decade he has worked closely with Professor Fiona Judd and Professor Leon Piterman, developing general practitioner training in psychiatry, including national and international conferences and developing a Masters of General Practice Psychiatry. He has been particularly inspired by his father Dr Tim Blashki, who undertook pioneering general practice psychiatry research in the late 1960s.

    Fiona Judd (MD, DPM, FRANZCP) is Professor of Rural Mental Health, School of Psychology, Psychiatry and Psychological Medicine at Monash University. Her interest in general practice psychiatry was kindled when working with Professor Brian Davies, the Foundation Professor of Psychiatry at the University of Melbourne, who emphasised in clinical work, teaching and research the key role played by general practitioners in the care of people with mental health problems and mental illness. Between 1986 and 1995 Dr Judd worked with Professor Graham Burrows in the organisation and delivery of the University of Melbourne's annual continuing education program, Psychiatry for Non-Psychiatrists. Subsequently, together with Leon Piterman and Grant Blashki, she was responsible for developing the General Practice Psychiatry Program, a joint initiative of the University of Melbourne and Monash University departments of Psychiatry and General Practice. Her other academwic interests are in medical workforce, anxiety and depression, rural mental health and help-seeking behaviours by those with mental health problems.

    Leon Piterman (AM, MMEd, MedSt, MRCP, FRACGP) is Professor of General Practice, Head of the School of Primary Health Care and Senior Deputy Dean of the Faculty of Medicine, Nursing and Health Sciences at Monash University. Having graduated in 1971 from the University of Melbourne, after a number of residency posts in Melbourne and London, he combined clinical general practice with a part-time academic career at Monash until 1993, when he took up the post of Director of Graduate Studies in the Department of General Practice. He is responsible for establishing Australia's largest and most successful university based Diploma/Masters in Family Medicine for general practitioners. This program has produced over 1000 graduates nationally and internationally. In 1996, along with Fiona Judd and Grant Blashki, he was responsible for establishing the General Practice Psychiatry Program, which led to the development of the Graduate Certificate and Masters in General Practice Psychiatry and laid the foundations for research in Primary Care Mental Health at Monash University. His other academic interests are in medical education, cardiovascular disease and chronic disease management.

THE CONTRIBUTORS

John Arranga MBBS, LLB, FACLM
Senior Claims Executive,
Medical Defence Association of Victoria,
Australia

Pamela Te Ara Bennett, BSc, MBChB, FRANZCP
Senior Lecturer
Te Kupenga Hauora Maori
(Department of Maori Health)
Faculty of Medical and Health Sciences
University of Auckland, New Zealand

Jo Buchanan
Australia

Nick Carr MA, MMed, MB, BChir, DCH, MRCGP, FRACGP
General Practitioner, Australia

Andrew Chanen MBBS, BMedSc, MPM, FRANZCP
Senior Lecturer,
ORYGEN Research Centre,
Department of Psychiatry,
The University of Melbourne;
Consultant Psychiatrist and Associate
Medical Director,
ORYGEN Youth Health,
Melbourne, Australia

Anthony M Cichello MPsych (Clin), BSc (Hons), MAPS
Senior Clinical Psychologist,
Centre for Rural Mental Health, Bendigo;
Clinical Psychologist, Australia

Lisa Ciechomski BA, GradDipEdPsych, MPsych, PhD
Psychologist and Research Fellow,
Department of General Practice,
Monash University, Melbourne, Australia

David M Clarke MBBS, MPM, PhD, FRACGP, FRANZCP
Associate Professor,
Department of Psychological Medicine,
Monash University, Melbourne;
Consultant Psychiatrist,
Monash Medical Centre,
Melbourne, Australia

Leanna Darvall LLB, PhD
Barrister and solicitor,
Supreme Court of Victoria;
Convenor,
Monash Medical Law Tutorial Program,
Faculty of Medicine, Nursing and
Health Sciences,
Monash University, Melbourne, Australia

Julian Davis MBBS, DGM, MPM, FRANZCP
Honorary Clinical Associate Professor,
School of Psychology, Psychiatry and
Psychological Medicine,
Monash University, Melbourne;
Consultant Psychiatrist,
Eating Disorders Services,
Bendigo Health Care Group,
Victoria, Australia

Maria Teresa Dawson BA, MA, PhD, MPH
Senior Project and Policy Coordinator
Health Issues Centre,
Melbourne, Australia

Steve R Ellen MBBS, MMed (Psych), MD, FRANZCP
Head, Consultation Liaison Psychiatry,
The Alfred Hospital, Melbourne;
Senior Lecturer,
Department of Psychological Medicine,
Monash University, Melbourne, Australia

Alan Gijsbers MBBS, FRACP, FAChAM, DTM&H, PGDipEpi
Medical Director,
Drug and Alcohol Liaison Service,
Royal Melbourne Hospital;
Medical Director,
Substance Withdrawal Unit,
The Melbourne Clinic, Australia

Dagmar Haller MD, PhD, GradDipAdolHealth
Academic GP,
Department of Community Medicine,
Geneva University Hospital, Switzerland;
Honorary Fellow,
Department of General Practice,
The University of Melbourne, Australia

Craig Hassed MBBS, FRACGP
Senior Lecturer,
Department of General Practice,
Monash University, Melbourne, Australia

Kelsey Hegarty MBBS, FRACGP, DipRACOG, PhD
Associate Professor,
Department of General Practice,
The University of Melbourne, Australia

Ian Bernard Hickie AM, MD, FRANZCP
Executive Director,
Brain and Mind Research Institute,
Sydney;
Professor of Psychiatry,
The University of Sydney, Australia

Barbara Hocking BSc (Hons), DipEd, DipHEd, GAICD
Executive Director,
SANE Australia, Melbourne, Australia

Gene Hodgins BA (Hons), DPsych (Clin), MAPS
Lecturer in Psychology,
School of Humanities and Social Sciences,
Charles Sturt University, Wagga Wagga;
Clinical Psychologist, Australia

Carol Hulbert, PhD
Senior Lecturer,
School of Behavioural Science,
The University of Melbourne;
Convenor,
Postgraduate Clinical Psychology Program,
The University of Melbourne, Australia

Leah Kaminsky MBBS, BA (Lit), Dip Prof Writing
General Practitioner, Australia

Nicholas Keks MBBS, MPM, PhD, FRANZCP
Professor of Psychiatry,
Monash University, Melbourne;
Mental Health Research Institute,
Delmont Hospital, Melbourne, Australia

Litza Kiropoulos BEdSc, BSc (Hons) Psych, MClinPsych, PhD
Senior Lecturer and Senior Research Fellow,
Department of General Practice,
Monash University, Melbourne, Australia

Steven Klimidis BSc (Hons) Psych, PhD (ClinPsych)
Associate Professor and Research Coordinator,
Centre for International Mental Health,
The University of Melbourne and
Victorian Transcultural Psychiatry Unit,
Melbourne, Australia

Michael Kyrios BA, DipEdPsych, MPsych, PhD, MAPS
Professor of Psychology,
Swinburne University of Technology;
Director,
Swin-PsyCHE Research Unit,
Melbourne, Australia

Anthony Love BA (Hons), MA (ClinPsych), DipEd, PhD, MAPS
Senior Lecturer
School of Psychological Science,
La Trobe University, Bundoora, Australia

Helen Malcolm MBBS, GradCertGPPsych, FRACGP, FACPsychMed
Senior Lecturer in Rural Medical Practice,
Rural Clinical School,
University of Tasmania, Australia

Jane H McKendrick MBBS, DPM, MD
Associate Professor,
Te Kupenga Hauora Maori
(Department of Maori Health),
Faculty of Medical and Health Sciences,
University of Auckland, New Zealand

Richard McLean
Australia

Pam McQueen MBBS, BSc (Med)
General Practitioner (retired), Australia

Graham Meadows MD, MPhil, MBChB, MRCP, MRCPsych, FRANZCP
Professor of Adult Psychiatry,
Monash University, Melbourne;
Director,
Southern Synergy,
The Sourthern Health Adult Psychiatry
Research, Training and Evaluation Centre,
Dandenong Hospital, Victoria, Australia

Michelle Menzel BSc (Hons), DPsych (Clin)
Senior Clinical Psychologist,
LCSM Eating Disorders Service,
Bendigo Health Care Group;
Senior Lecturer,
Department of Psychological Medicine,
Monash University, Melbourne, Australia

David Monash BMSc, MBBS, MastGPP, MastFM, FRACGP, FACRRM
Rural General Practitioner, Australia

Benny Monheit MBBS, MPH, FAChAM
Honorary Senior Lecturer,
Department of General Practice,
Monash University, Melbourne;
Addiction Medicine Consultant,
Southcity Clinic, Melbourne, Australia

Paul Nisselle AM, MBBS, MHlth&MedLaw, FRACGP
Senior Advisor, Risk Management,
Medical Defence Association of
Victoria, Australia

Trevor R Norman BSc (Hons), PhD
Associate Professor,
Department of Psychiatry,
The University of Melbourne, Australia

Richard O'Bryan MBBS, MGP Psych (Clin)
General Practitioner, Australia

Daniel O'Connor MD, FRANZCP
Professor of Old Age Psychiatry,
Monash University, Melbourne;
Director,
Aged Persons Mental Health Service,
Southern Health, Melbourne, Australia

**George C Patton MBBS, MD,
FRANZCP, MRCPsych**
VicHealth Professor/Director of
Adolescent Health Research,
Centre for Adolescent Health,
Royal Children's Hospital;
Murdoch Childrens Research Institute,
The University of Melbourne, Australia

**David Pierce MBBS, MGPPsych,
MMed, FRACGP, FACPsychMed,
Dip RACOG**
Research Fellow,
Department of General Practice;
Senior Lecturer,
School of Rural Health,
The University of Melbourne, Australia

**Hannah Piterman PhD, MEc,
BEc (Hons)**
Honorary Associate Professor,
Monash Institute of Health Services
Research,
Monash University, Melbourne;
Director,
Hannah Piterman Consulting,
Melbourne, Australia

Lena Sanci MBBS, PhD, FRACGP
Senior Lecturer,
Department of General Practice,
The University of Melbourne, Australia

**Andrew Stocky MBBS, MPM,
FRANZCP, MRACMA, GAICD**
Consultant Psychiatrist, Australia

**Bruce Tonge MD, DPM, MRCPsych,
FRANZCP, CertChildPsych RANZCP**
Professor of Psychological Medicine and
Head,
School of Psychology, Psychiatry and
Psychological Medicine,
Monash Medical Centre, Melbourne;
Clinical Advisor,
Southern Health MHP,
Melbourne, Australia

**Alasdair Vance MBBS, MMed, MD,
FRANZCP, Cert ACC Child Psychiatry,
LMusA**
Head Academic Child Psychiatry,
Department of Paediatrics,
The University of Melbourne,
Royal Children's Hospital,
Melbourne, Australia

**Kay Wilhelm AM, MBBS, MD,
FRANZCP**
Conjoint Associate Professor,
School of Psychiatry,
Faculty of Medicine,
The University of New South Wales;
Clinical Director,
Consultation Liaison Psychiatry,
St Vincent's Hospital, Sydney, Australia

CHAPTER 1
GENERAL PRACTICE PSYCHIATRY

F Judd, G Blashki and L Piterman

Goldberg's research has made it clear that mental disorder is so common that, no country, however rich it might be, can afford anything approaching sufficient specialist personnel to see and care for everyone with a mental disorder. Rather, most people with mental disorders will need to be seen and cared for by members of the primary health care unit…

R JENKINS, *1999*[1]

CASE STUDY

Leila is a 33-year-old mother of two young children who presents to surgery on a busy Monday morning with her active three-year-old, just 'to pick up a script' for the sleeping tablets your colleague prescribed for her two weeks ago. A brief history reveals two months of withdrawal from usual activities, occasional panic attacks, a persistent neck ache and spontaneous teariness, none of which has been relieved by either vitamins from the health food shop, or the three glasses of wine she's been drinking at night to settle herself. While her three-year-old proceeds to destroy your sphygmomanometer, and the computer software reminds you that her Pap smear is overdue, she asks if you could bulk bill today as she's had a falling out with her boss and has lost her job. As you begin to juggle the priorities in your mind for the remainder of the consultation, your receptionist beeps you to remind you that you are running late. Welcome to general practice psychiatry.

- General practitioners (GPs) are uniquely placed to work within the biopsychosocial model.

- GPs manage a broad spectrum of mental health problems and mental disorders, as well as 'normal' reactions to a range of stressors and traumas.

- Approximately 1 in 5 adults in the general population suffers from an anxiety, mood or substance use disorder.

- Approximately 1 in 7 children and adolescents have mental health problems.

- In the community many people with a mental disorder do not seek or receive help.

- Most people with a mental disorder seek treatment from their GP; very few are seen by specialist mental health services.

- Approximately 25% of patients seen by GPs have a mental disorder.

- Between one quarter and half of all patients with a mental disorder who are seen by a GP are not diagnosed for that mental disorder.

- Five of the ten leading causes of disability worldwide are mental disorders.

- Comorbidity—either two mental disorders and/or a mix of physical illness and mental disorders—is very common.

- Screening is an effective means of improving detection rates.

- Referral for specialist care should be driven by patient need and the GP's skills, experience and confidence.

INTRODUCTION

GPs conduct more psychiatric consultations than any other group of health care providers. Furthermore, GPs deal with a broad range of consultations, ranging from people before they become cases to those with chronic and severe mental illness. In this chapter we provide an overview of the scope, context and practice of general practice psychiatry.

THE NEED FOR PRIMARY CARE PSYCHIATRY

There are a variety of factors driving the development of primary care psychiatry services (see Figure 1.1). First, epidemiological studies have made it clear that mental disorders are so common that most people who suffer from these disorders will need to be seen and cared for in primary care. This driver for the development of primary care psychiatry has been strengthened by studies demonstrating high levels of unmet need in the community. For example, the Australian National Survey[2] found that only 38% of those with a disorder were seen by any health service provider. Most who sought help consulted their GP.

Over the past two decades, the disability and cost of mental disorders, and thus the importance of reducing the level of unmet need, has become increasingly evident.

The World Bank's Global Burden of Disease project[3] has convincingly demonstrated the importance of mental disorders as a cause of disease burden. Burden is the sum of premature death and years lived with a disability.[4] Mental disorders account for a quarter of the world's disability and 9% of the total burden. In established market economies such as the United States, the United Kingdom and Australia, mental disorders account for 43% of the disability and 22% of the total burden of disease. Five of the ten leading causes of disability worldwide are mental disorders—major depression, alcohol use, bipolar affective disorder, schizophrenia and obsessive-compulsive disorder. In established market economies, harmful drug use is also one of the ten leading causes of disability.

Consistent with the finding that most people who have a mental health problem see a GP, studies have shown that members of the community regard GPs as one of the most helpful sources of professional help for mental health problems.[5] However, there are a range of problems noted by those who seek care from a GP. These include difficulty finding a GP with the time, skill or commitment for mental health service provision, and a sense of not being taken seriously.[6] In addition, the general public has some reservations about the standard of management skills that GPs have in relation to mental illness.[7]

Another factor driving the development of primary care psychiatry has been the changes to mental health service delivery over the past few decades. In particular, there has been a move from institutional to community based care. In Australia, the National Mental Health Strategy, agreed to by all Health Ministers in 1992, heralded substantial change in the design and delivery of mental health services across Australia. Major service restructuring led to reduced reliance on stand-alone psychiatric hospitals, an expansion in the delivery of community based care, integration with acute inpatient care, and the mainstreaming of mental health services with other components of health care. These changes demanded an alteration in the way GPs interacted with psychiatric services, and increased the demand on GPs to care for individuals with mental illness.

FIGURE 1.1 Drivers of primary care psychiatry services

- Prevalence of mental disorders
- Burden of disease
- High levels of unmet need
- Consumer and carer preference
- Deinstutionalisation
- Mainstreaming of mental health service
- High rates of physical and psychiatric comorbidity

GENERAL PRACTICE PSYCHIATRY

It is generally accepted that mental health problems and mental disorders develop as the result of a combination of factors that predispose an individual to illness (underlying vulnerabilities) and precipitate the onset of illness (see Chapter 7). For example, a genetic predisposition (vulnerability) in combination with one or more stressors, such as unemployment, may lead to the onset of a mental disorder; this is called the 'stress-diathesis' model. It is important to note that the same stressor can have different meanings for different individuals. Thus, one person may develop a mental disorder following a stressor while another does not; understanding this difference requires an awareness of the underlying vulnerability (for example, genetic predisposition) and the meaning of the stressor for the individual. The biopsychosocial approach to understanding and treating individuals with mental health problems and mental disorder flows from this aetiological model (see Chapter 7).

GPs are uniquely placed to work in the biopsychosocial paradigm. The GP generally knows the patient, their family and often much about their social network. All too often family and carers report that their knowledge of the patient has not been sought by health providers. This is a lost opportunity, as they are usually a rich source of information that enables a greater understanding of an individual's vulnerability to illness. Often the GP has observed the patient, and those around them, negotiate life stages and developmental tasks, and is aware of any difficulties or traumas that the patient may have experienced. Thus, the GP can readily identify situations where present-day problems rekindle old traumas, and so understand the meaning of what may objectively be minor stressors.

GPs are also well placed to observe and understand the effects of an individual's illness on those around them. This enables the GP to provide or ensure the family has access to information and support. Furthermore, family and carers usually play a key role in a patient's recovery. The GP can readily facilitate and support this (see Chapter 3).

GPs deal with a broad spectrum of mental health problems. These will include normal responses to stress or trauma—for example, death of a loved one or difficulty coping with a diagnosis of a medical illness—that nevertheless may require assistance to prevent the development of a disorder and/or a functional impairment. GPs also see patients with a range of milder mental health problems, sometimes labelled 'sub-threshold' disorders. These frequently require short-term focused interventions to facilitate recovery. Finally, GPs are called upon to assess and manage patients with a range of mental illnesses, sometimes alone and sometimes in collaboration with specialist colleagues (see Chapter 22).

It is generally accepted that patients seen by GPs have a range of problems, 'comorbidity is the rule' and GPs are required to fill a number of roles simultaneously. For example, treating a patient's medical problems, then detecting and managing a depressive illness and attending to their adolescent daughter's drug abuse will require careful management of GP roles. Sometimes, the GP will need to inform the patient about aspects of their role, including any special limitations.

DIAGNOSIS AND CLASSIFICATION IN PSYCHIATRY

The term 'mental disease' was first used in the early years of the nineteenth century, emphasising the view that mental illnesses were diseases of the brain. While the territory of psychiatry is still described as mental illness or mental disorder, these terms now include a much broader range of conditions assumed to result from the complex interplay of biological, psychological and social factors. A commonly accepted definition of mental disorder that reflects this inclusive approach is:

> A clinically significant behavioral or psychological syndrome or pattern that occurs in an individual and that is associated with present distress (e.g. a painful syndrome) or

disability (i.e. impairment in one or more important areas of functioning) or with a significantly increased risk of suffering death, pain, disability, or an important loss of freedom. This syndrome or pattern must not merely be an expectable and culturally sanctioned response to a particular event, for example, the death of a loved one. Whatever its original cause, it must currently be considered a manifestation of a behavioral, psychological, or biological dysfunction in the individual. Neither deviant behavior (e.g. political, religious or sexual) nor conflicts that are primarily between the individual and society are mental disorders unless the deviance or conflict is a symptom of a dysfunction in the individual, as described above.[8]

While there is a diverse range of disorders and conditions in any classification system, the common disorders can be readily grouped into five main categories. These are:

- **Organic mental disorders** The aetiology of these disorders is either a structural brain lesion, a general medical condition, or a substance (for example, drug of abuse, toxin) or a combination of these. This group includes disorders such as dementia, delirium and amnestic disorders.
- **Psychotic disorders** This category includes schizophrenia and related disorders.
- **Mood disorders** Such disorders include depression, dysthymia and related disorders as well as bipolar disorder. When psychotic symptoms occur as part of a severe mood disturbance they are regarded as part of the spectrum of mood disorders.
- **Anxiety and stress related disorders** This group includes extremes of common emotional responses, psychophysiological reactions to stress and the range of anxiety disorders.
- **Personality disorders** These are enduring patterns of perceiving, relating to and thinking about the environment and oneself, exhibited in a wide range of personal and social contexts, which are inflexible and maladaptive, and cause significant impairment or subjective distress.[8]

The diagnostic task for GPs is often not straightforward; patients often present with a mixture of physical and psychological problems, or with sub-threshold syndromes. Nevertheless, making a diagnosis in psychiatry is important. Just as in physical medicine, diagnosis serves several purposes—descriptive, aetiological, therapeutic and prognostic. However, in making a psychiatric diagnosis, the GP is largely dependent on the clinical skills of history taking, mental state assessment and physical examination rather than on laboratory and other special tests (see Chapter 7).

There are two major diagnostic systems in use in psychiatry: one, developed by the American Psychiatric Association, the Diagnostic and Statistical Manual of Mental Disorders, 4th edition (DSM-IV);[8] and the other, developed by the World Health Organization, the International Classification of Diseases, 10th edition (ICD-10).[9] Essentially, these systems rely on grouping together similar psychiatric symptoms and signs and thus describing clinical syndromes (see Table 1.1). Therefore, unlike most diagnoses in physical medicine, diagnoses in psychiatry are symptomatically rather than aetiologically defined.

In the DSM-IV, a multiaxial system of description is used. This is a convenient method for categorising and communicating clinical information. It is commonly used for this purpose by psychiatrists. The axes are as follows:

- **Axis I** Diagnosed mental disorder or disorders.
- **Axis II** Disorders of personality or intellectual disability.
- **Axis III** Comorbid medical problems.
- **Axis IV** Acute stressors operative in the mental illness.
- **Axis V** The level of psychosocial dysfunction.

Summarising these domains of information requires the assessing clinician to look at both the immediate clinical presentation and at factors that are important in treatment planning. Thus, a biopsychosocial assessment can be concisely recorded and communicated, and a comprehensive treatment plan developed.

TABLE 1.1 Summary: current major classifications of psychiatric disorders

DSM-IV	ICD-10
■ Delirium, dementia, amnestic and other cognitive disorders ■ Mental disorders due to a general medical condition	■ Organic, including symptomatic mental disorders
■ Substance related disorders	■ Mental and behavioural disorders due to psychoactive substance use
■ Schizophrenia and other psychotic disorders	■ Schizophrenia, schizotypal and delusional disorders
■ Mood disorders	■ Mood (affective) disorders
■ Anxiety disorders ■ Somatoform disorders ■ Dissociative disorders ■ Adjustment disorders	■ Neurotic, stress related and somatoform disorders
■ Eating disorders ■ Sleep disorders ■ Sexual and gender identity disorders	■ Behavioural syndromes associated with physiological disturbances and physical factors
■ Impulse disorders ■ Factitious disorders ■ Personality disorders	■ Disorders of adult personality and behaviour
■ Disorders usually first diagnosed in infancy, childhood or adolescence	■ Mental retardation ■ Disorders of psychological development ■ Behavioural and emotional disorders with onset usually occurring in childhood and adolescence

REVISITING THE CASE STUDY

After assessing Leila briefly, you see her for a long consultation to further explore her problems. After this visit and after referring to notes of her previous visits, you make a diagnosis of depression with prominent anxiety features. There are multiple contributing factors and treatment will need to address several issues. The five axes from DSM-IV provide a useful way of summarising the situation:

- **Axis I** Major depression—moderately severe, with prominent anxiety (panic attacks) and somatic symptoms (neck ache); intermittent alcohol abuse (self-medicating).
- **Axis II** Problems with assertiveness.
- **Axis III** Lack of attention to preventive health measures.
- **Axis IV** Recent loss of job, financial difficulties; child with behavioural problems; marital conflict (husband cannot understand what is wrong).
- **Axis V** Moderate symptoms, with impairment in functioning, not managing her child at present, social withdrawal and difficulty with housework.

MENTAL ILLNESS IN THE COMMUNITY

Large epidemiological studies from a variety of countries have demonstrated that mental disorders are extremely common. For example, the Australian National Survey of Mental Health and Wellbeing[2] found that just less than 1 in 5 Australian adults (17.7%) had an anxiety, mood or substance use disorder (or more than one of these disorders) in the past year. Similar rates have been found in studies from the UK[10] and the US.[11–13]

In the Australian study, anxiety disorders were the most common: they affected just less than 1 in 10 adults (9.7%); substance use (predominantly alcohol) disorders affected 7.7%; and mood disorders affected 5.8% of adults. All three classes of mental disorder often occurred in persons who also had a chronic physical disorder, with just under half (43%) of those with any mental disorder having a chronic physical disorder. About 1 in 4 persons with an anxiety, mood or substance use disorder also had at least one other disorder—that is, they had two or more different classes of disorder, such as an anxiety and a mood disorder, or an anxiety and a substance use disorder.

A second part to the Australian study specifically examined the 'low prevalence disorders'.[14] This revealed that the prevalence of psychotic disorders in the adult population was 4 to 7 per 1000. Schizophrenia and schizoaffective disorder were the most common disorders identified. Comorbid substance use disorder ('dual diagnosis') complicated the course of the psychotic disorder in a substantial proportion of cases. Thirty per cent reported a history of alcohol abuse, 25% reported cannabis abuse and 13% other substance abuse.

Importantly, the Australian study also examined the prevalence of mental disorders among children and adolescents.[15] The study found 1 in 7 (14%) of children and adolescents in Australia have mental health problems. Among 6- to 12-year-olds the most common problem was attention deficit hyperactivity disorder (ADHD), followed by conduct disorder and depression. In those aged 13–17 years, the frequency of ADHD fell and that of depression increased.

MENTAL ILLNESS IN PRIMARY CARE
FREQUENCY AND DETECTION OF ILLNESS

The extent and nature of mental disorder in primary care settings has been explored using three strategies: identification of psychiatric disturbance by the attending GP;

evaluation of psychiatric 'caseness' by administration of screening instruments; and psychiatric evaluation using a diagnostic interview. Those studies relying on the GP in a primary care setting to identify the prevalence of mental disorders have yielded highly varying rates, from 5% to over 50%.[16] By contrast, studies using screening instruments such as the General Health Questionnaire (GHQ) to assess mental disorder generate prevalence figures of around 40% and those using structured psychiatric interview suggest a prevalence of 20–30%.[17] Overall, studies suggest that approximately 25% of patients in primary care have a mental disorder.

Studies have demonstrated that GPs vary considerably in their ability to detect mental disorders, and in general, they do not recognise a large proportion of these types of health problems. For example, Goldberg and Blackwell[18] found a quarter of patients with mental disorders went undiagnosed, while a World Health Organization multisite study found that about half of the psychological problems of patients were unrecognised.[19]

A variety of factors have been identified as barriers to the recognition and diagnosis of mental illness in primary care, and together they may contribute to the high level of unmet need. These factors include the following:

- Mental disorders are commonly associated with a physical disorder.
- The patient often has multiple presenting symptoms.
- The patient may selectively focus on somatic rather than psychological symptoms of a mental illness.
- The patient may present with physical complaints and a conviction of physical illness—for example, a patient with depression presents with chronic pain, or a patient with anxiety presents with palpitations or nausea.
- The patient's mental disorder may be long-standing, and the symptoms or effects accepted by the patient as 'just the way it is'.
- The patient may have atypical symptoms—for example, depression with overeating and oversleeping.
- The patient may be fearful of the stigma and discrimination.

In addition, studies have identified a range of GP behaviours that may influence the likelihood of detection of mental illness in patients. GP behaviours that increase the likelihood of cues being given by patients about their problems and thus increase the likelihood of detection of problems include: maintenance of eye contact with the patient, attentive posture, use of facilitating words, refraining from interrupting the patient or offering information early in the consultation, and an appearance of not being in a hurry. Cues from patients are reduced by certain GP behaviours such as directed questioning, questions without psychological content and interruptions to the patient's account of their problems early in the consultation.[20]

THE NATURE OF MENTAL ILLNESS

Goldberg and Gournay[21] have suggested that mental disorders encountered in general practice can be practically grouped as follows:

- Severe mental disorders, which tend to be relapsing and/or chronic and disabling. Patients usually require care from both the GP and specialist mental health services (see Chapter 22). The high rate of physical morbidity and premature mortality in patients with the severe mental disorders underscores the need for GPs to address medical and mental disorders.

- Well defined mental disorders for which there are effective psychological and pharmacological therapies—for example, depression and anxiety disorders (see Chapters 8, 9).
- Somatised presentations of distress such as prolonged fatigue, musculoskeletal aches and pains and gastrointestinal symptoms (see Chapter 11). These symptoms are most often associated with a diagnosis of depression or anxiety.
- Transient adjustment disorders, which tend to resolve spontaneously, and for which supportive and/or non-specific interventions such as stress management are usually sufficient.

GPs may assume a variety of roles in the assessment and management of patients with these disorders. In some circumstances, management will be provided predominantly or exclusively by the GP (for example, for transient adjustment disorders) while in others, shared care arrangements with specialist providers will be most appropriate (for example, for those with severe mental disorders).

PSYCHIATRIC EMERGENCIES IN GENERAL PRACTICE

In addition to providing diagnosis and care of acute and chronic illness, GPs may also be called upon to provide emergency care. Emergency presentations may include one or more of the following:

- Suicidal behaviour, which may be manifest as thoughts or intent to harm oneself or an attempt to self-harm. Often, but not always, this is associated with a mental disorder, most often depression (Chapter 8), substance abuse (Chapter 10), psychosis (Chapter 12) or personality disorder (Chapter 18).
- Acute behavioural disturbance—for example, aggression or self-harm resulting from the onset or exacerbation of a psychotic illness (see Chapter 12), an acute organic brain syndrome (delirium) (see Chapter 16), alcohol and/or drug intoxication or withdrawal (see Chapter 10).
- Acute disturbance in those with known chronic psychiatric illness such as psychoses—for example, an individual with persistent paranoid delusions and/or auditory hallucinations (see Chapter 12).
- Difficult or dangerous behaviour to self or others resulting from personality difficulties, or personality disorder (see Chapter 18).

GPs may be required to make a diagnosis, perform a risk assessment, and determine immediate management. The latter may involve a variety of other service providers, including ambulance, police, hospital emergency departments and community mental health teams. However, often the GP is the first person called upon and the person who determines immediate management. Important priorities for the GP include: determining that the presentation is due to a mental illness and not, for example, the result of physical illness or injury; ensuring the safety of the ill person and others; and if appropriate, organising inpatient treatment. The latter may include consideration of the need for compulsory treatment. A working knowledge of the relevant *Mental Health Act* is an important skill in general practice psychiatry (see Chapter 4).

PATHWAYS TO MENTAL HEALTH CARE

An important area for consideration and action by GPs is pathways to care. Most people with a mental illness do not seek or receive effective treatment. This situation has been elegantly described by Goldberg and Huxley[22] in a practical model outlining three distinct populations of subjects with mental illness: people in the community, people seen in primary medical care and people seen by specialist psychiatric services (see Figure 1.2). This model has been depicted as a 'cone of morbidity',[23] which emphasises that most people with mental health problems and mental illness are in the general community or are managed in primary care settings.

Importantly, Goldberg and Huxley identified a series of filters or barriers and enabling factors for passing from one level to the next. These filters provide a focus for understanding the key roles of the GP in the management of people with mental illness. Interventions at three key points (see Figure 1.3) may act to reduce the level of unmet need. Detection of illness is clearly a key step in the pathway to care.

Several strategies have been developed to support developments in primary care psychiatry. Overall these have been directed to three main areas: improved detection of those with a mental illness; support for GPs delivering treatment; and opportunities for appropriate referral—that is, interventions at Goldberg and Huxley's levels 2 to 4. Together, these strategies are designed to facilitate the pathways to care, thereby increasing the likelihood of symptomatic people receive the most effective treatment.

FIGURE 1.2 Cone of morbidity

Level 5	Psychiatric inpatients	People seen by specialist psychiatric services
Level 4	All patients seen by mental health services	
Level 3	Patients with mental illness detected and treated by family doctors	People seen in primary health care services
Level 2	People seen by family doctors	
Level 1	All people in the community with mental health problems and mental illness	The general community

FIGURE 1.3 Key points in the pathway to mental health care

- **HELP SEEKING** Moving from level 1 to level 2 is influenced by factors such as mental health literacy; attitudes of family, friends and the community about mental illness; severity and type of symptoms; and past experience of illness and help seeking.

- **DETECTION OF ILLNESS** Moving from level 2 to level 3 is determined by the doctor's ability to detect mental disorders among their patients, and this in turn is determined by characteristics of both the doctor and the patient.

- **REFERRAL TO SPECIALIST CARE** Moving from level 3 to level 4 will be determined by the nature and severity of the patient's problems as well as the knowledge, skills and confidence of the general practitioner.

IMPROVING DETECTION OF MENTAL DISORDERS

Many individuals with a mental disorder attend their GP for treatment of other problems and/or present with symptoms that are not recognised by the patient and/or the GP as symptoms of a mental illness. In order to progress up the cone of morbidity from level 2 to level 3, a variety of strategies have been suggested and/or implemented in general practice. These include:

- **Screening** The use of screening tools to aid detection is widely debated. Advocates highlight the benefits of early detection and treatment of mental disorder. Commonly used instruments include the Kessler-10 Questionnaire (K-10), the General Health Questionnaire (GHQ) and the Prime-MD. The last is reported to have doubled the detection rate of mental disorder when compared to GP assessment alone.[24] Those who argue against screening highlight the poor specificity of some screening instruments,[25] and high rates of 'false positives' for persons who are in temporary distress or who have significant physical health problems.[26]
- **Structural change** Relatively low patient load and longer than standard consultations are factors associated with improved detection of disorder. In Australia, recent changes to payment arrangements for GPs undertaking mental health assessments have enabled longer interviews and encouraged the use of screening instruments.[27]
- **Education and training** Improved GP training has been advocated as a way of improving recognition skills.[28] Skills based training programs can increase GPs' rates of diagnosing common mental disorders. However, intensive training and ongoing practice support are likely to have more significant effects than less intensive forms of education.[29]

SUPPORT FOR GPs DELIVERING TREATMENT

A variety of models have been developed to help GPs effectively manage mental disorders (see Chapter 22). These generally involve the provision of education to GPs who see patients with mental health problems and can provide direct treatment. They are also supported by opportunities for referral for patients with complex presentations or who do not respond to usual care and so require specialist care. This approach has been clearly articulated in a stepped collaborative care model.[30, 31]

For example, the stepped collaborative care model, developed in Seattle by Katon and colleagues, defines four levels of professional support for managing illness (see Figure 1.4). It allocates intervention resources in a stepwise fashion, which aims to match the intervention to patient preference and clinical need. Such a model also aims to enable effective treatment to be provided to a larger group of people.

This approach defines several key roles for the GP, including making the initial diagnosis, initiating treatment in less complex cases and ensuring overall continuity of care. Other important tasks for the GP, or other members of the primary care psychiatry team, include provision of education to patients, monitoring the adherence to treatment and outcomes, and counselling and support for behaviour change.

Specialist provider roles include the provision of consultation services to GPs when managing more complex cases, collaborative care or co-management of patients in the practice who do not respond to initial treatment provided by the GP, and ongoing speciality care for the most severe and complex cases.

A second development, complementary to and consistent with this, has been the adoption of a chronic disease management model for the treatment of relapsing or chronic mental disorders.[32] This includes components such as proactive care; patient education about signs and symptoms of the illness, treatments and early warning signs that herald relapse; and clear criteria for specialist consultation and/or treatment.

FIGURE 1.4 Stepped collaborative care model

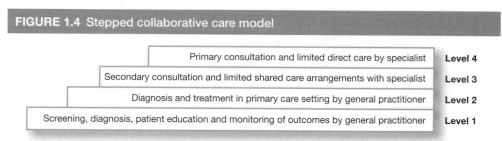

Primary consultation and limited direct care by specialist	**Level 4**
Secondary consultation and limited shared care arrangements with specialist	**Level 3**
Diagnosis and treatment in primary care setting by general practitioner	**Level 2**
Screening, diagnosis, patient education and monitoring of outcomes by general practitioner	**Level 1**

REFERRAL TO SPECIALIST MENTAL HEALTH PROVIDER OR SERVICES

Referral to a specialist provider may thus be made for advice about diagnosis and/ or management or for ongoing treatment. The decision about who should provide treatment and which treatments are most appropriate generally flows from the diagnostic assessment and formulation (see Chapter 7).

In essence, four main considerations should guide the decision to refer: diagnostic difficulty; clinical severity, as judged by symptom severity and disability; response to any treatment already initiated; and the nature of the service to which referral could be made—for example, referral for a particular type of treatment or therapy. It's worth noting that the GP may also refer for advice and/or reassurance that their planned management is appropriate.

REVISITING THE CASE STUDY

Having defined Leila's problems along the five DSM-IV axes, your role as the treating GP is to assess the severity of depression, in particular the level of suicidality, and develop a plan for appropriate intervention. This may involve you working directly with Leila, especially if you feel trained and competent to do so, or it may involve others, particularly if the problem is a major depressive illness. This may take the form of shared care or stepped care, using a local psychiatrist, psychologist and social welfare agencies.

CONCLUSION

General practice psychiatry has now been recognised as a core component of the mental health system. GPs see patients with a broad range of problems in a variety of circumstances. In recognition of this, new resources and supports have been developed in order to help GPs provide effective management to patients and their families/carers. It is hoped that recognition of the importance of the role of GPs, and supporting them so they can fulfill this role, will lead to more people with mental health problems seeking and receiving effective treatments.

REFERENCES

1. Jenkins R. The contribution of David Goldberg: a British perspective. In: Tansella M, Thornicroft G, eds. Common Mental Disorders in Primary Care. Essays in Honour of Professor Sir David Goldberg. London: Routledge, 1999;xvi–xxii.
2. Andrews G, Hall W, Teesson M, Henderson S. The Mental Health of Australians. Canberra: Mental Health Branch, Commonwealth Department of Health and Aged Care, 1999.
3. World Bank. World Development Report 1993: Investing in Health. New York: Oxford University Press, 1993.
4. Murray CJL, Lopez AD, eds. The Global Burden of Disease: A Comprehensive Assessment of Mortality and Disability from Diseases, Injuries and Risk Factors in 1990 and Projected to 2020. Cambridge, MA: Harvard University Press, 1996.
5. Jorm AF, Korten AE, Jacomb PA, Christensen H, Rodgers B, Pollitt P. 'Mental health literacy': a survey of the public's ability to recognise mental disorders and their beliefs about the effectiveness of treatment. Medical Journal of Australia 1997;166:182.
6. McNair BG, Highet NJ, Hickie IB, Davenport TA. Exploring the perspectives of people whose lives have been affected by depression. Medical Journal of Australia 2002;176(20 May 2002): S69–76.
7. Wirthlin Worldwide Australasia. National Mental Health Benchmark. Sydney: Royal Australian College of General Practitioners, 2001.
8. American Psychiatric Association. Diagnostic and Statistical Manual of Mental Disorders. 4th edn. Washington DC: American Psychiatric Association, 1994.
9. World Health Organization. The ICD-10 Classification of Mental and Behavioural Disorders. Geneva: WHO, 1992.
10. Jenkins R, Lewis G, Bebbington P, Brugha T, Farrell M, Gill B, Meltzer H. The national psychiatric morbidity survey of Great Britain—initial findings from the household survey. Psychological Medicine 1997;27:775–89.
11. Robins LN, Helzer JE, Weissman MM, Orvaschel H, Gruenberg E, Burke JD, Regier DA. Lifetime prevalence of specific psychiatric disorders in three sites. Archives of General Psychiatry 1984;41:949–58.
12. Kessler R, McGonagle KA, Zhao S, Nelson CB, Hughes M, Eshleman S, Wittchen H, Kindler KS. Lifetime and 12-month prevalence of DSM-III-R psychiatric disorders in the United States. Archives of General Psychiatry 1994;51:8–19.
13. Kessler RC, Chiu WT, Demler O, Walters EE. Prevalence, severity and comorbidity of 12-month DSM-IV disorders in the National Comorbidity Survey Replication. Archives of General Psychiatry 2005;62:617–27.

14. Jablensky A, McGarth J, Herrman H, Castle D, Gureje O, Morgan V, Korten A. People Living with Psychotic Illness: An Australian Study 1997–1998. Canberra: Mental Health Branch, Commonwealth Department of Health and Aged Care, 1999.
15. Sawyer MG, Arney FM, Baghurst PA, Clark JJ, Graetz BW, Kosky RJ, Nurcombe B, Patton MR, Raphael B, Rey J, Whaites LC, Zubrick SR. The Mental Health of Young People in Australia. Canberra: Mental Health and Special Programs Branch, Commonwealth Department of Health and Aged Care, 2000.
16. Goldberg DP, Lecrubier Y. Form and frequency of mental disorders across centres. In: Ustun TB, Sartorius N, eds. Mental Illness in General Health Care. An International Study. Chichester: Wiley, 1995.
17. Vazquez-Barquero JL, Herran A, Simon JA. Epidemiology of mental disorders in the community and primary care. In: Tansella M, Thornicroft G, eds. Common Mental Disorders in Primary Care. London: Routledge, 1999.
18. Goldberg D, Blackwell B. Psychiatric illness in general practice. A detailed study using a new method of case identification. British Medical Journal 1970;2:439–43.
19. Sartorius N, Ustun B, Costa e Silva J, Goldberg D, Lecrubier Y, Ormel J, Von Korff M, Wittchen H. An international study of psychological problems in primary care. Archives of General Psychiatry 1993;50:819–24.
20. Goldberg DP, Jenkins L, Millar T, Faragher EB. The ability of trainee general practitioners to identify psychological distress among their patients. Psychological Medicine 1993;23:185–93.
21. Goldberg D, Gournay K. The General Practitioner, The Psychiatrist and the Burden of Mental Health Care. Maudsley Discussion Paper No. 1. London: Institute of Psychiatry, 1997.
22. Goldberg D, Huxley P. Mental Illness in the Community. The Pathway to Psychiatric Care. New York: Tavistock Publications, 1980.
23. Henderson S. Conclusion: the central issues. In: Andrews G, Henderson S, eds. Unmet Need in Psychiatry. Problems, Resources, Responses. Cambridge: Cambridge University Press, 2000; 422–8.
24. Spitzer RL, Williams JB, Kroenke K, Linzer M, Verlion deGruy F, Hahn SR, Broady D, Johnson JG. Utility of a new procedure for diagnosing mental disorders in primary care—the PRIME-MD 1000 study. Journal of the American Medical Association 1994;272:1749–56.
25. Leon AC, Olfson M, Weissman MM, Portera L, Fireman BH, Blacklow RS, Hoven C, Broadhead WE. Brief screens for mental disorders in primary care. Journal of General Internal Medicine 1996;11:426–30.
26. McDowell I, Newell C. Measuring Health: A Guide to Rating Scales and Questionnaires. 2nd edn. New York: Oxford University Press, 1996.
27. Hickie I, Groom G. Primary care-led mental health service reform: an outline of the Better Outcomes in Mental Health Care Initiative. Australasian Psychiatry 2002;10:376–82.
28. Kroenke K, Taylor-Vaisey A, Dietrich AJ, Oxman TE. Interventions to improve provider diagnosis and treatment of mental disorders in primary care. A critical review of the literature. Psychosomatics 2000;41(1):39–52.
29. Naismith SL, Hickie IB, Scott EM, Davenport T. Effects of mental health training and clinical audit on general practitioners' management of common mental disorders. Medical Journal of Australia 2001;175:S42–7.
30. Katon W, Von Korff M, Lin E, Walker E, Simon GE, Bush T, Robinson P, Russo J. Collaborative management to achieve treatment guidelines: impact on depression in primary care. Journal of the American Medical Association 1995;273:1026–31.
31. Simon GE, Katon WJ, Von Korff M, Unutzer J, Lin EH, Walker EA, Bush T, Rutter C, Ludman E. Cost-effectiveness of a collaborative care program for primary care patients with persistent depression. American Journal of Psychiatry 2001;158(10):1638–44.
32. Andrews G. Should depression be managed as a chronic disease? British Medical Journal 2001;322:419–21.

CHAPTER 2
GP SELF-CARE

L Piterman, C Hassed and H Piterman

I thought doctors never got sick…   A PATIENT

Physician, heal thyself.   HIPPOCRATES, *c. 460–357* BC

CASE STUDY 1

John is a 68-year-old general practitioner (GP) who has chronic bronchitis and emphysema, a legacy of fifty years of cigarette smoking. Both his father and his brother died of bowel cancer in their early sixties. He has noticed intermittent rectal bleeding for six months but did not refer himself for colonoscopy until he developed abdominal pain. Investigation reveals carcinoma of the sigmoid colon with liver metastases.

CASE STUDY 2

Henry was a 42-year-old GP who had always been a high achiever and the 'life of the party'. In addition to being a partner in a busy general practice, he worked in the emergency department of a rural hospital in the town where he had a holiday residence. He served on numerous medical committees and was active on the local school council and in his old boys football club. Following a car accident, Henry developed headaches that he treated with Codral Forte. His marriage broke down when his wife discovered that he had been having a relationship with one of the clinic staff. Speculative share dealings in health related companies led to financial ruin. He was found dead in his garage from an overdose of codeine, alcohol and carbon monoxide.

- GPs are predisposed to a range of health problems—many of which have their roots in their student years—due to personality characteristics, and cultural and systemic issues.

- The most problematic areas for a doctor's health seem to be poor mental health and suicide, substance abuse and relationship breakdown.

- A GP's medical knowledge often does not translate into a healthy lifestyle.

- GPs often find it difficult to be patients and resist the role, and GPs often find it difficult to provide care for other GPs.

- Many GPs do not have their own GP, and often engage in inappropriate self-management and self-prescribing.

- Self-care for GPs requires attention to a range of domains, including personal care, care of colleagues and providing healthy environments within which to work.

- A holistic approach to self-care is most effective for prevention and management of illness.

- When dealing with workplace stress, the three key factors are: managing patient and staff demands; asserting control over hours and conditions; and seeking support from colleagues when difficulties arise. There are a range of physical, psychological, occupational, social, medicolegal and financial consequences if problems are ignored or intervention occurs too late.

- A range of confidential and expert services, dedicated to providing support to GPs, is available.

INTRODUCTION

Self-care is central to being an effective practitioner; however, this is often the last priority of GPs. The first step in improving self-care is raising self-awareness. This chapter will explore GPs' health and illness from a range of perspectives, including origin, recognition, prevention and management. It will also examine psychological, lifestyle and doctor–patient issues and provide useful references for further information. Hopefully, it will be a useful as well as thought-provoking resource.

GPs AND SELF-CARE

The two quotes at the beginning of the chapter encapsulate deeply rooted misunderstandings regarding the health and wellbeing of GPs. The first quote conveys an expectation, held by the community and frequently articulated by patients, that GPs should remain healthy in order to dispense care to those less fortunate than them. It also contains the presumption that GPs have the medical expertise to evade or avoid ill health. This is analogous to an expectation that a motor mechanic should always drive a well maintained car or a builder should live in a perfectly constructed house. Of course nothing could be further from the truth, as the spouses and partners of builders and motor mechanics will tell you.

The irony of the first quote is that, in the course of a consultation with an obviously sick doctor, a patient often expresses it. While the illness is most likely to be respiratory and usually self-limiting, the continued presence at work of the GP with an infectious condition is tolerated by colleagues and rarely questioned, despite the fact that rest hastens recovery.

The second quote can be both a positive and a negative. It can be a call to doctors to show the same appropriate care for their own health that they would wish for their patients, and to put their knowledge about the cause and prevention of disease to good use. On the other hand, it can be a further example of a mistaken belief that knowledge, or even insight, will lead to appropriate action. The expectation that physicians should dispense self-care is flawed, often with outcomes analogous to the 'lawyer who defends himself having a fool for a client'.

QUESTIONS AND ISSUES RAISED BY THE CASE STUDIES

The two cases illustrate a number of important issues about GPs' health and help-seeking behaviour, and raise many questions about the way GPs and their colleagues lead their personal and professional lives; this chapter will explore and attempt to answer some of these questions.

CASE STUDY 1

- Why did John smoke throughout his professional career, despite his knowledge of the harm it causes and his own personal experience of the devastating consequences of smoking?
- What did his patients think of him as a role model, and how effective was he in counselling patients to stop smoking?
- Given the terrible history of that disease in his family, why did he ignore advice from authoritative bodies regarding screening for colonic cancer?
- Why did he wait so long to seek help when obvious symptoms of colonic cancer were present?
- Why didn't he consult a GP when he first noticed symptoms?
- Why was denial of vulnerability to illness such a prominent feature of his psychological make-up?
- Can GPs who abuse their own physical and emotional wellbeing still be effective healers?

CASE STUDY 2

- Did Henry have any insight into his own hypomanic behaviour?
- Were the rewards and the accolades from peers and colleagues so great that they served to reinforce such behaviour?
- Why did he not seek help after the car accident?
- Did his family, friends and colleagues perceive him to be depressed and at risk of suicide, and could they, particularly his colleagues, have done more to prevent it?
- Did he have an undiagnosed bipolar disorder that was treatable?

WHAT DO WE KNOW ABOUT THE HEALTH OF DOCTORS?

The Standard Mortality Ratio (SMR) for all causes of death is 20% better for doctors than for the general population and also better for a number of conditions, in particular cancer and cardiovascular disease, than other professionals in Social Class 1.[1, 2] However, male doctors have much higher rates of depression and suicide than those in a comparable social class (see Table 2.1). Within the medical profession, solo GPs were found to have the highest SMR.[3] The benefits of autonomy do not seem to outweigh the difficulties that result from professional isolation. (The infamous Dr Harold Shipton case in the United Kingdom is a stark reminder of the potential danger of the combination of psychopathy and professional isolation.)

The findings in Table 2.1 are based on old data from the United Kingdom; however, similar trends in Australia have been found in Australian studies. For example, Schlicht and Gordon's study of 1453 Victorian male doctors[4] showed that the SMR for mental disorders, including drug and alcohol abuse, was higher for doctors than would be expected for a comparable social class.

TABLE 2.1 SMRs for UK male doctors (1979–83)		
MORTALITY CAUSES	**SOCIAL CLASS 1**	**DOCTORS**
All cancers	76	66
Lung cancer	50	33
Ischaemic heart disease	81	70
Cerebrovascular disease	77	71
Bronchitis, emphysema and asthma	39	28
Cirrhosis of liver	104	177
Suicide	88	172
Overall SMR	75	69

Source: Balarajan, 1989.[1]

LIFESTYLE FACTORS AND RISK-TAKING BEHAVIOUR

GPs are well aware of the relationship between lifestyle and disease, and most would counsel their patients on a regular basis on the importance of a healthy lifestyle. Ideally, doctors should provide a role model for their patients, unlike the doctor in the first case study.

SMOKING Over the past three decades there has been a progressive decline in smoking among health professionals (less so among nurses), which mirrors the decline in the general population; currently about 24% of the Australian population aged over 18 years of age smoke.[5]

A study by Chambers and Belcher[6] found that only 8% of GPs in the UK smoke, while in New Zealand it has been as low as 6.7% of GPs.[7] In Australia the number of GPs who smoke is even lower: 5.9% in Nyman's study in 1991[7] and 4% in McCall et al's study in 1999.[8] It would seem that when it comes to smoking, more and more GPs are heeding their own health messages.

DIET AND EXERCISE While the data on smoking is impressive, the same cannot universally be said for diet and exercise. Chambers found that only 9% of GPs in the UK exercised regularly.[6] Figures in Australia are more encouraging, with 45% of GPs in Victoria and 43% of GPs in Western Australia exercising regularly.[8] Richards[9] found that one-third of GPs surveyed in New Zealand were on a low fat/low cholesterol diet; this matched McCall's findings for GPs in Victoria.[8] Despite their dietary and exercise patterns, only 16% of GPs have been found to be overweight or obese, compared to 48% for the general Australian population.

PREVENTION AND IMMUNISATION Kay et al[10] reviewed the literature on the preventive health practices of doctors. For screening tests such as Pap smears, mammograms, blood pressure checks and lipids, most recent studies report frequencies of testing that are comparable to the general population. However, considering the level of awareness one would expect GPs to have about the importance of testing, it might be expected to be higher.

Doctors have an increased risk to infectious disease, some of which—such as HIV and hepatitis B, C—are blood borne. Kay et al[10] revealed unacceptable rates of vaccination among GPs for hepatitis B (49–87%) with McCall et al[8] finding that only 64% of GPs had a post-vaccination antibody test despite almost 50% reporting a recent needle stick injury.

WORK STRESS, MENTAL HEALTH AND WELLBEING Although the physical health and lifestyle of doctors deserves attention, failings in this area are often the consequence of, or are associated with, work related stress and poor emotional health. As such, much of the remainder of this chapter will be devoted to examining the causes and effects of work related stress and the psychological wellbeing of doctors. The pace of technological change and the widespread computerisation of the workplace have failed to deliver the promise of increased leisure time and improved quality of life. This has affected workers in many walks of life, but particularly those who are in senior management positions or self-employed. Computerisation has not alleviated the demands of red tape and increased administrative and bureaucratic requirements within general practice. In her book *Willing Slaves*, Madeline Bunting reports that:[11]

> For about one in three British workers, exhaustion, stress, or both have become inescapable parts of their working lives…The health of the overworked employee is hit twice—first by working too hard and second by not having the time to develop relationships, take exercise and pursue outside interests all of which strengthen resilience to pressure.

Medical practitioners, in particular GPs, experience high levels of stress in their work—a consequence of the nature of the work (high levels of demand, diagnostic uncertainty and lack of control), their personality (often obsessional, needing to be wanted and liked, unable to set boundaries, using denial as a defence against vulnerability) and inadequate organisational and emotional support at the practice level as well as from broader professional bodies.

Long working hours are well known to be associated with poor health outcomes, especially when the person finds the work stressful or demanding. Working more than ten hours per day on a long-term basis is associated with shorter life expectancy, independent of the effects that it also has on other health behaviours. Schattner and

Coman[12] showed that the time pressure of seeing enough patients was at the top of a list of ten most frequent stresses for GPs, whereas fear of litigation was the most severe source of stress (see Table 2.2).

TABLE 2.2 Top ten sources of stress for GPs	
MOST FREQUENT STRESSORS	**MOST SEVERE STRESSORS**
1 Time pressure to see patients	1 Threat of litigation
2 Paperwork	2 Too much work to do in a limited time
3 Phone interruptions during consultations	3 Earning enough money
4 Too much work to do in a limited time	4 Patients who are difficult to manage
5 Intrusion of work on family life	5 Paperwork
6 Patients who are difficult to manage	6 Intrusion of work on family life
7 Home visits (in hours)	7 The cost of practice overheads
8 Earning enough money	8 Time pressure to see patients
9 Intrusion of work on social life	9 Unrealistic community expectations
10 Unrealistic community expectations	10 Negative media comments

Source: Schattner & Coman, 1998.[12]

Since Schattner and Coman's study was conducted, litigation and the cost of medical defence insurance has increased significantly, making it too costly for GPs and some procedural specialists to perform often satisfying albeit demanding work, such as obstetrics. The need to maintain quality control procedures within the practice for accreditation purposes as well as the paperwork requirements of Commonwealth Government Practice Incentive Payments have added additional time management pressures for GPs, many of whom appear to be working longer on matters that are not directly related to patient care.

An ongoing imbalance between demands (professional, family and hidden personal), support and control over work life can lead to stress, burnout and a range of psychological morbidities. There is the potential for falling standards of care and the possibility of litigation, or even being brought before medical boards with the possibility of deregistration. Loss of control of their work environment or even of their professional destiny is an important issue for doctors, especially given their obsessive traits, high level of commitment and the fact the 'clinical buck' stops with them. This has been demonstrated in the United States where managed care has often resulted in a shift of control from doctors to administrators. With increasing numbers of junior GPs, both female and male, choosing part-time work and showing little interest in practice ownership, there is a danger that such loss of control may have similar psychological consequences on this generation of doctors in the years ahead.

PSYCHOLOGICAL MORBIDITIES

BURNOUT Burnout is a syndrome that consists of emotional and physical exhaustion, depersonalisation of others (including patients), low self-esteem, a negative attitude to work and a decline in work involvement and performance. Schattner and Coman[12] found that 53% of Australian GPs had considered leaving general practice. A study in

New Zealand found that 36% of rural GPs reported burnout;[13] British studies have reported similar findings.[14] Burnout seems more common for experienced full-time GPs, and its prevalence appears to have increased with greater organisational and administrative demands over which GPs have little perceived control. One of the most disturbing features of burnout is the depersonalisation or dehumanisation of patients and staff, for whom respect and understanding are lost. Most consultations become 'heart sink' encounters. Milton compared burnout to '...the long standing unhappy couple that have forgotten why they were drawn together in the first place; love is lost; they feel flat and disillusioned, bring out the worst in each other and grow to feel bad about themselves'.[15]

It seems that many factors within the medical culture and system that contribute to burnout are already entrenched by the time doctors come into private practice. Burnout is common in mid final year medicine, with 28% of students meeting the criteria for burnout; and during internship there is a steady increase in the prevalence of burnout, to a peak prevalence of 75% late in the intern year.[16] Of all interns, 73% met the criteria for psychiatric morbidity on at least one occasion.[16]

SUBSTANCE ABUSE Early studies, such as those reported in Table 2.1, revealed a higher SMR from alcohol related cirrhosis among doctors than in the general population; alcohol related problems with GPs are still a common reason for referral to medical boards for disciplinary action.[17] According to Warhaft's study of the Victorian Doctors Health Program,[18] drug related problems among doctors are now becoming more common Among the 220 participants in the Victorian Doctors Health Program (VDHP), 51 were for drug related problems and 41 for alcohol related problems. Psychiatric problems accounted for 82 of the contacts, with 50 of these being due to depression.

Many of the problems associated with substance abuse may begin early in a doctor's life. It is estimated that around 45% of medical students have abused alcohol and illicit substances.[19] It is also estimated that up to 22% of students have tried other illicit drugs; this has increased from just 3% ten years before.[20] Doctors often use these drugs to help them deal with stress and improve sleep, and many doctors started using while students [21] Other evidence suggests that usage rates increase as medical students move into their residency years.[21] With 66% of resident medical officers (RMOs) having less than six hours of sleep per night, the ready availability of sedatives may be difficult to resist.

Self-management of medical conditions and ready access to prescription drugs enables doctors to misuse these drugs more readily than other members of the community. The true prevalence of misuse is unknown; however, some studies report rates of 0.5–10%. In Warhaft's[18] study of 58 doctors involved in an intensive drug management program, 50 were men and 15 had a comorbid mental disorder, while the most commonly used prescription drugs were, in order of use: pethidine, codeine, benzodiazepines and amphetamines. GPs and anaesthetists seemed the most likely to misuse prescription drugs. Issues related to self-management of medical conditions will be discussed later in this chapter.

PSYCHIATRIC ILLNESS While there is no evidence that the prevalence of psychiatric morbidity is greater among doctors than in the general population, the management of these problems is often compromised by denial, delayed diagnosis, self-medication and drug abuse. This can sometimes result in suicide risks that are much higher than expected (see 'Case study 2').

Depression is the most common serious psychiatric problem, with reported lifetime prevalence rates of 12.8% for male doctors and 19.5% for female doctors, about the same as for the general population.[22] Schattner and Coman[12] further showed that 12.8% of Australian metropolitan GPs had a severe psychiatric disturbance (depression, anxiety or other) as demonstrated in the General Health Questionnaire.

SUICIDE Although suicide rates among doctors have progressively declined over the past twenty-five years, they are still disturbingly high when compared to other professionals and to the general population. In 1978 mortality from suicide among doctors in the UK was 335% greater than for the rest of the population. In 1989 Balarajan[1] reported an SMR for suicide of 172% for doctors in the UK compared to only 88% for other professionals. Suicide related deaths are proportionally considerably higher for females than males, despite Schlicht and Gordon's[4] finding that females have a greater willingness to discuss their emotional problems and seek help for them. This may, at least in part, reflect the difficulty of balancing work and family commitments and choices. Issues previously mentioned—such as avoiding help when needed, self-medicating, low awareness, low support and high demands—are among the factors that may predispose doctors to having a high suicide rate. Undergraduate and postgraduate education, which now includes information on self-care and other preventive strategies, may take a generation or more to have significant effects.

BOUNDARY VIOLATION Sexual boundary violations by health professionals with patients are an increasingly conspicuous problem in health care; this may be due to an increase in such incidents or it may reflect an increase in reporting and sensitivity to the problem. Some practitioners—for example, psychiatrists and psychotherapists—may be at greater risk for a range reasons, such as the therapeutic context, unresolved difficulties in relationships with their own partners, and the nature of the therapist–patient relationship. Assessing factors such as how long the therapeutic relationship has existed, how long since that relationship was terminated, the nature of the therapy, the vulnerability of the patient, the power relationships involved, the cultural context and gender issues can determine when a significant boundary violation might have occurred.

A number of factors have been identified by Gabbard as being important for preventing potential boundary violations among psychotherapists.[23] These include:

- the difference between conscious and unconscious intent;
- love as a defence against aggression;
- the confusion of supportive therapy and boundaryless therapy; and
- the perils of secrecy.

Prevention will always be better than cure. Important aspects of preventing the potential for doctor–patient boundary violation can be undergraduate and postgraduate training in ethics and psychology, adequate supervision and the positive mental, emotional and social health of the doctor. In the end there will never be a perfect strategy for preventing such transgressions. Each practitioner needs to acknowledge their potential vulnerability and be far-sighted enough to respond appropriately to potential problems if they do arise. Boundary violations are unacceptable in therapeutic relationships.

SELF-MANAGEMENT

While doctors are subject to the same ailments as all humans, with some variation in risk for occupational hazards (physical and emotional) and a heightened risk of suicide, what distinguishes them from the rest of the community is their ability to self-diagnose and self-manage. The consequences of both of these actions are often dire (as the case studies illustrate) and are determined by a range of complex psychological mechanisms, personality factors, upbringing, training and role modelling. Rogers[24] referred to the 3Ds (delusion, denial and delay) and the 4Ss (self-investigation, self-diagnosis, self-treatment and self-referral) approach by doctors to their health problems, which often leads to a fourth 'D'—disaster.

In McCall et al's study[8] it was found that of GPs in Victoria, 57% did not have their own treating GP, and among those who did, 13% nominated themselves as their GP and 31% nominated a colleague in their own practice. Similar findings were obtained in a New Zealand study,[25] which showed that when ill, 50% of surveyed GPs would treat themselves, 22% would ask a colleague and only 19% would formally seek treatment from another GP.

Self-medication is the troublesome consequence of self-diagnosis. Chambers and Belcher[6] reported that 83% of medications taken by GPs were self-prescribed. Although drugs commonly in this category include antibiotics, NSAIDs, H2 antagonists and so on, the less frequent reported usage of hypnotics, antidepressants and narcotic analgesics is nevertheless disturbing.[6–9]

Psychological problems, often accompanied by inappropriate self-medication, may produce personal, family, social and professional disintegration. The doctor in these circumstances is often labelled as 'impaired'. Impaired doctors may be brought before Medical Registration Boards for professional misconduct, such as unethical or illegal practices, negligent professional behaviour or sexual misdemeanours involving patients. It is in these circumstances that the underlying psychological problems, with or without associated drug and alcohol abuse, are discovered. Many of the Medical Registration Boards have established semi-independent or independent health advisory and medical treatment panels to assist and rehabilitate the impaired doctor. These will be discussed in more detail in the 'Management' section.

FACTORS UNDERPINNING DOCTORS' POOR HELP-SEEKING BEHAVIOUR

A doctor's personality is moulded in childhood and adolescence, and further developed in medical school and during vocational training. Personality traits such as obsessional attention to detail, intolerance of uncertainty, unwillingness to expose weaknesses or vulnerability and a certain level of neuroticism often underpin high achievement at school, particularly in science based courses. Hard work and in fact 'workaholism' are respected, and when they lead to examination success, these features are rewarded. Paradoxically, many of these personality traits are regarded as positive attributes for selection into medical school. The pressure to succeed can be both internal and external. Role modelling can reinforce behaviour—for example, during clinical training where consultants work long hours in a culture which rewards self-sacrifice and altruism. This can result in a denial of personal problems in order to maintain a façade of confidence and even omnipotence. Grateful patients, mentors and peers may provide further encouragement to continue the process of self-denial.

Clinical practice—in particular, general practice—is often characterised by high levels of complexity, ambiguity and diagnostic uncertainty. Doctors possessing the personality features outlined above may find it difficult to cope day-in-day-out in such an environment. This can lead to stress, and the physical and emotional consequences of that stress may require medical attention. In these circumstances doctors who thrive on a sense of control of their environment and their destiny may be unwilling to hand over their own care to a colleague, particularly a fellow GP. In their view, to do so would expose weaknesses and vulnerability. Self-management or self-referral to a specialist may be perceived as a better option. This behaviour is consistent with Rotter's theory of 'locus of control'.[26] Doctors who might normally have a 'high internal locus of control', based on their knowledge and experience, decompensate in the face of illness and behave in a fatalistic manner, leaving their destiny to chance through denial, delayed management or self-management.

UNCONSCIOUS DYNAMICS IN DENIAL OF VULNERABILITY

Understanding the unconscious motivations for actions can provide an important insight into reasons why some doctors have difficulty in seeking assistance during times of difficulty. Psychoanalytic theory provides a useful lens for hypothesising about observed behaviours through an exploration of some of the unconscious dynamics that may ensue in the doctor–patient relationship. The concepts of transference and countertransference provide a useful frame with which to investigate this area.

Sigmund Freud identified the psychological process of transference, which he described as the manifestation of unconscious mental activity that shapes our relations with others. Transference is the aspect of an interpersonal relationship in which a person's behaviour towards another is influenced by interactions with significant figures from childhood and infancy, usually parents. A patient's positive (negative) regard for the physician may have elements of transference feelings associated with authority and may be heightened in relationships of dependence, as in the doctor–patient relationship. The transference can, at the extreme, manifest in gross over-idealisation or demonisation, in which the doctor is idealised as the omnipotent healer, or demonised as the impotent, withholding and non-caring parent, respectively.

While patients' projections of positive feelings towards the doctor can assist the healing process, it is important that the doctor is able to detect these unconscious forces in both themselves and the patient and is aware of their own countertransference. Countertransference is the doctor's unconscious emotional response to the patient. For example, in response to a patient's feelings of dependency during a time of crisis, the doctor may respond in a way that mirrors patterns of behaviour that originate with significant others from their own past. They may have problems with managing dependency relationships and act this out in the therapeutic relationship, albeit unconsciously, by becoming overly critical, despondent, unduly protective, flattered or romantically interested. Unmanaged countertransference can lead to dysfunctional behaviour, whereas managed and understood countertransference can be a principal tool in managing difficult doctor–patient interactions.

The transferential frame can throw light on the phenomenon of a doctor's resistance to acknowledging and addressing their own health problems. Becoming a doctor involves a trajectory that is gruelling; getting through medical school and residency, let alone the exigencies of a medical career, demand excellence, perseverance, dedication, commitment and sacrifices. Doctors are held in high regard and still appear to maintain a special status in society. Doctors need to manage these societal expectations and be mindful of the impact of idealised societal projections. Unless countertransference is managed, there is a risk of unconsciously colluding with individual and societal projections and introjecting (internalising) societal adulation. This can manifest in feelings of either omnipotence or impotence, which renders a doctor resistant to their vulnerability. The doctor will use defensive behaviour to deny there is a problem and/or will attribute the problem to others. Failure to identify and to manage countertransferential feelings in response to patient and societal idealisation/demonisation of the doctor is detrimental to the doctor's psychological and physical health and the doctor's capacity as a professional.[27]

Resilience requires acknowledgment of one's vulnerability and the willingness to seek help when required. Appropriate attention to the psychological robustness of medical trainees through awareness, education, encouragement for self-reflection, and openness to one's potential frailty as a human being, can only enhance the sustainability of the medical profession in providing health care.

MANAGEMENT
PREVENTION

LIFESTYLE Just as the negative effects of stress, poor diet or inactivity can be felt in any and every system of the body, so can the benefits of managing stress and enjoying good nutrition and adequate physical activity be experienced in every system (see Chapter 17).

THE ESSENCE OF GOOD HEALTH[28] In taking a holistic approach to health, a systematic and comprehensive strategy is helpful. One way of thinking about this is the ESSENCE model. ESSENCE stands for:

- **Education** Education is useful in and of itself; however, medical education offers some extra benefits, such as knowledge about health behaviours, skills and attitudes.
- **Stress management** Managing stress and having good mental health will have flow-on effects to every other aspect of your health and lifestyle. Applying the skills outlined in the chapter on stress management may be helpful (see Chapter 17).
- **Spirituality** Spirituality is more than being religious. It can mean finding a sense of meaning and purpose in your life, taking time to reflect on your life philosophy and direction, and may even include your sense of creativity or altruism.
- **Exercise** Maintaining physical activity is hard for regularly desk-bound workers such as doctors; however, adopting regular but moderate physical activity at work and home has benefits for all aspects of mental and physical health.

■ **Nutrition** Good nutrition is more than a low-fat or low-salt diet. Healthy nutrition is preventive and therapeutic for nearly every conceivable condition.

■ **Connectedness** The role of social support and supportive relationships at work and home cannot be overstated. Learning how to build and maintain relationships and healthy communication is central to good health and happiness as is building strategies into our workplaces.

■ **Environment** A healthy environment is more than air, water and soil. It includes the mental and emotional environment we create, sensory stimuli, the places we choose to go and the people with whom we surround ourselves.

ESSENCE will be just as relevant for you as it is for your patients. It is possible to choose to reflect on, and work with, just one aspect at a time, or you may choose to address a number of aspects at a time.

CONTROL, SUPPORT AND DEMANDS Research on workplace stress and health by Theorell and Karasek[29] suggests that there are three main dimensions to workplace stress:

■ control;
■ support; and
■ demands.

Control has to do with both the external environment (the external locus of control) and, even more importantly, the internal environment (the internal locus of control). The external locus relates to you having control over the things around you, whereas the internal locus relates to you having control over your own responses, attitudes and yourself. Modifying the external environment, whether it be workplaces or the systems within which you work, can include things such as involving people in decision-making processes, developing systems based on co-operation (not competition), modifying the workplace to provide variety and offering choice, where possible, over things such as conditions and rostering.

Support can be built in—for example, as a formal process of debriefing, professional development and building effective communication strategies. Equally, if not more importantly, there is a need to build a 'workplace culture' that will sustain and support people. Having been raised in the furnace of competitiveness for many years, this is often a challenging shift in thinking for many doctors.

A mismatch between demands and performance can be moderated by reducing demands (for example, hours worked or number or type of patients seen), improving performance (improving systems and efficiency, dealing with stress) or moderating one's perception of demands where they are unrealistic. Thus, skills such as focusing, relaxation, training in time management and problem solving can be very helpful. Postgraduate education can help to provide these skills. Another solution, often easy to miss, is the ability to discriminate between real and perceived demands.

EARLY INTERVENTION Early intervention implies that there is an issue that requires further attention and action. Obviously a problem dealt with early will be simpler than one dealt with when it is more complex and entrenched, and also when other comorbidities may have evolved. Simple but important steps in intervening early with such problems can include the following:

■ Realise that to act now will save much more time and resources than it will cost to deal with or avoid a problem.

■ Speak about it to relevant people, including an independent GP or other primary health practitioner, who can give you independent and objective advice and possibly referral.

■ Put aside your own assumptions and be prepared to change roles from doctor to patient, at least for a time.

■ Be prepared to take time out if that is what is required. That may mean taking leave or just reducing your hours to allow adequate time for self-care activities on a daily basis.

■ Seek out reliable information sources, but avoid becoming your own therapist, especially when it comes to prescribing.

■ If necessary, contact one of the many doctor-support services whose job it is to help doctors in need. You can be assured the role of doctor-support services is not punitive.

■ Take some time to reflect on your values, priorities and direction rather than just push on unquestioningly.

LATER INTERVENTION The above guidance for early intervention also applies to later intervention, but more so. It's particularly important where relevant, such as when experiencing mental health problems or substance abuse, to seek the advice of the professional bodies that have the expertise and resources to specifically help doctors in these situations, especially before diminished performance and any potential medicolegal problems ensue.

ROLE OF MEDICAL REGISTRATION BOARDS AND DOCTORS' HEALTH PROGRAMS
The role of a Medical Registration Board is to protect the interests of the community while concurrently ensuring that doctors facing the Board receive natural justice.[30] To facilitate this separation of roles, a number of Medical Registration Boards have supported and funded Doctors' Health Programs, whose principal role is to ensure that the treatment and rehabilitation of impaired practitioners and medical students are performed in an appropriately supervised and confidential manner. The Doctors' Health Programs usually operate at arm's length from the Medical Registration Boards, with the Boards maintaining their independent power to deregister, suspend or place restrictions on practice.

In Victoria the VDHP was established in late 2000.[21] It serves 18 000 registered medical practitioners and 2500 medical students. From 2001 to 2004 it had 438 contacts—218 for advice and 220 requiring specific clinical services. Since the establishment of the VDHP, the number of practitioners referred by the Medical Registration Board to its own Health Committee has fallen from 50 to 23.[31]

LOOKING AFTER DOCTORS

DOCTORS AS PATIENTS Changing roles from doctor to patient does not come easily to most doctors. Loss of control, a desire to minimise the problem, thinking you know better and a lack of trust in your colleague's judgment can be some of the reasons for this. In playing the patient role, some guidelines might be useful:

■ Find a GP you trust and keep in regular contact. It can help if you do not have a working relationship with that doctor.

■ To some extent, you should put your medical knowledge aside. Trying to second-guess diagnoses, filtering information you give to the doctor, and trying to influence treatment decisions can negatively impact upon the consultation, making it very difficult for the treating doctor to play their role.

■ Comply with treatment and recognise that adverse events and response to treatment will need to be monitored by the treating doctor.

■ Respect the professional boundaries of the consultation; you are now a patient.

BEING A DOCTOR FOR OTHER DOCTORS Treating other doctors can be one of the most challenging clinical encounters for any doctor. Some GPs and specialists specialise in this work and have clear guidelines and long experience in the field and know how to go about this. Some useful points for undertaking this work include the following:

■ It is easier to treat doctors with whom you do not have a long-standing personal or professional relationship. Where this is not possible, perhaps in rural settings, it will be doubly important to pay attention to the following guidelines and to recognise that during consultations there is the potential for professional and personal roles to become mixed and complicated.

■ Understand the boundaries of the consultation.

■ Put the professional labels aside and treat a doctor like other patients, while at the same time acknowledging they have experience and knowledge. Try not to assume anything.

■ Consider referring if you are out of your depth or the relationship is not productive. Advise your patient to seek help from professional bodies when it is appropriate to do so.

■ Take care that you are not prompted by the GP patient to make a clinical judgment with which you are unhappy, especially when it comes to prescribing or potential medicolegal problems.

■ Be meticulous with confidentiality and clear in your reassurances to the GP patient about this.

■ As with any other patient, do not necessarily take the façade that the GP patient presents as a reliable indication of what is underneath, especially considering how hard it can be for a doctor to adapt to the potentially more vulnerable patient role.

■ Try not to impose suggestions, but let explanations and reasoning be explicit and clear.

■ Avoid the tendency to undertreat or overtreat.

REVISITING THE CASE STUDIES

There are a number of potential points of intervention in the case studies that may have resulted in less unfortunate outcomes, and some of these will be briefly considered below.

CASE STUDY 1

SELF-CARE

- If the GP had heeded the non-smoking message it would have been positive.
- It would have been beneficial if he had paid attention to screening procedures and to other lifestyle risk factors for colorectal cancer, such as alcohol use and nutrition—just as he would have with one of his patients.
- Being aware of using denial as a defence against the anxiety of a potentially upsetting diagnosis would have helped.

COLLEAGUES

- The scenario does not say whether he worked in a solo or group practice, but there may have been a chance for colleagues to prompt healthy behaviours, perhaps by knowing his family history or by observing a deterioration in his health.

SYSTEM

- There is an increasing number of programs run by Divisions of General Practice that target doctor health. Unfortunately, it is often the doctors who need these most who are the last ones to attend.
- Considering the low number of doctors who have their own GP, there may come a time when doctors are legally required to have health checks and personalised advice on screening; this is often the case in other professions with a high level of responsibility.

CASE STUDY 2

SELF-CARE

- In this case, where insight was poor as result of an underlying psychiatric condition, self-care would have been rather difficult.
- An inappropriate form of self-care was expressed in self-prescribing, especially for a chronic pain condition and with potentially addictive drugs.
- Not recognising the early stages of bipolar disorder is common to doctors and non-doctors alike. The lack of care in relationships and business dealings is problematic because of the lack of insight associated with the condition.
- Denial may also have been used as a defence against the anxiety of a potentially upsetting diagnosis.

COLLEAGUES

- There may have been a chance for colleagues to prompt an assessment, especially observing Henry's recent behaviour and the deterioration in his health.
- There may have been a level of denial among colleagues wishing to avoid dealing with a potentially emotional and disruptive workplace situation.
- There may have been a need for more support from colleagues both before and after his health problems.

SYSTEM

- Henry may have benefited from the programs run by the Divisions of General Practice that target doctor health, although he may not have perceived he had a problem until late in the process.

- The various organisations set up to deal with such problems can only assist if they are notified and their help sought.
- Being a doctor in a rural area, where there may be relatively little support, may have exacerbated the problem.

CONCLUSION

Professionally charged with a duty of care to their patients, doctors also have a duty of care to themselves. While the physical wellbeing of GPs is comparable to that of other professionals, the same cannot be said of their mental wellbeing. Stress, anxiety, depression, drug and alcohol related problems, a tendency to self-medicate and avoidance of help-seeking behaviour remain significant issues within the profession. Systemic change, beginning in medical school and reinforced through vocational training and accompanied by available support systems during active practice, are needed to overcome ingrained negative attitudes towards vulnerability.

REFERENCES

1. Balarajan R. Inequalities in health within the health sector. British Medical Journal 1989;299:822–5.
2. Doll R, Peto R. Mortality among doctors in different occupations. British Medical Journal 1977;1:1433–6.
3. Carpenter L. Swerdlow A, Fear N. Mortality of doctors in different specialties: findings from a cohort of 20 000 NHS consultants. Journal of Occupational and Environmental Medicine 1997; 54:388–95.
4. Schlicht SM, Gordon IR. Suicide and related deaths in Victorian doctors. Medical Journal of Australia 1990;153:518–21.
5. NBS National Health Survey. Summary of Results. Canberra: Australian Bureau of Statistics, 2001.
6. Chambers R, Belcher J. Comparison of the health and lifestyle of general practitioners and teachers. British Journal of General Practice 1993;43:378–82.
7. Nyman K. The health of general practitioners: a pilot survey. Australian Family Physician 1991;2:637–45.
8. McCall L, Maher T, Piterman L. Preventive health behaviour amongst general practitioners in Victoria. Australian Family Physician 1999;28:854–7.
9. Richards JG. The health and health practice of doctors and their families. New Zealand Medical Journal 1999;112:96–9.
10. Kay MP, Mitchell GK, Del Mar CB. Doctors do not adequately look after their own physical health. Medical Journal of Australia 2004;181:368–70.
11. Bunting M. Willing Slaves. London: HarperCollins, 2004.
12. Schattner P, Coman G. The stress of metropolitan general practice. Medical Journal of Australia 1998;169:133–7.
13. Jenkins D. Burnout in rural general practice. New Zealand Medical Journal 1998;111:328.
14. Kirwan M, Armstrong D. Investigation of burnout in a sample of British general practitioners. British Journal of General Practice 1995;45:259–60.
15. Milton J. Stress, strain and burnout: support and supervision. In: Elder A, Holmes J, eds. Mental Health and Primary Care. London: OUP, 2002.
16. Willcock SM, Daly MG, Tennant CC, Allard BJ. Burnout and psychiatric morbidity in new medical graduates. Medical Journal of Australia 2004;181(7):357–60.
17. Wilhelm KA, Reid AM. Critical decision points in the management of impaired doctors: the New South Wales Medical Board program. Medical Journal of Australia 2004;181:372–5.
18. Warhaft N. The Victorian Doctors Health Program: the first 3 years. Medical Journal of Australia 2004;181:376–9.

19. Newbury-Birch D, White M, Kamali F. Factors influencing alcohol and illicit drug use amongst medical students. Drug and Alcohol Dependence 2000;59(2):125–30.

20. Ashton CH, Kamali F. Personality, lifestyles, alcohol and drug consumption in a sample of British medical students. Medical Education 1995;29(3):187–92.

21. Newbury-Birch D, Walshaw D, Kamali F. Drink and drugs: from medical students to doctors. Drug and Alcohol Dependence 2001;64(3):265–70.

22. Center C, Davis M, Detre T, Ford DE, Hansbrough W, Hendin H, Lazlo J, Litts DA, Mann J, Mansky PA, Michels R, Miles SH, Provjansky R, Reynolds CF III, Silverman MM. Confronting depression and suicide in physicians. Journal of the American Medical Association 2003;289:3161–6.

23. Gabbard G. Lessons to be learned from the study of sexual boundary violations. Australian and New Zealand Journal of Psychiatry 1997;31:321–7.

24. Rogers T. Barriers to the doctor as patient role. A critical construct. Australian Family Physician 1998;27(11):1009–13.

25. O'Hagan J, Richards J. Doctors and Their Health. A Handbook for Medical Practitioners and Other Health Professionals, Their Partners and Their Families. Wellington, NZ: Doctors Health Advisory Service, 1998.

26. Rotter JB. Generalised expectancies for internal versus external control of reinforcement. Psychological Monographs 1966;80(1):609.

27. Goldberg PE. The physician patient relationship. Archives of Family Medicine 2000;9(10):1164–8. www.archfammed.com

28. Hassed C. Unit Study Guide. Monash University: Health Enhancement Program, 2005.

29. Theorell T, Karasek RA. Current issues relating to psychosocial job strain and cardiovascular disease research. Journal of Occupational Health Psychology 1996;1(1):9–26 Erratum in: Journal of Occupational Health Psychology 1998;3(1).369.

30. Breen KJ, Court JM, Katsoris J. Impaired doctors: the modern approach of medical boards. Australian Family Physician 1998;11:1005–8.

31. Medical Practitioners Board of Victoria. Annual Report. Medical Practitioners Board of Victoria, 2003: http://medicalboardvic.org.au/content.php?sec=67 (last accessed February 2006).

CHAPTER 3

CONSUMERS AND FAMILY CARERS' VIEWS OF GP PSYCHIATRY

MT Dawson, B Hocking, R McLean and J Buchanan

We would like to believe that insanity happens only in other people's families and never to us. But any one of us can brush wings with madness.

ANNE DEVESON, *Tell Me I'm Here, 1998*

CASE STUDY 1

Joe comes to see you because he has been finding it increasingly hard to feel motivated to do anything; even getting up in the morning is hard. He has started taking days off work over the past weeks and his boss is now making comments about his job performance. He has no interest in playing with the kids or doing any work around the house. Joe has also been thinking about suicide a lot. After reading a magazine article about mental illness, his wife insisted he call the SANE Helpline. He was then referred to you for assessment and treatment for depression.

Joe has heard and read about potential problems with medication and is reluctant to try antidepressants. He cannot afford to pay to see a psychologist. However, his wife has said she's had enough and if he does not get treatment she will have to consider leaving him; she says she will take the children with her.

KEY FACTS

- Many consumers and family carers consider the care provided by the general practitioner (GP) to be holistic, and appreciate the fact that GPs often know the family situation as a whole. (The term 'consumer' is used as a generic term to refer to 'patients', 'users of health services', 'potential users of health services' or 'clients'.)

- Many consumers and family carers consider general practice to be more accessible and less stigmatising than specialist mental health services. It is often the first port of call for anyone concerned about their mental health.

- Where possible, GPs should look after not only the person with a mental illness but also *all* family members and carers, as they too are potentially affected by the situation.

- The stigma and discrimination often associated with having a mental illness have distressing personal and social impacts on the daily lives of consumers and family carers. It is important that GPs also consider their own attitudes and behaviour in this regard.

- Actively involving consumers and carers in illness management is important, as they are more expert than anyone else about how the illness affects them.

- User-friendly education and self-help material have been shown to be effective in helping consumers and carers to better understand and manage mental illness.

- Consumers and carers will benefit if GPs know what mental health and community treatment and support services—such as accommodation, rehabilitation and family education and support programs—are available in their local area.

- If consumers and family carers are unable to access comprehensive and effective treatments and support in their local area, GPs are well placed to lobby for these services.

INTRODUCTION

It is well known that most people go to see a GP as the first port of call for anything related to their health. Those who are concerned about their own or a family member's mental health are no exception, usually approaching a GP for help with identifying and treating a mental illness. In fact, because the main focus of specialist public mental health services is on the treatment and care of people with long-term psychotic illnesses, such services are unable to help people with mild to moderate depression or anxiety. Consequently, most people with these conditions will turn to a GP for ongoing treatment or for referral to a private mental health specialist.

Therefore it is necessary for GPs to have a good understanding of common presentations, assessment and current treatments of the high prevalence mental health disorders. An understanding of drug abuse and of suicidal thinking and behaviour is also important, as these often mask and/or complicate the presentation of mental illness. Intuition plays a critical role, as often people with mental illness will present quite 'normally', and the full discordance of their illness is not apparent in a short consultation. It is important to take a person's concerns seriously as they need to feel they can trust their GP when raising sensitive mental health issues. Family carers, often the first to raise concerns with the GP, should also be listened to carefully and respectfully, as their knowledge of the person and observations about their changes in behaviour are often extensive.

Consumers and carers will go to GPs because they know and have confidence in them; they believe that the GP can look into their problems holistically, helping them to address a range of issues affecting their everyday life. The role that the GP plays can influence the degree of ease or difficulty faced by consumers and family carers in the overall management of mental illness. It is helpful then if consumers and family carers are actively engaged with the GP wherever possible, in all decisions related to the management of mental illness.

CONSUMER AND CARER PARTICIPATION

The conceptual background for consumer participation in health care is to be found within the principles of primary health care, as defined by the World Health Organization (WHO). The International Conference on Primary Health Care (PHC), held in Alma-Ata (formerly in the USSR, currently in Kazakhstan) in 1978, stated that primary health care was the key to attaining health for all. Primary health care requires and promotes maximum community and individual self-reliance, and community participation in the planning, organisation, operation and control of primary health care, using local, national and other available resources.[1]

In Australia, in 1993, the National Health Strategy established that consumer participation in health implies that:

- all citizens have a democratic right to participate in their own health care and the organisations that provide care;
- participation produces better health outcomes and improves the quality of health; and
- most people would like to have information about their own health and the processes involved in the delivery of health services.[2]

An extensive body of literature suggests that consumer, carer and community participation in health is beneficial for all those involved in the provision and use of health services.[3] It has been suggested that active participation in care and self-management of illness, education and written action plans leads to reduced hospital admissions, reduced visits to emergency departments, fewer unscheduled visits to the doctor and fewer days off work or school.[4] A randomised control trial showed that chronic disease self-management can improve health status and reduce hospitalisations.[5] Another study demonstrated that active involvement of patients in the management of their diabetes leads to more effective control of blood sugar levels.[6]

The principles of consumer participation seem to be agreed upon; however, some discussions have been held with regard to the terms 'consumer' being used in place of 'patient' or 'client'. It has been proposed that the concept of consumer represents an attempt to reconceptualise the relationship between health providers and those treated by the health system. The change in word usage from patient to consumer was an attempt to establish that users of the health system were individuals with rights, preferences and responsibilities. 'Consumer participation' has become a generic term that is used to indicate that consumers (either those using the health system directly or potential users)[7] and carers (those looking after consumers)[8] should be actively involved in all levels of health care. This includes participation in strategic planning, service planning, service delivery and evaluation of health services as well as in decision making about individual health care planning, treatment and rehabilitation.[9]

PROVISION OF MENTAL HEATH SERVICES BY THE GP

A study on service delivery and pathways to mental health care models showed that consumers and carers experience greater satisfaction when the GP acts as a gatekeeper to support and provide referrals to secondary consultations with specialist mental health services.[10] To be able to do this, GPs need to be well informed about the full range of treatments and to be aware of what local services are available in their community. Nevertheless, many GPs do not have this information and some do not yet have either the skills or confidence to identify and deal with mental health disorders. Time constraints and financial disincentives to providing long consultations also affect their capacity to provide mental health care.[10] It has been reported that the discriminatory behaviour of some GPs towards patients with mental illness, especially those with schizophrenia, combined with a tendency to ignore their physical health needs, may result in the patients' premature death (mainly from cardiovascular disease). Longer consultations and early diagnosis and treatment of both mental and physical illness should ensure a better outcome.[11]

Regional and rural areas often miss out on the full range of treatment options and services, thus making illness identification and treatment and support for consumers and family carers even more difficult.[12] Effective service delivery and good mental health care relies on a multi-pronged approach, including:

■ developing trust between services (for example, integrating the GP into strategic planning for specialist mental health services);
■ acknowledging that there are multiple pathways to recovery;
■ engaging consumers and their family carers in care and treatment plans;
■ viewing help seeking as part of treatment and recovery;
■ acting at multiple levels in multiple sectors (for example, integration of primary care, community support services and specialist mental health services); and
■ developing agreements and protocols for collaboration[10] (for example, this is especially important between the diagnosing psychiatrist and the GP who is providing ongoing support).

Encouraging the person affected by mental illness to take an interest in their own recovery is also important, as those patients who develop a better insight into their illness and an interest in their own recovery usually have a better long-term prognosis.

CASE STUDY 2

Nicky, aged 43, is worried. She's visiting her sister but hasn't slept for 48 hours; she has racing thoughts and fears she's heading for another manic episode. She agrees to visit her sister's GP. Nicky tells the GP that three weeks ago she stopped taking her medication,

---

as she was concerned about her 10 kg weight gain over the previous months. This was distressing her, as none of her clothes fitted and her job requires a smart appearance. She had mentioned her worries to her own GP but felt these were dismissed and that the GP was only interested in the symptoms of her bipolar disorder.

She decided to stop the medication for a while to see how she would go. Since then, she has lost 4 kg and was feeling much more energetic and happy until now. She was pleased when this GP sympathised about her weight gain and suggested that she consider taking a lower dose of medication to see if her symptoms could be managed with lower weight gain. Nicky agreed to consider doing regular exercise and to review her diet with a dietician. Nicky also agreed to take the medication again, feeling reassured that if the weight gain continued in spite of lifestyle and medication dosage changes, there were other possible medication options.

CONSUMERS AND FAMILY CARERS: AN INSIDER'S PERSPECTIVE

People seeking help for mental health disorders consider access, cost,[13] the physical characteristics of treatment settings and the integration of medical and psychological care to be the most relevant factors—factors that the health care system does not usually consider.

Consumers and family carers usually have concerns about issues such as the role and use of medication (including potential side effects), difficulties in keeping treatment schedules or appointments, waiting for long periods in waiting rooms, and not having access to community treatment and support services. Being able to discuss these concerns with their GP will often improve the management of their mental illness.[11]

Consumers and family carers feel that the management of mental illness should take account of the history of the illness, any associated disability and their ongoing personal and social needs as well as their access to a range of community treatment, accommodation, rehabilitation and support programs. It has also been suggested that some people need access to services that focus on reducing the danger of self-harm, rather than those that promote notions of personal recovery, long-term outcomes and a return to social participation.[12]

The stigma associated with mental illness is also distressing for consumers and family carers as it contributes to loneliness and discrimination. A recent study in Australia of people with mental illness and their families reported that 'less stigma was the number one thing that would make their lives better'.[11] People pleaded for a community that would understand that they are not 'lazy or weak' and that treatment is not just a matter of 'pulling oneself together'; they also asked for health professionals to treat them with respect and kindness. Discrimination towards people with mental disorders means that people are reluctant to seek help and are disadvantaged when looking for work, housing or education; such discrimination may contribute to suicidal thoughts or behaviour, self-loathing or feelings of hopelessness, which may lead to substance abuse or self-harm.

The level of knowledge and understanding of mental illness by consumers and carers also affects their decisions about seeking treatment. Many people do not understand or recognise the early signs of mental illness and are not unaware of what constitutes good treatment or who can provide it. People need information about mental illnesses, their symptoms and early intervention strategies as well as the available services and resources in their community.[10] As community awareness of mental health in general improves, however, it is important that those who do take a 'leap of faith' and confide in the GP about these issues are met with support, empathy and effective treatment. This may save a lot of suffering as well as financial burden on both the consumer and the health providers.

In consultation with consumers and carers affected by depression, a 'consumer's agenda for health care services' was produced. This agenda includes:

- more responsive primary and specialist care sectors;
- education of professionals to ensure they do not contribute to the stigmatisation of people with depression;
- development of improved treatment and services information;
- advocacy for improved access to non-pharmacological forms of care at low cost;
- advocacy for better professional based responses to the uneven distribution of specialist services;
- support for the development of accessible self-help, mutual support and other non-professional care agencies;
- promotion of the key role of carers;
- promotion of broader models of recovery from illness;
- development of novel measures of service quality and the mechanisms for collecting such data; and
- development of measures on consumer based and carer based concepts of clinical recovery to be incorporated in treatment and services research.[12]

Collaboration with consumers and family carers can improve both the process and structure for the delivery of mental health services. It is important therefore that GPs, other health professionals and community support services make every effort to co-ordinate their services to deliver effective treatment and rehabilitation to those with a mental illness.

CASE STUDY 3

Gary, aged 30, is worried. He has now been sleeping badly and feeling tired and irritable for about three months. To top things off, he has just developed an unsightly skin rash. He is having problems at work; he is a store manager in a music shop and last week a complaint was made about him to his line manager. Following this, he had to take two days off work, as he felt so hopeless and could not get out of bed. Gary has not seen a GP before as he felt his irritability, poor sleeping and lack of energy were 'not worth worrying the doctor about'. However, he feels that the skin rash is a valid reason to go.

He was annoyed by the first GP, who was in a rush, hardly asked any questions, and just wrote out a script for skin ointment. Gary had been ready to talk with the GP about the other things happening in his life and how he sometimes feels like ending it all, but during this consultation he could not even make a start. When the rash did not go away, Gary saw another GP who was much more helpful and who asked questions. He found himself talking about the other issues in his life. It was a great relief. Gary is now seeing a psychologist.

WHAT CAN GPs DO?

GPs have a pivotal role in increasing community awareness of mental illness, reducing any stigma and discrimination within their own practice, improving co-ordination of services and lobbying for additional and more effective community treatments and supports for consumers and their family carers.

It is important that, wherever possible, GPs provide long-term support for both consumers and family carers. This can include complementary support when a psychiatrist or specialist mental health services are involved. GPs can refer patients to other specialist services and programs, such as cognitive therapy, social skills training, vocational rehabilitation and group therapy.[14] The GP is well placed to encourage consumers to continue with treatment for their mental illness while promoting good physical health through support for a reduction of smoking, alcohol and other substance misuse. GPs can also provide accurate and culturally sensitive information about mental illness.

It is helpful if GPs have training in the use of psychological treatments in conjunction with (or sometimes instead of) medication for the treatment of mental illness. Randomised control trials have demonstrated the effectiveness of a combination of antidepressant medications with cognitive behavioural therapy and interpersonal psychotherapy. Programs based on the use of interpersonal counselling, cognitive behaviour therapy and problem-solving therapy are examples of psychological therapies being trialled in Australia (see Chapter 17).[15–17]

It is also helpful if GPs update their knowledge about the range and availability of community rehabilitation and support services available to consumers and carers. Some of the available services include social and vocational skills training programs and on-the-job support; housing; further education and employment information; respite care; recreation; and carer and consumer support groups and networks. Telephone help lines, such as the SANE Helpline, provide information and can also put callers in touch with services and supports in their local area. Increasingly, consumers and family carers are formally involved in health services through advisory or reference groups, and GPs would benefit from knowing about these so they can refer to them as appropriate.[18]

The GP also has a critical role in supporting family carers, who often feel isolated, neglected, confused and stressed by their caring role. This support role for the carer should be in place regardless of whether or not the person with a mental illness is a patient of the GP. In some situations families may be pre-judged as 'dysfunctional' and it is tempting for all problems to then be attributed to this. It is important to be open to seeing the presenting 'dysfunction' as a consequence of the difficult behaviour associated with untreated illness rather than the cause.

It can be helpful and reassuring if GPs can put families and carers in touch with carer consultants in the local mental health service area and with mental health support groups and education programs for carers. Some carers who visit the GP themselves when they feel extremely stressed comment that medication, which may indeed help calm them down, also makes them feel 'dazed' and not as alert as they should be for their caring role. Spending time, expressing interest and understanding and acknowledging the difficult time they are having can all make an enormous difference to the carer. If the GP is unable to provide the time or expertise for this, then a referral to someone who can is important.

Practical support—such as the provision of respite care, befriending programs for the ill person, referral to community day programs and supported accommodation—may contribute enormously to the wellbeing of both consumer and carer.

A difficult and very distressing issue for some carers is that the person they care for has an illness that has resulted in loss of insight into their own behaviour and they are therefore unable or unwilling to seek help. In these situations the GP is sought for advice and guidance on the best way to get appropriate assessment and treatment, as well as to be a source of understanding and support for their difficult situation. For these families and for those where the ill person is disabled by their illness, commonly there is a devastating 'grief' reaction to the 'loss' of the child/sibling/partner, who has been replaced by a stranger. It is helpful for the GP to acknowledge this and to deal with the situation accordingly. Referral to a carer support service is particularly valuable in these instances.

In some cases there will be consumers who have no family support. For a variety of reasons, the ill person may no longer wish to have contact with the family, or the family may have 'given up' and distanced themselves from the ill person. In the latter situation, consumers may feel they are being punished further for their illness. The GP is therefore in an important position as a person of trust for the consumer, and/or to ensure that they are linked into local community support networks.

When medication is prescribed, it is important that this be monitored and reviewed regularly and that consumers are encouraged to report any problems or concerns they may have. In some cases consumers may practise 'doctor shopping': in their constant search for relief, they may seek out different doctors, and they may receive different diagnoses and prescriptions for a range of different medications. This may lead to a situation where it is hard to distinguish between the original mental illness and prescription medication abuse.

In crisis situations the GP may play an important role in helping consumers reach specialist psychiatric care. It is important at these times to acknowledge the terror and distress of the consumer and of the accompanying carer. It is unhelpful and insulting for the person to be told to stop 'catastrophising' and be sent home without support or validation of their distress; this is a high-risk time for suicidal behaviour.

For those consumers whose illness is managed by public mental health services or private psychiatrists, the GP can still play a role in ongoing maintenance treatment of the illness. It is important that in these situations there is open communication between the treating psychiatrist and the GP about the nature of the illness and prescribed treatment. The GP will still be providing care for any physical health problems the person may experience, and therefore an understanding of the mental illness and its impact on their lives is extremely important.

In its *Standards for General Practice*, The Royal Australian College of General Practitioners has developed indicators relevant to consumer interests. It states: 'Patients should be encouraged to participate in their own health care and in each consultation' and 'the practice provides opportunity for, and responds to, patient feedback'. It is acknowledged that the unique information provided by patients about their illness and care needs will enhance a GP's quality of care.

Ideally the relationship between the GP and the consumer and their family carers includes:

- a patient-centred, and where possible, 'family-centred' approach;[19, 20]
- the provision of accurate and accessible information about the illness and its treatment;
- a clear and agreed plan about what to do in an emergency; and
- referral to ongoing support for practical problems, such as employment, finances and accommodation.[21]

CASE STUDY 4

Maria is at her wit's end. Her son George, 18 years, has been acting aggressively at home, throwing saucepans around and making weird comments to his 13-year-old sister, who is becoming distressed. He also laughs at serious reports on the television news, giggles at sculptures he creates from mashed potato at meal times and occasionally either takes his showers fully clothed or stands naked under it without turning on the tap.

George refuses to see a GP as he does not agree there is a problem. Maria's sister has schizophrenia, so she visits a GP herself, recognising that George needs help. After describing what's happening at home, she feels very frustrated when the GP says she can do nothing unless George comes in himself. After some persuasion George agrees, as he can 'snap out' of an episode. To the GP he appears quite 'normal' and he leaves after just a short chat.

Nothing changes at home, and Maria again visits the GP, who then prescribes a sedative for her. This makes her feel very spaced out and does nothing to help her family or George's situation. Maria wishes the GP could arrange for someone to do a home visit to assess George before a crisis occurs. She would also like to talk with someone who has been in a similar situation.

CONCLUSION

The GP has a vital role to play in the overall management of mental illness. An interested and supportive GP, with knowledge of psychological therapies as well as medication, who knows about the available community support services, and who has a holistic view of the situation, will make a great difference to the lives of people affected by mental illness. In some cases, the GP may also support their clients by referring them to community support services. For example, if the person wishes to return to work after a period of unemployment due to their illness, the GP can refer them to a rehabilitation program (to improve social and work skills) or to an employment support service. The GP can also help family carers by expressing interest in how they are coping and referring them to a carers' support group or to respite care provided by a non-government organisation or their local council. Understanding the needs of and supporting family carers as well as consumers strengthens the whole family unit. A support network for the GP will enhance their ability to do this. Thus, effective co-ordination with specialist mental health services, other health professionals and the community sector will make it easier to care effectively for, and improve the lives of, people with mental illness and their family carers. This is a rewarding and fulfilling activity that goes beyond the narrow role of dispensing medication, often attributed to clinicians.

REFERENCES

1. World Health Organization. A Global Review of Primary Health Care. Emerging Messages. Geneva: WHO, 2003.

2. National Health Strategy. Healthy Participation: Achieving Greater Public Participation and Accountability in the Australian Care System. Background Paper No. 12. Canberra: Treble Press, 1993.

3. Consumer Focus Collaboration. The Evidence Supporting Consumer Participation in Health. Canberra: Consumer Focus Collaboration, 2000.

4. Lahdensuo A. guided self-management of asthma: how to do it. British Medical Journal 1999;319:759–60.

5. Lorig K, Sobel D, Stewart A, Brown B, Bandura A, Ritter P, Gonzalez V, Laurent D, Holman H. Evidence suggesting that a chronic disease self-management program can improve health status while reducing hospitalization—a randomised trial. Medical Care 1999;37(1):5–14.

6. Kaplan S, Greenfield S, Ware J. Assessing the effects of physician–patient interactions on the outcomes of chronic disease. Medical Care 1998;27(3):S110–27.

7. Department of Health, Flinders University, South Australian Community Health Research Unit. Improving Health Services through Consumer Participation. A Resource Guide for Organisations. Canberra: Consumer Focus Collaboration and Commonwealth Department of Health and Aged Care, 2000.

8. Carers Victoria (2004): www.carersvictoria.org.au

9. Draper M. Involving Consumers in Improving Hospital Care: Lessons from Australian Hospitals. Canberra: Commonwealth Department of Health and Family Services, 1997.

10. Keleher H, Keks NM, Pietsch J. Models of shared care for depression and related disorders. Central East. http://www.centraleastpcp.infoxchange.net.au/news/items/2004/09/00274.shtml (accessed 27/9/2004).

11. Hocking B. Reducing mental illness stigma and discrimination—everybody's business. Medical Journal of Australia 2003;178:S47–8.

12. McNair B, Highet N, Hickie I, Davenport T. Exploring the perspective of people whose lives have been affected by depression. Medical Journal of Australia 2002;176(10):S69–76.

13. Walker C, Tamlyn J. The Cost of Chronic Illness for Rural and Regional Victorians. Melbourne: Chronic Illness Alliance, 2004.

14. Blashki G, Keks N, Stocky A, Hocking B. Managing schizophrenia in general practice. Australian Family Physician 2004;33(4):21–7.

15. Judd FK, Piterman L, Cockram AM, McCall L, Weissman MM. A comparative study of venlafaxine with a focused education and psychotherapy versus venlafaxine alone in the treatment of depression in general practice. Human Psychopharmacology: Clinical and Experimental 2001;16:423–8.

16. Mynors-Wallis LM, Gath DH, Day A, Baker F. Randomised controlled trial of problem solving treatment, antidepressant medication, and combined treatment for major depression in primary care. British Medical Journal 2000;320(7226):26–30.

17. Gregory RJ, Canning SS, Lee TW, Wise JC. Cognitive bibliotheraphy for depression: a meta-analysis. Professional Psychology: Research and Practice 2004;35:275–80.

18. For more information about these, contact Department of Health and Ageing—National Mental Health Strategy, SANE Australia, beyondblue, Carers Australia, Chronic Illness Alliance, Australian Council of Community Services (ACCOS).

19. Little P, Everitt H, Williamson I, Warner G, Moore M, Gould C, Ferrier K, Payne S. Preferences of patients for patient centred approach to consultation in primary care: observational study. British Medical Journal 2001;322:468–72.

20. Stewart M. Towards a global definition of patient centred care—the patient should be the judge of patient centred care. British Medical Journal 2001;322:444–5.

21. The Royal Australian College of General Practitioners. Draft Standards for General Practices. 3rd edn. Royal Australian College of General Practitoners, 2004.

CHAPTER 4
MENTAL HEALTH, THE LAW AND GENERAL PRACTICE

P Nisselle, J Arranga and L Piterman

A man without privacy is a man without dignity; the fear that Big Brother is watching and listening threatens the freedom of the individual no less than the prison bars.

SIR ZELMAN COWEN, *The Right To Be Let Alone: The Private Man*, Boyer Lecture, 1969

CASE STUDY

The Thomas family is well known to you. Mr Thomas is a 67-year-old retired engineer who has significant heart problems. His wife, 15 years his junior, is a history teacher. They have two sons. The younger one William, aged 19, performed brilliantly at school but has struggled in the first year of his science/engineering course. He spends considerable periods of time in his room on the computer and on the internet, and his mother feels that he is using large quantities of cannabis. She also feels that he is taking other drugs, including anabolic steroids, as his body has changed shape over a very short period of time. She tells you this in a phone conversation, having convinced William to come in for a check up.

During the consultation William admits to using cannabis and says that Xenon rays have interfered with his pituitary gland, reducing his growth hormone and testosterone levels, and he would like you to prescribe replacement therapy. He claims that other doctors have done this. Your refusal and suggestion that he may need psychiatric help are met with hostility. Two months later his mother calls you to the house. William has smashed all the windows in a fit of rage and cut his hands. He claims that unless the energy company stops emitting Xenon rays through his computer, he will kill their CEO and himself.

■ What is the most likely diagnosis?
■ What is your most appropriate course of action?

- What are William's rights?
- How can they be protected?
- What is your ongoing role in this case?

KEY FACTS

- General practitioners (GPs), the professionals most likely to be responsible for early diagnosis and ongoing management of patients with mental illness, should have considerable knowledge of the laws relating to the management of the mentally ill.

- Laws governing the management of the mentally ill may vary somewhat from state to state, but they are underpinned by principles adopted by the United Nations in 1991 and endorsed by the Commonwealth Government in its 1992 National Mental Health Policy.

- The policy adopted by the United Nations calls for 'rigorous criteria to be met before involuntary hospitalisation should be considered and wherever possible treatment should be provided with the consent of the patient'.[1]

- The laws are enshrined in the state *Mental Health Acts*, which are designed to balance the need to protect the rights of the individual against the requirement to ensure that both the individual and society are protected from possible harm.

- The details of *Mental Health Acts* vary from state to state. For example, in Victoria, if a major psychiatric illness has been diagnosed and the patient refuses psychiatric treatment then, using appropriately prescribed forms, the GP can make a request for certification. This remains valid for 72 hours, during which time the patient may be transported against their will to an approved mental health service or be assessed in the community by a mental health practitioner employed by an approved mental health service.

- The circumstances in which recommendation to certify may occur include the following:
  — where the patient is or appears to be mentally ill;
  — where a patient poses a significant risk of causing harm to themselves or to others; or
  — where a patient is exposed to non-deliberate harm through neglect or forgetfulness or harm by others through exploitation or abuse (guardianship orders rather than certification may apply in these circumstances).

- Progressive deinstitutionalisation over the past twenty-five years has resulted in Community Treatment Orders, with tightening of the criteria for involuntary admission. In Victoria a Community Treatment Order, valid for up to 12 months and enabling treatment to be provided in the community on an involuntary basis, may be made.

- In each state Mental Health Review Boards are in place to hear appeals by patients against involuntary admission.

- GPs are often called upon to witness signatures to important documents, such as wills. Under these circumstances, doctors should not consider themselves 'passive witnesses', but must be able to reassure themselves of the 'testamentary capacity' of the person signing the document. This requires assessment of cognition and mental capacity and may include performance of a Mini Mental State Examination (MMSE).

continued overleaf

■ GPs should exercise extreme caution in disclosing information regarding a patient's mental illness to a third party, even when it may appear to be in the interests of public good. Legal advice from a relevant medical defence organisation should be sought in these circumstances.

INTRODUCTION

While there are both public and private specialist services that assist in the management of psychiatric illness, GPs are not only the most common first contact of a person with such an illness but they are also most commonly responsible for the continuing care of such patients. This requires the clinical skills involved in diagnosis and treatment as well as considerable knowledge of the law as it relates to mental health and mentally ill people.

Most mental illness is diagnosed and treated in general practice. Support is available, but mental health resources are limited. The Australian Institute of Health and Welfare reported in 2004[2] that in 2002–2003, there were an estimated 1030 full-time equivalent psychiatrists in private practice—914 in metropolitan areas (6.9 per 100 000 population) and 116 (1.1 per 100 000 population) in rural and remote areas. In 2002–2003, psychiatrists provided some 2 million services while community mental health care services provided about 4.2 million, almost half of which involved management of schizophrenia or related disorders. GPs provided over 100 million consultations in the same year, of which a substantial percentage were solely or partly for management of a mental illness.

Australia is a country ostensibly united by an act of Federation in 1901, but still governed by different laws in each of the six states and two territories and by laws enacted by the Commonwealth government.

Zifcak has outlined the origin and core principles of mental health law in Australia.[3] In his paper, he details how Australia responded to the General Assembly of the United Nations' adoption, in 1991, of 'Principles for the Protection of Persons with Mental Illness'.[1] These principles were endorsed by the Commonwealth government in its National Mental Health Policy (released in 1992) and detailed in the National Mental Health Statement of Rights and Responsibilities.[4]

The United Nations' Principles stated that people with mental illness should:

> ...be treated with dignity and humanity...be free from exploitation, abuse and degrading treatment...as far as possible continue to exercise their civil, political and economic rights...be provided with information about and explanations of their rights...have the right to privacy [and]...be entitled to care and treatment at the same standard as other people who are ill.[1]

The United Nations document also dealt with the protection of people hospitalised against their will—involuntary patients, admitted following 'certification'. The policy called for 'rigorous criteria to be met before involuntary hospitalisation should be considered' and stressed that 'wherever possible, treatment should be provided with the consent of the patient'. It said that protective law should:

...contain restrictions on the use of particularly invasive forms of treatment including medication...[and]...provide for appeal and review both of detention and certain forms of treatment by an independent reviewing authority...[as well as] establish rights to representation, advocacy and procedural fairness.[1]

While there is considerable variation in the wording of the relevant legislation in the Australian states and territories, Zifcak wrote, citing a 1993 analysis,[5] that 'it may fairly be said that this legislation complies substantially with the international standards outlined'.

Why was and is there a perceived need for specific mental health legislation, for safeguards for mentally ill patients over those already available under common law and by statute for all patients? For most of recorded history 'madness' has been considered a medical problem. In the seventeenth century, religious influences altered perceptions of the cause of mental illness, leading to increased persecution of the mentally ill.[6] This is not to imply that prior to this time the mentally ill were viewed with equanimity; however, the perception of mental illness as a sin requiring punishment derived largely from this period. Later, madness again became a medical matter and, with the progress of the Industrial Revolution, asylums were developed to both confine the mentally ill and attempt to treat them. A consequence of this was the separation of mental illness from the medical mainstream and the mentally ill from society.

Thus the mentally ill acquired the stigma of sin and were feared because of their isolation from society. As a consequence of this, legislation that protects the rights of the mentally ill while balancing societal concerns to protect society was developed.[7]

In Australia, legislative responses to mental illness have existed since the nineteenth century. By the mid-twentieth century there was a push to highlight individual rights. The growth of 'consumerism', which empowered consumers and enabled them to bring providers of goods and services more readily to account, spread to medicine generally and psychiatry in particular. In the last third of the twentieth century, Australia became a more 'rightsist' society. There was no longer a need to rely on the Law of Contract and Negligence to pursue redress through Common Law; legislation such as the *Trade Practices Act 1974 (Cwlth)* and legislation establishing and empowering a range of ombudsmen services provided statutory redress.

Politicians did not drive this movement, however; they responded to it by introducing legislation to enhance consumers' rights. It was no coincidence that the enactment of legislation that established medical ombudsmen services, such as the Health Care Complaints Commission in NSW and the Office of the Health Services Commissioner in Victoria, occurred at much the same time as an overhaul of mental health legislation and the introduction of entities such as the Mental Health Review Board to provide statutory protection for the rights of the mentally ill.

Between 1986 and 2000, each state and territory has passed *Mental Health Acts* incorporating relevant legislation to protect the rights of the mentally ill.

The development of mental health law over the last quarter of the twentieth century embraced the concept of less restrictive management of the mentally ill with treatment in the community rather than in an institution; this has been encouraged by the development of concepts such as Community Treatment Orders.

Further, these statutes imposed strict criteria for involuntary admission to a psychiatric hospital, introduced independent external review of involuntary admissions and imposed strict conditions on the provision of electroconvulsive therapy (ECT) and psychosurgery. Doctors are now more aware of the legal framework and limitations within which they can provide psychiatric care. However, Zifcak points out, citing the Burdekin Report,[8] that:

> The contribution of the rights strategy to improving access to and standards of treatment, increasing the resources available for community mental health, decreasing social stigmatisation and engendering more informed policy debate and development, among other things, has been a dispiritingly negligible one.

There are two core reasons for this, one practical and one philosophical. Philosophically, a move to a 'rightsist' society assumes that each individual has the capacity to use their rights rationally—that they, better than the State, know, and will act, in their own best interests. The most fundamental 'right' is the right to be left alone and to decide for ourselves what we wish to do in and with our lives. Justice Benjamin Cardoza most eloquently expressed this in 1914 when he said: 'every human being of adult years and sound mind has a right to determine what shall be done with his own body'.[9]

Championing each individual's right to autonomy and self-determination ignores the reality that sometimes society needs to usurp that autonomy in a person's best interests. The nub is the process by which 'best interests' are determined. It may be difficult to agree on the point where compassion ends and paternalism starts, but the right of autonomy and self-determination needs to be balanced against the right to become and remain well, by receiving appropriate care, even when an individual does not agree that they are 'sick'.

In practical terms, the latter part of the twentieth century saw a massive shift in the care of chronic psychiatric patients away from hospital care to care provided in the community. Was this to protect liberty or to save money? Either way, it has had a negative effect. An economics writer, Kenneth Davidson, wrote in *The Age* in Melbourne in 2003 that 'The policy of closing mental institutions was well meant. But it should be reviewed.'[10] He went on to write:

> The failure to provide for these people outside the institutions has resulted in many of those with more severe mental illness becoming feral psychotics, recycled through the acute psychiatric wards of public hospitals and even the criminal justice system—when a sensible, as well as humane society, should still be offering asylum for those who need it.

To the extent that they receive any ongoing care, many of those chronic 'feral psychotics' now end up in GPs' consulting rooms, between endless episodes experiencing the revolving door of very short-term public care.

COGNITION AND MENTAL CAPACITY
DOCTORS ARE *NEVER* JUST WITNESSES TO DOCUMENTS

Medical practitioners are usually high on the list of people approved to witness signatures on a range of documents. The list varies according to the type of document, but usually includes professional and other groups of high standing and reputation in the community, such as justices of the peace, authorised notaries, solicitors and pharmacists. However, doctors are set apart from the rest of the approved classes of witnesses by their medical knowledge. When a doctor is asked to witness a signature, even if they are reassured that they are simply being asked to act as a witness and not to form any professional view on the competency of the signatory, it may be assumed that in signing a document as a witness to a signature, the doctor has, in effect, certified that the signatory was 'competent' at the time.

ISSUE When asked to witness a signature—whatever the setting, personal or professional—doctors should assume that it is possible they will be asked some time in the future for their view as to the signatory's mental state. If the person is not well known to the doctor—for example, they are a relative of a known patient or friend—the doctor should perform, perhaps by casual conversation, a limited mental state examination, sufficient to come to a reasonable conclusion as to competency. It is strongly recommended that GPs make a diary note about having witnessed a document, and record some notes on the signatory's demeanour and mental state at the time. If the signatory is an established patient, enter such notes in that patient's medical record.

Particular care should be taken if you are asked to witness a will. Arguing that you simply acted as a witness to a signature and did not form a view as to competency or capacity will not go down well if you are cross-examined when the will is contested.

When you are only certifying a person's identity (such as when signing passport photographs and applications), it is clear what you are attesting to, and there is no presumption that you formed a view regarding competency.

The law requires that a person making a will, or giving power of attorney to a third party, must, at the time they sign the document, have 'testamentary capacity' for the document to be effective. This means that the person must have a sound mind, a reliable memory and an understanding of the purpose and content of the document. All persons are considered to be of sound mind unless there is evidence to the contrary.

The sentinel legal principles of testamentary capacity with regard to signing a will have not changed since they were first enunciated, in the language of the time, in an 1870 English decision.[11] Cockburn CJ said:

> It is essential to the exercise of testamentary power that a testator shall understand the nature of the act and its effects; shall understand the extent of the property of which he is disposing; shall be able to comprehend and appreciate the claims to which he ought to give effect; and with a view to the latter object, that no disorder of the mind shall poison his affections, pervert his sense of right, or prevent the exercise of his natural faculties—and that no insane delusions shall influence his will in disposing of his property and bring about a disposal of it which, if the mind had been sound, would not have been made.

Thus there are four principal legal requirements for capacity when assessing whether a person is competent to make or sign a will.[12] The testator, the person signing the will, must:

- understand the purpose of a will, and that the document being signed is a will;
- be aware of the assets to be distributed and deal with them with 'understanding and reason' ('sound disposing mind');

- be aware of those who might reasonably expect to be beneficiaries; and
- be able to consider the options for distribution of assets in a rational way.

Further, for a will to be valid, the testator must have made their decisions freely, without coercion or undue influence.

'Testamentary capacity' is a legal term. Medical practitioners cannot certify testamentary capacity (for example, they cannot certify that there was no coercion or undue influence), but they can provide medical evidence as to a person's mental state.

There are no specific agreed or prescribed tests of mental state and capacity that should be performed when making a formal assessment of a person's mental state and capacity. However, when asked to give evidence, doctors will have been expected to take a reasonable history, and to have conducted an appropriate physical and mental state examination. The doctor should document any condition that might affect a person's mental state as well as any medication being taken by the patient. If, at the time of the assessment, the doctor cannot come to a firm conclusion, specialist neuropsychiatrist assessment should be arranged.

Sometimes the doctor will have performed no formal assessment proactively; however, some time after a patient's death, when (for example) a claim has been lodged, seeking to have a late will set aside and an earlier one put in its place, the doctor will be asked for an opinion as to the patient's mental competence at the time of signing the later will. Doctors are duty bound to assist patients and their families, and on occasions, their legal representatives. Doctors can be compelled by subpoena to attend court. However, once asked to give an opinion or to attend court and give evidence, the doctor's duty is to the court, not to the party who sought the opinion. The doctor must not assume a role as a medical advocate. The doctor's evidence should be entirely non-partisan. If you have no evidence on which to base an opinion, it is entirely appropriate, both in a written report and in verbal evidence, to say just that. When a barrister says, 'But surely, doctor…', you might feel pressured to offer a view, but unless that opinion is supportable by reliable clinical evidence, the opposing barrister will quickly demolish it. Much better to say 'I don't know' and stick to it, if that is truthfully the case.

It is also essential that the doctor have no conflict of interest in making an assessment of competence.[13] To quote from a Policy Statement of the Medical Practitioners Board of Victoria:

> [T]he doctor in question must not knowingly have a conflict of interest at the time of certifying capacity. That is, the doctor should not personally be a beneficiary of the will in question nor should he or she be a member of an organisation that stands to benefit. In such a situation the doctor would do well to suggest than an independent doctor be asked to document the person's capacity to make a will.[14]

Of course, you are not obliged to perform an assessment of mental state and capacity. As with any other medical procedure, if you are asked to assess a patient's capacity, you are entitled to say that such an assessment is outside your technical competence, and to encourage whoever is asking you to seek an independent medical assessment.

ASSESSMENT OF CAPACITY

A number of guidelines on the assessment of mental capacity have been published, including a recently issued Australian book[15] and a book co-issued by the British Medical Association and the Law Society.[16] Another useful reference is a paper, 'Psychiatric assessment in community practice',[17] published in 1998 by Yellowlees. In an attachment, he outlines an approach to mental state assessment.[18]

ISSUE

If you are asked to assess a person's mental capacity, and if, as a result of simple observation, you are in any doubt, a formal assessment, such as the Mini Mental State Examination (MMSE)[19] is a useful starting point (see Chapter 16). It should be stressed that the MMSE is a screening tool for the presence of cognitive impairment. A person could score 30 out of 30 on the MMSE and still be incapable of managing their own affairs. Clearly, however, a score suggestive of cognitive impairment is good objective evidence of the need for further assessment to determine mental capacity.

CAPACITY TO REFUSE TREATMENT

When you are assessing a patient's capacity to consent to or refuse treatment, similar criteria also apply. In Victoria, for example, under the *Medical Treatment Act 1988*, a person can issue a refusal of treatment certificate for a 'current condition'. The *Enduring Power of Attorney (Medical Treatment) Act 1990* (EPA), together with the *Medical Treatment (Agents) Act 1992* (MTAA), enables an adult person of sound mind to appoint an agent (or alternate agent) who can refuse medical treatment for a 'current condition' on behalf of the patient when he or she becomes incompetent.[20] Again the issue of the mental competency of the person at the time they signed the documents may become relevant.

There is a reverse subtlety—the patient who agrees to have treatment but lacks the capacity to give lawful consent. This may occur with the 'compliant elderly'—patients who accept whatever the doctor (or other health care provider) recommends. These are also the people who are preyed upon by unscrupulous salesmen. Doctors may be involved in actions to break contracts on the grounds that the person who entered into the contract was not mentally competent at the time they signed it.

The law on these issues, and related guardianship issues, varies in each state and territory. It is beyond the scope of this chapter to detail all the law.[21]

LACK OF CAPACITY TO REFUSE TREATMENT— THE INVOLUNTARY PATIENT

Mental health legislation focuses on diagnosis and risk of harm as well as the individual's capacity to make competent decisions.

When a doctor has diagnosed a major psychiatric illness in a patient, this will often require the doctor to assess whether the patient poses a risk to himself or herself, or the community, and whether the patient should be detained, involuntarily, in a mental hospital for either or both their and the community's protection. A doctor will need to consider the following issues:

- Is there a significant risk of deliberate harm to self or to others?
    — To self—has the patient expressed thoughts or plans of suicide?
    — To others—has the patient expressed threats to others? These often result from paranoid delusions.
    - Are they exposed to non-deliberate harm?
    — By neglect—has the patient's psychiatric condition caused neglect of their own care (for example, are they not eating or drinking)?
    — By forgetfulness—for example, is their dementia causing them to leave the gas on or the oven door open?[22]
- Are they exposed to being harmed?
    — By intent of others—are there signs of 'elder abuse'?
    — By exploitation (especially financial)?

There are lawful processes by which mentally ill patients can be admitted to hospital, and treated, against their will. These processes are now tightly regulated, and there are substantial rights of review and appeal. The various Mental Health Review Boards are statutory tribunals established to conduct reviews of, and hear appeals by, psychiatric patients being treated involuntarily, either as inpatients or on Community Treatment Orders.

Statutory criteria for involuntary treatment are highly specific. For example, paragraph (1) of section 8 of Victoria's *Mental Health Act 1986*[23] tightly defines the criteria to be that:

(a) the person appears to be mentally ill; and
(b) the person's mental illness requires immediate treatment and that treatment can be obtained by the person being subject to an involuntary treatment order; and
(c) because of the person's mental illness, involuntary treatment of the person is necessary for his or her health or safety (whether to prevent a deterioration in the person's physical or mental condition or otherwise) or for the protection of members of the public; and
(d) the person has refused or is unable to consent to the necessary treatment for the mental illness; and
(e) the person cannot receive adequate treatment for the mental illness in a manner less restrictive of his or her freedom of decision and action.

Subsection 1(A) loosely defines a mental illness as: '…a medical condition that is characterised by a significant disturbance of thought, mood, perception or memory'.

Perhaps in the knowledge of the abuse of psychiatric certification in other countries, paragraph (2) of that section explicitly defines circumstances that cannot be cited as evidence of mental illness:

A person is not to be considered to be mentally ill by reason only of any one or more of the following—

(a) that the person expresses or refuses or fails to express a particular political opinion or belief;
(b) that the person expresses or refuses or fails to express a particular religious opinion or belief;

(c) that the person expresses or refuses or fails to express a particular philosophy;

(d) that the person expresses or refuses or fails to express a particular sexual preference or sexual orientation;

(e) that the person engages in or refuses or fails to engage in a particular political activity;

(f) that the person engages in or refuses or fails to engage in a particular religious activity;

(g) that the person engages in sexual promiscuity;

(h) that the person engages in immoral conduct;

(i) that the person engages in illegal conduct;

(j) that the person is intellectually disabled;

(k) that the person takes drugs or alcohol;

(l) that the person has an antisocial personality;

(m) that the person has a particular economic or social status or is a member of a particular cultural or racial group.

Paragraph (3) makes clear that (2)(k) 'does not prevent the serious temporary or permanent physiological, biochemical or psychological effects of drug or alcohol taking from being regarded as an indication that a person is mentally ill'.

GPs themselves cannot 'certify' patients; they can only recommend certification. Again, taking the *Mental Health Act 1986 (Vic)* as an exemplar, once a 'request for certification' has been made 'in the prescribed form and containing the prescribed particulars' and a recommendation made by a medical practitioner, again 'in the prescribed form and containing the prescribed particulars', it is valid for 72 hours. Within that time the patient can be transported against their will and held at an 'approved mental health service' where they must be reviewed within 24 hours by a psychiatrist. Alternatively, they can be assessed in the community by a mental health practitioner, who must determine whether the person needs to be taken to the Mental Health Service. If it is determined they do not, an Involuntary Treatment Order (ITO) is made, the person is not detained, but must be seen within 24 hours by the Authorised Psychiatrist who must confirm the ITO and either make a Community Treatment Order (CTO) for the person or detain them in the Mental Health Service, or discharge the person from involuntary status. Thus the GP's only power, in this regard, is to ensure the patient is held in a secure setting pending formal psychiatric assessment. Even then, that power is not exercised alone. Another person must have signed a request for certification.

Once the person has been admitted to the Mental Health Service, they must be seen and assessed by an authorised psychiatrist within 24 hours. If the psychiatrist does not agree that there is a need for an ITO, then the patient may either remain as a voluntary patient or be discharged/allowed to leave. If the psychiatrist confirms the ITO, the patient can be detained against their will. If the patient is unable or unwilling to consent to treatment, the authorised psychiatrist can provide such consent.

Once an ITO has been confirmed, the person can be treated as an inpatient or managed in the community. If the latter, a CTO, valid for up to 12 months, may be made.

The patient may appeal any order to the Mental Health Review Board.

DUTY OF CONFIDENTIALITY VERSUS DUTY TO PREVENT FORESEEABLE HARM

Legislation has been enacted by the Commonwealth (*Privacy Act 1988*, as amended in 2001), and some states (Victoria's *Health Records Act 2002*, NSW's *Health Records and Information Privacy Act 2002* and the ACT's *Health Records (Privacy and Access) Act 1997*) to protect the confidentiality of health information, but each piece of legislation allows disclosure to prevent harm.

In the *Privacy Act 1988*, this is outlined in Principle 11, 'Limits on disclosure of personal information':

1. A record-keeper who has possession or control of a record that contains personal information shall not disclose the information to a person, body or agency (other than the individual concerned) unless:

    ...(c)   the record-keeper believes on reasonable grounds that the disclosure is necessary to prevent or lessen a serious and imminent threat to the life or health of the individual concerned or of another person.[24]

Note that disclosure is permitted without the patient's consent only if three criteria are satisfied:

- 'serious and imminent threat'—not medium or longer term;
- 'life or health'—not, for example, a potential pecuniary loss; and
- 'the individual concerned or of another person'.

Similarly, in Victoria's *Health Records Act 2002*, Privacy Principle 2(h) uses similar language to allow disclosure of health information without the patient's consent if the holder of the information:

(h)   ...reasonably believes that the use or disclosure is necessary to lessen or prevent—
   (i)   a serious and imminent threat to an individual's life, health, safety or welfare; or
   (ii)   a serious threat to public health, public safety or public welfare...[25]

In a recent article,[26] the author canvassed the ethical and legal dilemma posed when a doctor's duty of confidentiality to a patient appears in conflict with a duty to prevent foreseeable harm to another. When dealing with a disturbed, mentally ill patient who states threats, a GP may feel alarmed that the patient poses a credible risk to either a person nominated by the patient or to the community at large. If the patient satisfies the criteria for involuntary admission to and detention in a secure mental hospital, the obvious course of action is to obtain the forms necessary to request certification and, if necessary, seek the assistance of the police to transport the person to secure detention in a psychiatric hospital.

Whether or not the patient satisfies the criteria for certification, can the doctor breach confidentiality and notify those at whom the threats were directed? There is legal support for that view. In 1969, Lord Denning, the great English judge, said: '[T]here are some things which may be required to be disclosed in the public interest, in which event no confidence can be prayed in aid to keep them secret.'[27]

When a doctor provides information in a 'Recommendation for Certification', that clear breach of confidentiality is not only sanctioned by law, but also protected by law. The doctor cannot be sued for compliance with a statutory duty.

There is one Californian judgment that goes directly to the issue of breaching confidentiality to warn of a risk posed by a mentally ill patient.[28] In the 1970s, Tatiana Tarasoff, a student at the University of California, was murdered by a mentally disturbed fellow student, Prosenjit Poddar. He had earlier discussed his intention to kill her with a University Health Service psychologist, who felt bound by his duty of confidentiality not to report this threat to Ms Tarasoff directly. However, the psychologist did tell his supervising psychiatrist, who reported the matter to the campus police, who in turn interviewed Mr Poddar, but they let him go. After the murder, the girl's parents sued the psychologist (or, rather, his employer) for 'failure to warn', in that no warning was conveyed to their daughter. The trial court held that no such duty to warn existed but, on appeal, the Californian Supreme Court disagreed and found for the parents of the dead girl.

However, at a Medical Board hearing in 2004 in Western Australia, a finding of 'gross carelessness and improper conduct' was made against an Australian Defence Force doctor who had, according to the Board, 'improperly referred [a senior officer] to a psychiatrist in the absence of any symptoms' and 'acted against [the officer's] trust and confidence' when he conveyed his concern about the officer's mental state to her commanding officer.

It was alleged that the doctor had written inaccurate reports about the patient, that he had sent a referral to a psychiatrist without the patient's consent, and that he had breached his duty of confidence by discussing the patient's condition with the commanding officer. This precipitated a wave of concern, as there was a general assumption, indeed an expectation, that doctors would breach patient confidentiality if they believed, on reasonable grounds, that there was a significant chance that others could be put at risk by a patient's illness— especially in the armed forces, where the patient could have access to weapons.

There is no question that, even in the armed forces, doctors have a duty of confidentiality to their patients. People do not give up their right to medical privacy just because they have enlisted. But sometimes, when there is a conflict between their duty of confidentiality to the patient and their duty to prevent foreseeable harm to others, doctors must decide which duty should prevail. It is certainly wrong, but can breaching patient confidentiality be seen as the lesser of two evils? In 1991, the abduction and murder of a 13-year-old Melbourne schoolgirl, Karmein Chan, was thought to be the work of a serial offender, dubbed 'Mr Cruel' by the press. A letter was sent to all Victorian doctors by the Medical Board and Victoria Police, detailing a profile that was thought would apply to the offender and asking doctors to disclose the identity of any patient they suspected might fit the profile.[29] The then President of the Medical Practitioners Board of Victoria, Dr Bernard Neale, stated in the letter that in his view breaching patient confidentiality was in this instance justified by the better interests of the community—that is, the prevention of harm to other children at the hands of 'Mr Cruel'.

The attitudes of the Western Australian Medical Board and the Victorian one seem diametrically opposite, at least in 2004 and 1991, respectively.

Faced with that dilemma today, a GP caught between the needs and rights of a mentally ill patient and a duty to prevent foreseeable harm should seek legal advice, usually through their medical defence organisation. It would seem unlikely that any criticism could attach to a GP who acted on reasonable grounds, without malice, in accord with competent advice, and where the situation accords with the special circumstances broadly outlined in the *Privacy Act 1988*, viz:

- a 'serious and imminent threat';
- to the 'life or health'; and
- of 'the individual concerned or of another person'.

REVISITING THE CASE STUDY

William is most likely to be suffering from an acute psychotic episode, probably schizophrenia with paranoid delusions. The onset of psychosis may have been triggered by overusing cannabis. He has significant associated somatic delusions that may prove difficult to manage in the long term, although the prognosis in relation to the acute episode may be good.

Every effort should be made to convince William to accept admission to a mental health facility as a voluntary patient. In the event that this is not possible, given the serious nature of his delusions with associated threats to kill himself and the CEO of the energy company, there are sufficient grounds to recommend certification as an involuntary patient. Appropriate documentation will therefore need to be prepared and the Crisis Assessment Team called, as well as the police if necessary, to transport William to the local psychiatric facility.

In Victoria, the request and recommendation for involuntary treatment are valid for 72 hours, but need to be ratified within 24 hours of admission through assessment by a mental health practitioner or by the authorised psychiatrist. Should William wish to challenge this involuntary treatment order, he may do so through the Mental Health Review Board, which has been established to protect his rights in this case.

Your role as a family doctor in this case is, of course, rather complex. Following William's discharge from the psychiatric hospital, in addition to supporting the family, you may also need to play a continuing role in supporting him in a difficult setting in which he knows you were responsible for his involuntary admission if that was the outcome of your earlier management. Generally speaking, once in remission, a patient in these circumstances will accept ongoing care from their GP even though the doctor may have played a role in their involuntary hospitalisation (see Chapter 12).

CONCLUSION

As in other interactions with the law, GPs need to balance their role as patient advocates against their duty of care to protect the community. In dealing with mental illness, this may be challenging. The rights of patients are enshrined in a number of *Mental Health Acts* and guardianship laws. GPs should be familiar with these, especially or particularly when it comes to involuntary admission of patients to institutions and to assessment of testamentary capacity.

REFERENCES

1. Principles for the Protection of Persons with Mental Illness and for the Improvement of Mental Health Care, United Nations General Assembly (1991), 46th Session, Item No. 98(b).
2. http://www.aihw.gov.au/publications/aus/ah04/ah04-c12.pdf (accessed 3 July 2005).
3. Zifcak S. Towards 2000: Rights, Responsibilities and Process in the Reform of Mental Health Law. Australian Journal of Human Rights: http://www.austlii.edu.au/au/other/ahric/ajhr/V4N1/ajhr413.html#fn1 (accessed 3 July 2005). An earlier version of this article was delivered as the keynote address to the conference 'Mental Health: Where's the Vision', The First National Conference of Mental Health Review Tribunals and Guardianship Boards, Centre for Health Law, Ethics and Policy, University of Newcastle, February 1997.
4. Australian Health Ministers National Mental Health Policy (Commonwealth of Australia, 1992). Australian Health Ministers National Mental Health Statement of Rights and Responsibilities (Commonwealth of Australia, 1991).
5. Human Rights and Mental Illness, Report of the National Inquiry into the Human Rights of People with Mental Illness, Human Rights and Equal Opportunity Commission (the Burdekin Report). Canberra: AGPS, 1993.
6. James N, Barrett R. A Historical Context. In: Bloch S, Singh B, eds. Foundations of Clinical Psychiatry. 2nd edn. Melbourne: Melbourne University Press, 2001:4–5.
7. James N, Barrett R. A Historical Context. In: Bloch S, Singh B, eds. Foundations of Clinical Psychiatry. 2nd edn. Melbourne: Melbourne University Press, 2001:6–7.
8. Human Rights and Mental Illness, Report of the National Inquiry into the Human Rights of People with Mental Illness, Human Rights and Equal Opportunity Commission (the Burdekin Report). Canberra: AGPS, 1993:Chapter 30.
9. *Schloendorff v The Society of New York Hospital* (1914) 211 N.Y. 125 (at 129–30), 105 N.E. 92, 93.
10. Davidson K. What about the disabled. The Age, 19 June 2003 http://www.theage.com.au/articles/2003/06/18/1055828379282.html (accessed 3 July 2005).
11. *Banks v Goodfellow* (1870) 5 QB 549.
12. Peisah C, Brodaty H. Dementia and the will-making process: the role of the medical practitioner. Medical Journal of Australia 1994;161:381–4.
13. http://www.mdasa.com.au/files/BulletinDec04.pdf (accessed 9 July 2005).
14. http://medicalboardvic.org.au/content.php?sec=38 (accessed 9 July 2005).
15. Collier B, Coyne C, Sullivan K. Mental Capacity: Powers of Attorney and Advance Health Directives. Sydney: Federation Press, 2005.
16. British Medical Association and the Law Society. Assessment of Mental Capacity—Guidance for Doctors and Lawyers. 2nd edn. London: BMJ Books, 2002.
17. http://www.mja.com.au/public/mentalhealth/articles/yellowlees/yellowlees.html (accessed 9 July 2005).
18. http://www.mja.com.au/public/mentalhealth/articles/yellowlees/yelbox3.html (accessed 9 July 2005).
19. Folstein M, Folstein SE, McHugh PR. 'Mini-Mental State': a practical method for grading the cognitive state of patients for the clinician. Journal of Psychiatric Research 1975;12(3):189–98.
20. Mendelson D. The Medical Treatment (Enduring Power of Attorney) Act and assisted suicide: the legal position in Victoria. Bioethics News 1992;12(1):34–9.
21. A useful summary can be found at pages 57–9 and 83–5 in: Medicine and The Law—A Practical Guide for Doctors. Medical Defence Association of Victoria, 2005. See: http://www.mdav.org/Content.asp?Document_ID=664
22. This is unlikely to be grounds for certification under the *Mental Health Act* but may be grounds for seeking placement under a guardianship order.
23. The whole Act can be found at http://www.austlii.edu.au/au/legis/vic/consol_act/mha1986128/ (accessed 9 July 2005).
24. http://www.austlii.edu.au/au/legis/cth/consol_act/pa1988108/s14.html (accessed 16 July 2005).
25. http://www.austlii.edu.au/au/legis/vic/consol_act/hra2001144/sch1.html (accessed 16 July 2005).

26. Nisselle P. Can you tell? Should you tell? ADF Health 2005;6(1):9–11.
27. *Fraser v Evans* (1969) 1 All ER 8, 11.
28. *Tarasoff v regents of the University of California* (1974) 529 P 2d 253.
29. Mendelson D. 'Mr Cruel' and the medical duty of confidentiality. Journal of Law and Medicine 1993;120.

CHAPTER 5
CROSS-CULTURAL ISSUES IN GP PSYCHIATRY

L Kiropoulos, S Klimidis and G Blashki

The characteristics of a people should find expression in the frequency as well as the shaping of the manifestations of mental illness in general; so that comparative psychiatry shall make it possible to gain valuable insights into the psyche of nations and shall in turn also be able to contribute to the understanding of pathological psychic processes.

KRAEPELIN, 1904[1]

CASE STUDY

Anh is a 45-year-old Vietnamese woman who has limited English skills and presents with sore legs, back and neck pain and a range of other muscle pains. Anh states that these muscle pains sometimes become unbearable, that she is always fatigued and that lately her sleep has been disrupted. This is the tenth time Anh has seen the GP; she is always accompanied by her husband in the consultation room. Anh endured her symptoms for a couple of years and has consulted with 'traditional' healers prior to seeing the GP. Anh only speaks when she is spoken to and avoids eye contact with the male GP. Often her husband, whose English is more fluent, answers questions that the GP has directed to Anh. Tests have shown no diagnosable physical disorder. Anh was sponsored by her husband and migrated here when she was 16 years old. She has been working in the same factory job for years and has two children who are studying at university. Anh also manages the household. She has no other family here in Australia and has limited contact with her parents and siblings in Vietnam. Due to financial reasons, Anh and her husband have not been able to visit her family in Vietnam, and this has always been a stress for Anh.

- Exclusive somatic presentation and frequent attendance in people of culturally and linguistically diverse (CALD) background may suggest the presence of psychological problems.

- The stigma of mental illness is especially prominent in people of CALD and refugee background, and may affect symptom disclosure.

- Traditional collectivistic values and beliefs, such as gender roles based on patriarchal values, may be held by CALD patients, and these may affect the GP–patient interaction.

- Language issues such as limited English skills, lack of equivalent emotional concepts across cultures and loss of meaning, information and understanding upon translation may affect the presentation by CALD and refugee patients as well as the detection of mental disorder by GPs.

- Cultural health belief systems or explanatory models differ in CALD populations.

- Understanding CALD and refugee patients' social and pre-migratory circumstances may aid in the detection, diagnosis and management of mental disorder.

- Awareness of what CALD and refugee patients see as appropriate doctor–patient dynamics will facilitate the GP–patient interaction.

- Pharmacological effects (dosage requirements and side effects) may differ in patients from CALD backgrounds, especially Asian patients.

- Identifying negative attitudes and perceptions regarding medication use in CALD patients within the clinical context may improve therapeutic alliance, compliance and treatment completion.

- Frequent presentation of symptoms such as sleep disturbance, nightmares, anxiety, panic attacks, phobic reactions, irritability and aggressiveness may suggest a psychosomatic basis to mental illness in refugee patients as a result of torture and trauma.

INTRODUCTION

Emil Kraepelin, the father of modern Western psychiatry, suggested a new specialty—comparative psychiatry—be created within psychiatry to study cultural differences in psychopathology. This evolved from his journeys from his home in Germany to Asia and North America, where he noted differences in the frequency and expression of mental disorders compared to Germany and Northern Europe. Following from Kraepelin's work, the last few decades have seen psychiatry and other mental health professions acknowledge the critical importance of cultural factors in mental disorders. This has led to an emerging conceptual and methodological framework that views cultural factors as integral determinants of the onset, expression, course and outcome of mental disorders. In accord with this framework, this chapter will discuss cultural factors that may influence the presentation, diagnosis, treatment and disorder in culturally and linguistically diverse (CALD) patients in general practice. These factors will be illustrated by reference to Anh as a case study that will be referred to throughout the chapter.

Australian general practitioners (GPs) are often the first point of call for people, including those of CALD backgrounds, seeking mental health care. Typically the GP is confronted with the more complex problems in assessing and treating mental disorder in CALD people, and this is further complicated by the presence of physical comorbidity. The case study of Anh typifies some of the cultural issues that have been shown to influence the presentation of mental illness in general practice as well as the assessment, treatment and management of mental illness in patients of CALD background by GPs. Effective care of this patient group requires that GPs are aware of and understand how cultural issues may influence the presentation of mental illness and the recognition, diagnosis and management of mental illness for CALD patients. Specifically, the factors that have been shown to be influenced by culture—including somatisation, stigma of mental illness, values and beliefs, language, beliefs about illness, explanatory models, a patient's social context, power dynamics and attitudes towards GPs, and medication compliance—will be discussed. In addition, there are other cultural factors influencing refugee patients in general practice.

WHAT IS CULTURE?

In this chapter we refer to culture as the world views of particular groups of people defined by commonalities in language, religion, traditions, values, attitudes, beliefs, rules guiding behaviour, modes of dress, relationship to the physical and metaphysical environment, relationship to time, physical appearance and race, and interpersonal behaviour. These are usually but not exclusively related to historical and geographical determinants. There may be 'within-group' variance present in a group of people who have the same birthplace or ethnicity, and this 'within-culture' variance may, in fact, be larger than any 'between-cultures' variance.[2] This implies that GPs should be cautious in using cultural stereotypes as a means of interpreting any patient's behaviour (normal or otherwise). Culture is both an ascribed and subjective phenomenon, and there may be discontinuity between the two. Based on knowledge of birthplace, ethnic group and religious orientation, among other indicators, culture may be ascribed to members of a group (in-group members) by those outside the group (out-group members). Those from the out-group may hold assumptions (stereotypes) about particular groups that may or may not be accurate, that may be held strongly or weakly (as preliminary 'working' definitions), and these assumptions come to influence the nature of their interactions with in-group members. Subjective culture is an individual phenomenon where certain attributes of the culture are more emphasised and valued than others in defining personal identity and how the self should interact with others as well as the physical and metaphysical environments. Culture differs from ethnicity—the latter is considered to be self-defined and corresponds to an individual's self-perceived identity (see also Chapter 6 for a discussion of the importance of GPs identifying the cultural identity of patients, particularly those from indigenous populations).

FACTORS AFFECTING MENTAL HEALTH CONSULTATIONS WITH CALD PATIENTS IN GENERAL PRACTICE
STIGMA OF MENTAL ILLNESS

The stigma associated with having a mental disorder is present in many CALD populations, and this influences symptom disclosure and appropriate help seeking for mental health problems. This may in turn influence the detection and diagnosis of mental illness in patients. Stigma relates to an attribute that is socially discrediting.[3] Cultural beliefs and the cultural environment influence a person's and a community's view or attitudes regarding mental illness. In collectivistic groups (see below), such as many of the CALD groups, the social stigma of having a mental illness may be more likely to spread to other in-group members[4] than is the case in more individualistic communities, such as the Anglo-Australian. Stigma therefore poses real threats of social exclusion and cultural discontinuity in members of CALD communities, including family members.

The stigma attached to psychiatric disorder and emotional distress stems from many sources. For example, the content of symptomatic experience and behaviour may be viewed as strange or bizarre; others may fear the unpredictability and real or imagined violence from the individual; or the sufferer may constitute a drain on limited material or psychological resources within the group. According to certain ethnopsychological ideas, there may also be a fear of contagion. If the disorder is thought to be hereditary or to reflect moral wrongdoing, there may be 'guilt by association'. In addition, the individual with a mental illness may remind others of their own vulnerability. It has been suggested that these multiple sources ensure that the stigma associated with mental illness will be a problem in most societies.[5, 6]

In the case study, Anh, who may be experiencing depression and/or anxiety, has presented to the GP with somatic symptoms perhaps because these may be relatively more socially benign than psychological symptoms. In Vietnamese culture, depressive symptoms may be seen as socially disadvantageous and may lead to diminished social status and self-esteem, impacting on a person's ability to perform effectively in society.[7] In comparison, a diagnosis of a physical disorder may serve to avoid the stigma of mental illness. A diagnosis that is culturally 'sanctioned', such as a physical diagnosis, may provide validation of Anh's suffering to her family and the broader Vietnamese community, of which she is a member. In addition, compared to patients from individualistic cultures, CALD patients who come from collectivistic cultures are less likely to disclose emotional and psychotic symptoms to a doctor.[8] Hence, the stigma of having a mental illness may be a powerful barrier affecting the presentation and disclosure of mental health problems in CALD patients in general practice. A strong implication of this is the need for GPs to establish a trusting relationship with the patient and the family, and to give repeated assurances regarding the confidentiality of the doctor–'consumer' relationship.

SOMATISATION

Cultural variations in the expression and presentation of mental disorders in general practice have been regularly noted.[9] Patients from a CALD background who have a mental disorder are likely to present more often with somatic rather than psychological symptoms to their GP.[10, 11] This has been termed 'somatisation', and for many patients it may be a culturally appropriate way of expressing distress in their culture.[10, 12, 13] One of the implications of cultural variations in the expression and presentation of emotional distress by CALD patients is that they may lead to underdetection and misdiagnosis of mental disorder by GPs. This is because they direct attention away from emotional and behavioural symptoms that are critical for a mental health diagnosis. Throughout her ten visits to the GP, Anh only reported somatic symptoms such as muscular, back and joint pains and sleeping problems (which were inconsistent with a specific physical diagnosis) rather than presenting with negative thoughts or complaints of lowered mood. This is consistent with Australian research results that have suggested that hypertension, acute upper respiratory tract infection, diabetes and lipid disorder (which are all physical problems) were all managed more frequently for CALD patients than Anglo-Australian patients, and also that psychological problems were less likely to be managed.[14]

It should be noted that the phenomenon of somatisation has been widely reported; one of the repeated explanations has been that somatisation is a way to avoid social stigma.[15, 16] An example of somatisation is neurasthenia (*Shenjing, Shuairuo* or weakness of nerves) within Chinese communities. It is a syndrome of sleeplessness, physical exhaustion, headache, poor memory, distractibility and dizziness. It enables the expression of mental distress and the labelling of minor mental illness without incurring the stigma of a psychiatric diagnosis. In this context, somatisation can be a morally acceptable way of legitimising psychosocial problems.[16] In Anh's case, the stigma attached to mental illness in her culture may have forged the expression of a mental condition to a more physical/somatic expression. In addition, some of the other reasons suggested to explain why CALD patients somatise include: differential responsiveness to the situational cues (demand characteristics) involved in the doctor–patient situation;[8, 17] and biased information processing (the degree and nature of attention to the self have been cited as a potentially important factor in mediating certain dysfunctional processes in psychological disorders).[8, 18]

For further information on somatisation, see Chapter 11.

COLLECTIVISTIC VALUES AND BELIEFS

In collectivistic cultures, where people are integrated from birth into strong and cohesive in-groups, family relationships are central.[19] Collectivistic cultures often have traditional sex roles based on patriarchal values that include high parental control of children and control of the wife by the husband.[20] Cultural values reveal the dynamics operating in interpersonal relationships. In collectivistic cultures, a form of control of the wife by the husband may include making the key decisions relating to his wife's and family's health and wellbeing. This is illustrated in Anh's case, as she is always accompanied to the GP's surgery by her husband, who often responded to the GP on behalf of his wife. This is not simply due to the differences in English proficiency. In some cultural groups, such as those from Iraq, there are taboos imposed on male doctors examining female patients, especially in the absence of the husband. This implies that the GP must forewarn the patient and gain permission to conduct physical examinations or, alternatively, make arrangements for appropriate gender compatible examinations.

Some patients of CALD background present to the GP at a later stage of their mental disorder, tolerating a great deal of emotional and psychological distress before seeking professional assistance. In addition to stigma, this may be due to cultural character factors such as stoicism as well as collectivistic values that dictate a focus on not disturbing family harmony and coherence.[21] Hence, collectivist values and beliefs may impact on the GP–patient interaction by influencing the communication and disclosure of symptoms by the patient, which in turn will affect the GP's diagnosis and treatment.

LANGUAGE

A number of language difficulties may affect the presentation, detection and diagnosis of mental health problems in CALD patients. Communicating symptoms and experiences across linguistic and cultural boundaries may result in a loss of meaning, information and understanding that may affect the detection and diagnosis of a mental disorder.

Assessing a bilingual patient or a patient for mental disorder such as Anh, who has limited English, may prove difficult, because emotion and mental health terms are much harder to express in a second language. Even if the patient is able to conduct a simple conversation in English, they may not be sufficiently proficient in English to discuss their psychological state or to understand and participate in a clinical discussion of diagnosis and treatment.[22] Furthermore, expressing emotion in one's second language is often associated with a lack of emotionality—this should not be confused with affect being blunted or inappropriate (which is a clinical sign of mental disorder).

Ideally, non-bilingual GPs should use a trained interpreter who is fluent in the language of the patient to ensure a meaning oriented translation of what is being said during the consultation. This will help avoid mistranslations of biomedical concepts, errors of omission and having a three-way conversation where the translator is inserting their version of the material being discussed. An interpreter is preferred over a family member, as the patient may not want to disclose information in front of their family. Indeed, use of informal interpreters such as family members can lead to major distortions and perhaps dangerous outcomes for the patient. For instance, Anh has not seen her GP without her husband, and this may affect her ability to openly discuss her concerns. It is also important to ensure patient confidentiality regarding the interpreter's role, especially when discussing mental health issues. Many patients from small communities fear a loss of confidentiality with such highly stigmatised conditions and this therefore inhibits their communication with the GP.

Another language issue that Anh may be facing is that her language may lack particular terms—for example, Vietnamese has no direct translation for the word 'depression'. Different cultures do not necessarily have the equivalent emotional concepts found in the English language; in fact, emotional concepts are particular to culture and language—that is, patients from a CALD background will learn and inherit concepts such as sadness from their culture, and CALD people will also differ in terms of what they feel emotion about.[23] Different cultures emphasise different emotions and these have different values and meanings attached to ostensibly similar terms.[24] Furthermore, in many Asian groups excessive expression of emotion is not condoned because it is seen to disrupt social harmony and cause sickness. Hence, it cannot be assumed that emotions are the same or represent the same values and meaning across cultures. Therefore, it should not be assumed that CALD patients will present in general practice with the typical Western-style emotion nor that the emotional disorder will be similar to that experienced by Western patients.

EXPLANATORY MODELS

Explanatory models may play a role in the presentation, detection, diagnosis and treatment of mental disorders in general practice.[25] An explanatory model, or the way that an illness is conceptualised, relates to the meaning of illness—specifically, what constitutes the views of causes, important symptoms, course, consequences and treatments or remedies.[9] All aspects of the explanatory model are influenced and shaped by cultural and social factors, such as socioeconomic status and education,[17] and can influence help seeking, compliance with treatment and patient satisfaction.[26]

Cultural variation in explanatory models is particularly relevant to causal attributions of mental illness. For example, non-Western theories of natural causation include concepts such as inbalance in the qualities of *yin* and *yang* (in Chinese medicine) and *am* and *duong* (in Vietnamese culture), and also nerve weakness (as in neurasthenia), where there is inadequate physical energy in the central nervous system.[27] Supernatural theories of causation of mental illness—such as fate, magic or 'evil eye'—are also prevalent in many cultures. For example, in Vietnamese culture, mental illness may be viewed as being caused by a supernatural agent, such as a soul, ghost or god. Violation of a taboo or a moral wrongdoing is also seen to cause mental illness.[24] Hence what a CALD patient views as the causes or important symptoms of a mental disorder may influence whether or not mental disorder is presented to a GP. Beliefs about the nature and cause of a particular mental disorder will determine when and from whom people will seek help.[28] Clearly conceptualising experience as something other than a mental illness often results in help seeking from alternative sources (for example, priests, traditional healers, prayer, herbal remedies) as well as delays in appropriate access to care. This may result in the patient presenting to a GP at a point where the mental illness is in a late phase and more difficult to treat.

Different presentations of mental illness by CALD patients—for example, symptoms may be mainly physical or patients may be hearing voices that they may consider culturally appropriate—may result in misdiagnosis by the GP and inappropriate treatment, failure to co-operate with treatment or refusing treatment. GP consultations with patients of CALD background may require a 'negotiation of explanatory models' between the GP and the patient, where both the patient and the GP acknowledge differences in belief systems, and the GP makes attempts to reconcile these differences.[29] Part of this process requires the GP to be aware of his or her own ethnocentric and professional biases[29] and for the GP to demonstrate awareness of, and respect for, their patient's health and illness beliefs. Questions around the patient's view of mental disorder will elicit information about their explanatory model. Figure 5.1 provides a summary of questions, based on Kleinman's[17] original concepts of health and sickness and the short explanatory model interview,[30] which can be used by GPs to elicit CALD patients' explanatory models relating to mental disorder.

In Anh's case, information about her help seeking and any alternative treatments she may be receiving concurrently may be helpful in designing a treatment and management plan that is both acceptable to her and will facilitate treatment compliance. For example, negotiation between the GP and a CALD patient's explanatory models—that is, display of understanding and respect for Anh's health beliefs by the GP—may result in the GP working collaboratively with a traditional healer in order to provide the most effective treatment and management plan for Anh.

FIGURE 5.1 Eliciting explanatory models of illness in CALD patients

1 NATURE AND CAUSES OF THE PROBLEM

- When did you first notice that there was a problem?
- Why do you think that the problem began when it did?
- What do you call this problem? What is its name?
- How long ago did you first notice this problem?
- What do you think caused this problem?
- Do you think that this problem is an illness?

2 IMPORTANT SYMPTOMS OF THE PROBLEM

- What do you think are the most troublesome aspects of this problem?
- Which symptoms trouble you the most?

3 DEVELOPMENT AND COURSE OF PROBLEM

- How did the problem develop with time up to now?
- How do you think this problem may develop and progress over time in the future?
- Do you think the condition will become worse, improve, stay the same or come and go over time?

4 SEVERITY AND CONSEQUENCES OF THE PROBLEM

- How serious do you think this problem is?
- What are the most and least troublesome aspects of the problem?
- What are the main difficulties your problem has caused you?
- How does the problem affect your relationships, your work/study, your family role and responsibilities, attending to your daily needs and so on?

5 TREATMENT AND HELP SEEKING FOR PROBLEM

- Is there a particular way that people in your culture/ethnic group deal with this type of problem? What is usually done?
- Is this treatment relevant in your case?
- What treatment do you think will be effective with this problem?
- What do you think you yourself can do to help with this problem?
- How do you think I can help with this problem?
- [If medicine is asked for] Do you think the medicine will cure the problem or just help to control it? How quickly do you expect the medicine to do this?

PATIENT'S PAST AND CURRENT SOCIAL CONTEXT

Mental illness may be strongly influenced by adverse social circumstances, and these may alert the GP to the possibility of a mental disorder.[31] For example, factors affecting the clinical presentation may include the political context of arrival, reasons for migration (political, economic), level of contact with the Australian majority group, level of exposure to high risk industries and lower post-migration employment status relative to education and experience of discrimination. Research has indicated that recent adverse life events (more than one in the past year) together with multiple visits to the GP (greater than ten visits in a year) increased the odds for the presence of a mental disorder forty-fold.[32] Opening a discussion to one's more recent life difficulties may be one way GPs could begin to explore the possible presence of a mental disorder.

REVISITING THE CASE STUDY Anh arrived in Australia as a migrant sponsored by her husband. It would be worthwhile asking her what pre-migration factors may have had an impact on her current emotional state (see 'Cultural factors influencing mental health consultations with refugee patients'). She has limited contact with the majority Anglo-Australian culture, perhaps because of her limited English skills. Anh and her husband usually perform heavy manual work and have been under constant financial strain; they are also supporting their two children at university. This financial stress has meant that she also has limited contact with her family in Vietnam.

Depending on several factors, such as family expectations of a continuing role in supporting the family in Vietnam, the issue of separation from the family may also be significant for Anh. It is important to understand her current level of contact with other Vietnamese (especially women), her level of social support, opportunities for socialisation and any means of redressing social or psychological difficulties.

Anh's social context (pre-migration and post-migration) puts her potentially in the high risk category for developing a mental disorder. Her frequent visits to the GP may also indicate some underlying mental health problem. Hence, an awareness of the CALD patient's past and their current social context, particularly patients who have experienced recent adverse life events or who attend the GP frequently, may aid GPs in the detection of mental disorder as well as support the diagnostic decisions regarding mental health problems. Patients may also consult a GP after consulting a number of other culturally appropriate healers, or they may be using other culturally sanctioned remedies and rituals for their mental health.[17] For example, Anh carries amulets with her and frequently prays, and prior to seeing a GP she had consulted her herbalist, who suggested that she needs to rebalance the energy (*am* and *duong*) in her body by taking herbal medications.

INTERPERSONAL DYNAMICS AND ATTITUDES TOWARDS GPs

Power distance between the CALD patient and the GP has important implications for the detection, diagnosis, treatment and management of mental disorders. Power distance is the extent to which relationships are structured hierarchically. In high power distance societies, those in power are respected and obeyed, while those not in power can expect the powerful to look after their interests and protect them. It is important to be aware that within any society there may be different definitions of status. In many high power distance cultures, those in positions of status, such as doctors, carry power. Subordinates in high power distance cultures expect to be told what to do by those in authority. Subordinates are expected to show respect and deference to their superiors and this sets the tone of many relationships, including the doctor–patient relationship.

In the high power distance culture, such as in the Vietnamese culture, professionals are viewed and accepted as superior, and they expect to be treated with respect and deference. This is shown in Anh's behaviour, which is characterised by a less direct and assertive manner, overt passive acceptance of the treatment and low expressed demand for education by the GP regarding the problem and its treatment. Limited eye contact, not addressing the doctor by his first name, speaking only when she is asked specific questions and not asking any questions are typical expressions of the patient's perception of the relative status of the doctor. These should not be interpreted as signs of psychopathology necessarily. Indeed, in this situation, Anh is faced with two power distance issues that may influence her decision to disclose relevant symptoms. Abiding by the high power distance rule, she may regard both the doctor and her husband as superior, to be treated with respect and deference. In Anh's case, her husband is present during all consultations and often speaks to the male GP on her behalf.

Patients from a CALD background may have different expectations, concerns, meanings and values about GPs. People of CALD background may view the GP as the expert on physical illness while their role as the patient is to present and describe their physical illness.[17, 33] This may explain, in part, the higher rate of somatic presentations to GPs (despite the presence of a psychological disorder) as is the case with Anh. It may also partly explain why emotional, social and psychological difficulties are less often reported to a GP, because the problem may not be considered relevant or appropriate for such reporting.[17, 33]

MEDICATION COMPLIANCE

Non-compliance appears to be more problematic and prevalent in some non-Western cultures.[34] GPs may need to be aware of a number of factors that influence medication use and compliance in CALD patients. Some of these factors include attitudes towards, and expectations of, drug effects as well as bona fide differences in the effects of psychotropic medication that then influence attitudes.

ATTITUDES, EXPECTATIONS AND RELIGIOUS BELIEFS Attitudes towards, and expectations of, drug effects are often shaped by the patient's cultural origin and past experiences, and this influences medication use and compliance.[34] Non-Western CALD patients commonly perceive Western medicines to be more potent and to have greater adverse side effects than herbal or traditional therapies, often with good reason.[35] Cultural differences in the expectation and the interpretation of drug effects can also significantly influence the acceptance and adherence to pharmacological treatment. So much of modern medicine and its means of use is incongruent with traditional healing.[35] These considerations may require the GP to more vigorously educate the patient about the nature and the use of medications. Careful monitoring of attitudes to drug treatment is of particular relevance to the ongoing acceptance of medications and compliance in CALD patients.

It is also worth noting that attitudes in the patient's social network can also influence the patient's compliance with the recommended treatment.[36] In collectivistic societies, it is generally expected that other family members will be intensively involved in the treatment, administration of medicines and decisions to continue or not with treatment. This highlights the need to negotiate treatment with the wider family system and particularly with those who have power over important decisions.

Religious beliefs may also affect compliance with medication in people from CALD backgrounds. For example, some Muslim patients have been known to make changes to medication intake time and dosing during Ramadam, often without seeking GP advice.[37] As the efficacy and toxicity of psychotropic medications can vary, depending on the time of administration and their interaction with food intake, GPs must consider religious beliefs and practices when advising patients. This is even more relevant for drugs with a narrow therapeutic index, as the risk of toxicity or side effects is higher.

DIFFERENCES IN THE EFFECTS OF PSYCHOTROPIC MEDICATIONS In recent years, research has found significant differences among ethnic groups in their response and propensity to side effects of medications related to genotypic variations in drug-metabolising isoenzymes.[38–40] These differences lead to variability in pharmacokinetics (absorption, distribution, metabolism and excretion) and pharmacodynamics (biological mechanisms whereby psychotropic agents generate therapeutic and side effects).[41] Metabolism is regarded as the most significant factor in determining interindividual and interethnic differences.[42] Research has found that a greater proportion of some patients of Asian background require lower dosages of neuroleptics than Caucasians or European patients.[43] For example, in one study, compared to Caucasians and African Americans, Asian patients who were prescribed antipsychotic medication were found to have a greater incidence of extrapyramidal side effects.[44] Another study found that, compared to Caucasians, patients of Asian background responded therapeutically to a lower dosage of lithium.[40] In addition, patients of Asian background tend to require lower doses of tricyclic antidepressants.[45] The implications of this are that GPs need to stringently monitor drug effectiveness and toxicity, and be guided by their clinical observations rather than by dosage recommendations alone.

CULTURAL FACTORS INFLUENCING MENTAL HEALTH CONSULTATIONS WITH REFUGEE PATIENTS

In Australia, GPs provide the majority of health care to refugees and asylum seekers, most of whom have come from Yugoslavia, the Middle East, South-West Asia and Africa. Refugees and asylum seekers differ from migrants in that they have different pre-arrival experiences and needs to most other migrants, in particular because they may require counselling for torture or trauma, secure housing and medical care. Refugees are people who have been persecuted and forced to leave their country. Asylum seekers are people arriving without a valid entry permit or on a temporary visa who subsequently apply for refugee status.

These immediate settlement and mental health needs impact on the treatment and management of refugee patients in primary care. GPs may have difficulties identifying refugee patients and establishing whether these patients have experienced torture and other traumatic experiences. As a consequence of these experiences, refugees may be at great risk of a range of psychological problems, including post-traumatic stress disorder, depression, anxiety, stress related psychosomatic symptoms and greater 'self-medication' through the use of alcohol or other drugs. With this patient group, GPs need to be aware of cultural issues (similar to those of CALD patients) that may affect assessment, diagnosis, treatment and ongoing management, including: limited English skills, the sociocultural context at pre-migration, the patient's cultural and religious beliefs, somatisation and the stigma of mental illness. Reluctance to discuss trauma is common, and there may be additional fears of deportation due to poor health—both of which may limit the GP's ability to understand the patient's mental health status.

CULTURAL FACTORS INFLUENCING THE ASSESSMENT AND PRESENTATION OF REFUGEE PATIENTS

As many refugees do not speak fluent English, this may pose a problem when working with this patient group. Family members and friends may often act as interpreters, and this may affect the quality and range of conveyed information about mental health status. The potential for miscommunication between the GP and the refugee patient is heightened by the impact of psychological trauma that may be evident in the refugee patient. In those with post-traumatic stress disorder, there may be substantial avoidance of discussion of trauma and reminders of traumatic experiences, a common feature of the syndrome. As with CALD patients, professional interpreters are recommended, and it is important that GPs be aware that in certain circumstances political, religious or cultural sensitivities may influence an interpreted interaction. Further, it is important to establish whether the patient prefers a male or female interpreter.

As refugees have commonly suffered abuse and persecution, sensitivity regarding different religious or ethnic groups may also be needed, including in choosing an interpreter. Those who have experienced torture and other traumatic experiences may display distrust and suspicion of authority figures as well as of services and people they do not know, and may be reluctant to seek help outside their family. Moreover, the GP needs to avoid consultation conditions that may imply 'interrogation'. Patients may be reluctant to sign documents, including consent for medical procedures. In some cases a patient may fear deportation on the basis of their poor health status; the GP should vigorously reassure patients about the use of the information gained during the consultation.

Assessing refugees for mental illness in general practice may pose other difficulties for GPs. For example, refugee patients may be reluctant to tell their GP about their pre-migratory experiences, which may include torture or traumatic experiences. Refugees may avoid discussing these issues with the GP due to mistrust, fear of reprisal towards themselves or their family, fear of humiliation and stigmatisation and fear of re-living the experience. In addition, in their culture it may be inappropriate to discuss these issues with a GP, who may need to be aware of certain symptoms and signs that may suggest that the refugee patient has experienced trauma or torture. These include multiple physical complaints that seem unresolved, complex injuries and unusual or complex real or psychosomatic problems. Common presenting symptoms of mental health problems by refugees to GPs may include: sleep disturbance, nightmares, anxiety, panic attacks, phobic reactions, irritability, aggressiveness, sadness, poor concentration or memory problems, dissociation, paranoid ideation and drug and alcohol abuse. Presentation of these symptoms may suggest a psychosomatic basis to the illness as a result of experiences of torture and trauma, especially if there is frequent presentation in general practice of these symptoms with no physical basis.

CULTURAL FACTORS INFLUENCING THE MANAGEMENT OF REFUGEE PATIENTS

Management of refugee patients may be complicated by cultural and/or religious differences between the GP and the patient. For example, some refugees may have come from cultures in which patients were not provided with opportunities or encouraged to ask questions or seek clarification about issues discussed in consultations. Refugees may also have a distrust of authority figures (these authority figures may have been involved in perpetrating or supervising torture in the refugee's country of origin). Overall, the GP needs to be aware of and assess issues related to the torture and trauma of the refugee patient—for example, whether the patient and GP are ready to discuss and deal with these issues in the consultation and what the refugee patient's expectations of the GP are. It may also be appropriate for GPs to explore the patient's explanatory model (causes, important symptoms, appropriate treatment and expectations of treatment).

As with CALD patients, GPs should implement a management plan jointly with the refugee patient in order to facilitate treatment compliance. The refugee patient's cultural and religious beliefs and practices may have an impact on treatment options. For example, refugees may come from areas where medications may be poorly regulated, and refugees may not be aware of the consequences of inappropriate doses. Compliance with medication may also be influenced by the refugee's lack of English skills and understanding of the effects of the medication.

GPs need to be aware that many refugee patients may not be familiar with counselling for mental health problems in their culture, and that they often have different coping mechanisms for dealing with psychological trauma. For example, refugees from the Horn of Africa have described 'forgetting' or 'active forgetting' as their usual means of coping with psychological difficulties.[46]

In management it may be important to attend to pragmatic issues of support for housing, work and social connectedness, as problems in such areas serve to heighten the propensity for traumatic syndromes. A referral to appropriate trauma counselling is a necessity in indicated cases.

CONCLUSION

Through the discussion of the various cultural factors presented in our case study of Anh and other examples, we have demonstrated that underdetection, misdiagnosis and inappropriate treatment of mental health problems can be avoided if GPs embark on an exploration of the cultural and social background of each patient. A comprehensive exploration of cultural issues will enable an in-depth understanding of a patient whose cultural background is different from their own. We have also attempted to illustrate how the immediate settlement and mental health needs of refugees also affects the GP–refugee patient interaction. Adopting a conceptual and methodological framework that views cultural factors as integrated in the expression, assessment and treatment of mental disorders will help GPs to provide the most appropriate and acceptable management for CALD and refugee patients.

REFERENCES

1. Kraepelin E. Vergleichende psychaitrie. Zentralblatt fur Nervenherlkande und Psychiatrie 1904;15:433–7.
2. Triandis H. Cross-cultural perspective on personality. In: Johnson JA, Hogan R, eds. Handbook of Personality Psychology. San Diego: Academic Press, 1997;439–64.
3. Goffman E. Stigma: Notes on the Management of Spoiled Identity. Englewood Cliffs, NJ: Prentice Hall, 1963.
4. Gudykunst WB, Ting-Toomey S, Chua E. Culture and Interpersonal Communication. Thousand Oaks, CA: Sage Publications, 1988.
5. Kirmayer L. Cultural variations in the response to psychiatric disorders and emotional distress. Social Science and Medicine 1989;29:327–39.
6. Fabrega H. Psychiatric stigma in non-western societies. Comprehensive Psychiatry 1991;32:534–51.
7. Hsiao F-S. Chinese-Australian Families' Help-seeking Behaviours for Mental Illness. Melbourne: Department of Psychiatry, University of Melbourne, 2002.
8. Kiropoulos L. Psychosocial Mechanisms Underlying Cultural Differences in Depressive and Anxiety Illness Symptom Reporting and Presentation: A Comparison of Greek-born Immigrants and Anglo-Australians. Melbourne: Department of Psychiatry, University of Melbourne, 2004.
9. Bhui K, Bhugra D. Explanatory models for mental distress: implications for clinical practice and research. British Journal of Psychiatry 2002;181:6–7.
10. Chan B, Parker G. Some recommendations to assess depression in Chinese people in Australasia. Australian and New Zealand Journal of Psychiatry 2004;38:141–7.
11. Gater R, De Almeida E, Sousa B, Barrientos G, Caraveo J, Chandrashekar CR, Dhadphale M, Goldberg D, al Kathiri AH, Mubbashar M, Silhan H. The pathways to psychiatric care: a cross-cultural study. Psychological Medicine 1991;21:761–74.
12. Gureje O, Simon GE, Ustun TB, Goldberg DP. Somatization in cross-cultural perspective: a World Health Organization study in primary care. American Journal of Psychiatry 1997;154:989–95.
13. Comino EJ, Silove D, Manicavasagar V, Harris E, Harris MF. Agreement in symptoms of anxiety and depression between patients and the GPs: the influence of ethnicity. Family Practice 2001;18:71–7.
14. Knox SA, Britt H. A comparison of general practice encounters with patients from English-speaking and non-English speaking backgrounds. Medical Journal of Australia 2002;177:98–101.
15. Cheung F. Facts and myths about somatization among the Chinese. In: Lin TY, Tseng WS, Yeh EK, eds. Chinese Societies and Mental Health. Hong Kong: Oxford University Press, 1995;156–66.
16. Cheung F, Lau BWK, Waldman E. Somatization among Chinese depressives in general practice. International Journal of Psychiatry in Medicine 1981;10:361–74.
17. Kleinman A. Patients and Healers in the Context of Culture. Berkeley, CA: University of California Press, 1980.
18. Kiropoulos L, Klimidis S. A self-focused attention scale: factor structure and psychometric properties. Cognitive Therapy and Research 2006;in press.
19. Hofstede G. Culture's Consequences: International Differences in Work-related Values. Beverley Hills, CA: Sage, 1980.
20. Georgas J, Berry JW, Shaw A, Christakopoulou S, Mylonas K. Acculturation of Greek family values. Journal of Cross-Cultural Psychology 1996;27:329–38.
21. Loo C, Tony B, True R. A bitter bean: mental health status and attitudes in Chinatown. Journal of Community Psychology 1989;17:283–94.

22. Westermeyer J, Janca A. Language, culture and psychopathology: conceptual and methodological issues. Transcultural Psychiatry 1997;34:291–311.
23. Triandis HC. The Analysis of Subjective Culture. Canada: John Wiley and Sons, 1972.
24. Andary L, Stolk Y, Klimidis S. Assessing Mental Health Across Cultures. Qld: Australian Academic Press, 2003.
25. Goldberg DP, Huxley P. Mental Illness in the Community. London: Tavistock, 1980.
26. Carillo JEA, Green AR, Betancourt JR. Cross-cultural primary care: a patient-based approach. Annals of Internal Medicine 1999;30:829–34.
27. Kleinman A. Rethinking Psychiatry: From Cultural Category to Personal Experience. New York: Free Press, 1988.
28. Angel R, Thoits P. The impact of culture on the cognitive structure of illness. Culture, Medicine and Psychiatry 1987;11:465–94.
29. Kleinman A, Eisenberg L, Good B. Culture, illness and care: clinical lessons from anthropological and cross-cultural research. Annals of Internal Medicine 1978;88:251–8.
30. Lloyd KR, Jacob KS, Patel V, St Louis L, Bhugra D, Mann AH. The development of the Short Explanatory Model Interview (SEMI) and its use among primary-care attenders with common mental disorders. Psychological Medicine 1998;28:1231–7.
31. Maginn S, Boardman AP, Craig TKJ, Hadad M, Heath G, Stott J. The detection of psychological problems by general practitioners: influence of ethnicity and other demographic variables. Social Psychiatry and Psychiatric Epidemiology 2004;39:464–71.
32. Klimidis S, Cao H, Chiang S. Patient Factors Associated with Doctor- and Patient-reported Mental Disorders in a General Practice for Mainland Chinese Patients: Part 3. Melbourne: Centre for International Mental Health, University of Melbourne, 2004.
33. Parker G, Gladstone G, Chee KT. Depression in the planet's largest ethnic group: the Chinese. American Journal of Psychiatry 2001;158:857–64.
34. Li KM, Poland RE, Nakasaki G. Psychopharmacology and Psychobiology of Ethnicity Washington, DC: American Psychiatric Press, 1993.
35. Lee RP. Perceptions and uses of Chinese medicine among the Chinese in Hong Kong. Culture, Medicine and Psychiatry, 1980;4:345-75.
36. Mantonakis J, Markidis M, Kontaxakis V, Liakos A. A scale for detection of negative attitudes towards medication among relatives of schizophrenic patients. Acta Psychiatrica Scandinavica 1985;7:186–9.
37. Aadil N, Houti IE, Moussamih S. Drug intake during Ramadan. British Medical Journal 2004;329:778–82.
38. Ng C-H, Schweitzer I, Norman T, Easteal S. The emerging role of pharmacogenetics: implications for clinical psychiatry. Australian and New Zealand Journal of Psychiatry 2004;38:483–9.
39. Matthews HW. Racial, ethnic and gender differences in response to medicines. Drug Metabolism and Drug Interactions 1995;12:77–91.
40. Pi EH, Gray GE. A cross-cultural perspective on psychopharmacology. Essential Psychopharmacology 1998;2:233–59.
41. Lin K-M. Biological differences in depression and anxiety across races and ethnic groups. Journal of Clinical Psychiatry 2001;62:13–19.
42. Sjoqvist F, Borga O, Dahl M-L, Orme MLE. Fundamentals of clinical pharmacology. In: Speight TM, Holford NHG, eds. Avery's Drug Treatment. Auckland: Adis International, 1997;1–73.
43. Lin K-M, Finder EJ. Neuroleptic dosages in Asians. American Journal of Psychiatry 1983;40:490–1.
44. Lin K-M, Poland RE, Nuccio I, Matsuda K, Hathuc N, Su TP, Fu P. A longitudinal assessment of haloperidol doses and serum concentrations in Asian and Caucasian schizophrenic patients. American Journal of Psychiatry 1989;146:1307–11.
45. Yamamoto J, Fung D, Lo S, Reece S. Psychopharmacology for Asian Americans and Pacific Islanders. Psychopharmacology Bulletin 1979;15:29–31.
46. British Medical Association. Asylum Seekers: Meeting Their Healthcare Needs. London: British Medical Association Publications Unit, 2002.

CHAPTER 6
INDIGENOUS ISSUES IN GP PSYCHIATRY

J McKendrick and P Te Ara Bennett

Te whare e kitea, te kokonga ngakau e kore e kitea
Things are not always as they seem

ANCIENT MAORI PROVERB

KEY FACTS

- Indigenous peoples have been defined as original inhabitants, people who have a long-standing close relationship to a specific area of land (in the case of Aboriginal Australians, it's tens of thousands of years). There are over 500 groups of indigenous people throughout the world. Indigenous peoples have diverse cultures, but are linked by the fact that they have all been colonised.

- Through their experiences of colonisation, indigenous peoples are exposed to the risk factors for the development of mental health problems at much higher rates than other people.

- Indigenous peoples have shown great resilience in the face of colonisation. Australian Aboriginal people and New Zealand Maori have retained strong identities and connectedness to kinship groups, culture and land. If recognised by the general practitioner (GP), these strengths can assist in the development of the therapeutic relationship with indigenous patients as well as their assessment and management.

- Language misunderstandings between Western clinicians and indigenous patients impact on the therapeutic relationship, diagnosis, management and compliance.

- Indigenous cultural values and beliefs differ from Western values, and this factor can influence the therapeutic relationship, and also compliance with management plans. Indigenous cultural beliefs can be misinterpreted as being indicative of psychopathology.

KEY FACTS *continued*

- Indigenous people often have different views of wellbeing and illness, including different views of the ways in which illness should be managed.

- The Western GP should take time to get to know the indigenous patient and also let the patient get to know the doctor.

- Careful, interested listening is an important technique to develop for all patients, but especially those from indigenous backgrounds.

- The assessment, diagnosis and management of indigenous patients are often complicated by cultural and social factors that are not obvious to the clinician. Cultural consultants with specific knowledge of the culture and circumstances of the patient and their community can advise on such factors. Cultural consultants may be members of the patient's extended family, indigenous health workers from the local Aboriginal health service or Maori health provider, or indigenous liaison workers in the local mainstream health service.

- The indigenous patient may prefer to see the GP in the company of a family member, friend or a worker from the local Aboriginal health service or co-operative or Maori health provider. This method of consultation usually has a positive impact in terms of accuracy of assessment, compliance with treatment and the ongoing therapeutic relationship.

INTRODUCTION

In this chapter, we focus on the indigenous peoples of Australia and New Zealand. It is necessary to examine their histories and current status to understand the mental health problems they experience and how we as clinicians can help them in attaining wellbeing. Living as they do in environments ranging from temperate to tropical, coastal to desert, mountains to plains, Australian Aboriginal people have always been diverse—in lifestyle as well as culturally and linguistically. In contrast, New Zealand Maori share a common language, customs and key cultural concepts. However, there is also significant diversity. Recognition of this diversity is important in the clinical setting—for example, in selecting the most appropriate cultural consultant.

Aboriginal people comprise 1% of the total Australian population, although in parts of the north, central and west of Australia, Aboriginal people form the majority of local populations. Fifteen per cent of the New Zealand population identify as Maori; however, in some regions, Maori are in the majority.

Colonisation of indigenous peoples has invariably had negative consequences, including multiple losses (land, family, wellbeing, life), rapid changes in lifestyles, and assaults on the physical, psychological, spiritual and social wellbeing of individuals and communities. Most indigenous peoples are marginalised and excluded from participation in the majority culture. However, indigenous peoples around the world have continued their relationships with the land and their ancestors, from which their identities spring. Where necessary, they have made changes to the ways in which they live and practise their cultures so that their cultures can survive.

The processes of colonisation, to which the Aboriginal people of south-eastern Australia were subjected, were replicated throughout the country. Aboriginal people were forced from their traditional lands by settlers, thus deprived of their sources of food, shelter and spirituality. Starvation, introduced diseases and violence perpetrated by settlers resulted in a rapid decline in Aboriginal populations. The remnants of Aboriginal tribes were sent to missions, where their lives were controlled by European managers. The official view was that Aboriginal people would gradually die out, and that the role of the missions was to 'smooth the dying pillow'.[1] However, Aboriginal populations began to increase in the early twentieth century, and active assimilation policies were pursued in all states and territories, with the ultimate aim of having Aboriginal people merge with Europeans, and disappear as a separate group.[1, 2] The most devastating policy was that of taking Aboriginal children from their parents and extended families, a policy that continued into the 1970s.[2] It is estimated that one-third of Aboriginal people were removed from their families during the twentieth century. Many suffered emotional, physical and sexual abuse at the hands of their carers in foster homes and children's homes.[2] Aboriginal musician Archie Roach and his siblings were taken from their parents in the 1960s. Like so many members of the 'Stolen Generations',[1–3] Archie was never to see his parents again. Archie tells the story of his life through his music. His song 'Took the Children Away' captures the pain and hurt that spans generations.

New Zealand was colonised later than Australia, although trade between Australian settlers and Maori flourished from the late 1700s onwards. Maori societies were self-sufficient in resources and had well developed systems of knowledge and learning. The maintenance of good health was the responsibility of the individual, the family and the tribe, and depended upon the integrity of these networks and culture.[4] In 1840, the Treaty of Waitangi was signed by tribal chiefs and the Crown. Among other things, the Treaty guaranteed Maori the right to control their own lives and *taonga* (treasures, including lands, forests, rivers and health) as well as equal rights with British subjects. The numbers of European settlers in New Zealand increased rapidly in the latter half of the nineteenth century and in the early twentieth century. In contravention of the Treaty, Maori lands were taken initially by force and later through legislation, with ownership transferred to Europeans for farming and other developments. By the middle of the twentieth century, so much land had been taken that to survive, Maori had to move from rural areas to the towns and cities where work was available. Many Maori now lived far away from their extended family and tribal networks. The resultant breakdown of some Maori family and tribal networks was accompanied by a reduction in the health status of Maori.

Today, Australian Aboriginal people and New Zealand Maori are the most socioeconomically deprived groups in their respective countries. They have lower school completion rates than other Australians and New Zealanders, respectively, and higher rates of unemployment, and are over-represented in the criminal justice systems. Australian Aboriginal people have a life expectancy that is twenty years less than other Australians while New Zealand Maori have one that is ten years less than other New Zealanders. The excess morbidity and mortality among Australian Aboriginals and Maori is due to early onset of, and mortality from, cardiovascular disease, diabetes, respiratory disease and cancer. There has been little change for the better in these health statistics over the past four decades.[1, 3–5] However, both Aboriginal people and Maori reject a deficit approach to the health of their communities.[6] Instead they recognise the resilience of their people and the strength of cultural beliefs, which have facilitated survival, recovery and development in the face of the marginalisation, socioeconomic deprivation and poor health—physical, psychological and spiritual—which impinge on their everyday lives.[1, 4–6] Aboriginal and Maori communities emphasise the good of the collective, which in turn ensures that individuals within the collective are supported. In Australia, Aboriginal people have established community based and controlled health services, legal services, child care agencies and co-operatives to meet the needs of their people.[1, 3] Maori iwi (tribes) have established health services, including mental health services, and social services to provide an alternative to, and to work in cooperation with, mainstream health services.[5] These initiatives on the part of Aboriginal people and Maori can provide assistance to GPs working with indigenous patients. Time spent establishing co-operative relationships with local indigenous services is time well spent.

In this chapter we identify key factors that can promote positive outcomes in clinical encounters between the primary care physician and indigenous patients in mental health. The model allows for the incorporation of both indigenous and Western knowledge in the clinical setting.

COMMON MENTAL HEALTH PROBLEMS AMONG ABORIGINAL PEOPLE AND MAORI

Clinical experience and research in general practice and the community shows that Aboriginal people experience higher rates of psychiatric morbidity than the general community.[1, 3] The excess morbidity is due to higher rates of depression and post-traumatic stress disorder. A study of a randomly selected sample of Aboriginal adults attending a GP with a physical complaint found that two-thirds were depressed.[1, 7] Similarly, a random community sample of Aboriginal adults found that 50% of respondents were depressed.[3] Diagnoses of depression were associated with the experience of multiple losses (especially the deaths of close family members), removal from their Aboriginal family during childhood, poverty, the experience of racism and dislocation from traditional lands.[1, 7, 8] Evaluation of the first Aboriginal specific mental health programs[8] found that women were more likely to attend as outpatients than men, with the most common reason for presentation being depression associated with a variety of life stressors. Men were more likely to be admitted to an acute inpatient psychiatric service with psychotic symptoms often associated with heavy substance use. Most mental health service users also had a coexisting chronic physical illness (diabetes, respiratory disease and cardiovascular disease). Those who had been separated from their Aboriginal families during childhood were over-represented in both inpatient and outpatient groups.[8] GPs, especially those working in remote or rural areas, may be confronted with high rates of suicide and attempted suicide among young indigenous people.[3, 9] Young men are more likely to complete suicide, and young women are more likely to make suicide attempts.

In New Zealand, there is little evidence from community or general practice studies about the patterns of mental health problems among Maori. New Zealand's pre-eminent psychiatrist and Maori academic Professor Mason Durie, drawing on his decades of

---

FIGURE 6.1 Key factors pertaining to mental health problems among Aboriginal people and Maori

1 Depression and post-traumatic stress disorders, associated with loss, poverty, lack of educational opportunity and adverse life experiences (exclusion from full participation in wider society; experience of racism; dislocation from extended family support networks; dislocation from traditional lands) are the most common mental health problems among Aboriginal people and Maori.

2 Misdiagnoses can occur unless symptoms and signs are viewed in a cultural context and a good therapeutic relationship is established. Two of the most common errors are:

   (a) Symptoms of grief and depression, including communicating with ancestors, are misinterpreted as symptoms of psychosis.
   (b) The patient provides little information (verbal and non-verbal) and is (mistakenly) said to have no psychiatric disorder.

3 People with mental health problems often present to the GP with a physical health problem, either their own or that of their child or grandchild. Details of the mental health problem are often left to last, emerging only when the physician has established a relationship of trust.

4 Aboriginal people and Maori may consult an indigenous healer before consulting the Western clinician, or may seek advice from both at the same time.

5 Aboriginal people and Maori with a mental health problem often also have a chronic physical illness, such as diabetes, cardiovascular disease or respiratory disease. These illnesses occur at earlier ages among Aboriginal people and Maori than other Australians and New Zealanders, respectively.

---

experience working in the area of Maori mental health, believes rates of depression are high, especially among Maori women. Much of this depression is unrecognised and so untreated.[10] A qualitative study of the views of Maori mental health providers and Maori community members about mental health[11] found that both groups saw depression as being very common and 'part of life'. Most community members said they would follow healing practices, passed down through the generations, before consulting a Western clinician. Rates of admission of Maori men and women to psychiatric hospitals with a diagnosis of schizophrenia have remained higher for Maori than non-Maori over the past decade; the reasons for this are being investigated.[11, 12]

There are many reports in the psychiatric literature of differing symptomatology among indigenous peoples compared with non-indigenous peoples and of factors associated with mental health problems that are specific to indigenous peoples.[1, 10, 12–14] In a longitudinal study of a cohort of Aboriginal general practice attendees, where over 90% of diagnoses were of depression, many respondents had high scores on the paranoid and psychotic dimensions of the Symptom Checklist.[1] It may be that symptoms labelled as 'psychotic' in Western cultures can be normal expressions of grief and depression among some indigenous people, raising the possibility of misdiagnoses in cross-cultural clinical settings.

CASE STUDIES

The following case studies of Ellen and Matiu describe two common mental health problems among Australian Aboriginal people and Maori people: one of depression and one of psychosis. Each illustrates aspects of mental health problems among Aboriginal people and Maori and of best practice in consultation, diagnosis and management when working with Australian Aboriginal people and Maori with mental health problems.

CASE STUDY 1: ELLEN

Ellen is a 48-year-old Aboriginal woman. She lives in a country town, and has come to the city to visit her sister. She visits your surgery with her sister, who is a long-term patient of yours. You ask Ellen and her sister into your office for the consultation and notice immediately that Ellen is trembling. Ellen's sister makes introductions, then urges Ellen to 'tell doctor what has been happening'. She tells you she needs some blood pressure tablets, having left hers at home.

You take a history. Ellen is not very forthcoming, although she does say she has been told she has a problem with 'sugar', but she is not on any medication and does not monitor her blood glucose. She does not move when you ask her to go to the examination couch and she refuses to have her blood pressure taken. She cannot remember the name of her antihypertensive medication. You ask if you can telephone her usual doctor. At this she becomes very upset and starts to cry. She says she does not go to see him any more, and she has in fact been taking her husband's blood pressure tablets because she has been feeling a bit 'giddy' lately and they seem to help. You persuade her to let you take her blood pressure and find her to be normotensive. When you tell her this, Ellen starts to sob and, with her sister's encouragement, she begins to slowly tell you her story.

Five years ago her 18-year-old son committed suicide by hanging himself in a police cell. He had been gaoled overnight for being drunk. There had been an inquiry, but Ellen was not happy with the findings—her son's body was badly bruised and she believed he had been beaten in the cell. Furthermore, he had been a champion footballer and held down a steady job with the local Aboriginal co-operative. He had always been a happy, outgoing person and Ellen tells you there is no way he would have killed himself. Ellen said she had never been the same since her son's death. She has lost interest in everything, has given up her job at the local Aboriginal co-operative and rarely leaves the house. She has also stopped being a regular at the local football team's matches and training; her son had been one of the team's best players.

To make matters worse, Ellen's husband has started drinking heavily and refuses to talk about their son. Ellen's other four children are married with their own families and have moved away from their home town. Ellen rarely sees her grandchildren, although her daughters ring her several times a week. Lately, Ellen says, she cannot even be bothered to get out of bed. She has stopped shopping and preparing meals, and has no interest in keeping house. She and her husband cannot speak to each other without becoming sad or angry. Ellen denies feeling suicidal, but admits she has not been sleeping and has lost 12 kg over the past couple of months.

You ask if anyone in her family has had a mental health problem. She says no. 'In fact,' she says, 'my father was a "clever man" [an Aboriginal doctor] who had special powers and could cure all sicknesses.' She says he had taught her some of the things he knew. Ellen says she has been hearing her father's voice lately and he has come to her when she is in her house (she had inherited the house from her father). He told her he was looking after her son, and not to worry. He told her that she could become well by preparing the 'bush remedies' he had taught her. When she went into the forest to collect the plants from which she would prepare the bush medicine, Ellen says she clearly saw the 'old people', in their possum cloaks and carrying their digging sticks, walking past her. She says her son was with them, but they disappeared when she tried to catch up with them. Ellen rushed home to tell her husband. He told her to stop speaking nonsense, and became enraged and tried to hit her.

Ellen went to the local doctor—he wanted her to go to the psychiatric hospital. She refused, and went home and rang her sister, who immediately drove up and brought Ellen to her home in the city. Ellen often starts crying during the telling of her story and is comforted and reassured by her sister. The sister tells you she has often had experiences similar to those Ellen has described, and that the people in their home community believe such experiences to be normal, especially for someone like Ellen, who is known as a 'clever woman'. Ellen's sister tells the doctor that Ellen will stay with her until she feels better—'as long as it takes'.

You make an appointment for Ellen and her sister the next day, asking them to ring the emergency number if there are any problems. After several more consultations with Ellen's sister present, you have ruled out diabetes and hypertension; Ellen is very healthy physically. As you get to know Ellen and her sister, you are confident that the psychiatric diagnosis is one of mild to moderate depression following the death of her son. Ellen agrees to a trial of antidepressants and to come in regularly 'for a chat'. Ellen's sister agrees to help with the medication and sometimes comes in with Ellen to let you know how things are going from her perspective. You notice improvement in Ellen's mental state within ten days and her improvement continues over the next few weeks. One day Ellen brings her husband with her to the consultation. He, Ellen and Ellen's sister have been talking together about their son's death. The husband has stopped drinking and is back at work. He thanks you very much for all your help. Not long after, Ellen moves back home. Her sister comes to let you know, and asks you to write a letter to the doctor at the local Aboriginal co-operative to tell her Ellen's story.

CASE STUDY 2: MATIU

Matiu comes into your office. He is accompanied by his Auntie Estelle and his older brother Manu. Matiu is a tall handsome teenager, who immediately sits down in the chair furthest from you and looks at the ground. He is obviously not happy and says nothing, nor does he look at anyone. Auntie introduces herself and her two nephews, and tells you she is a retired social worker who spent many years working in one of the large hospitals in the city. She indicates there are more family in the waiting room and asks if they may come in. When everyone is settled, she asks if you would mind if the family start the meeting with a *karakia* (prayer). You agree, and an older man gets to his feet and says a short prayer in Maori. Everyone introduces themselves, and you introduce yourself from a professional perspective: 'I am Dr McDonald and I have been working as a GP in this practice for the last six years and before that I spent three years working on the West Coast down South in Hokitika.' Auntie Estelle begins Matiu's story. Matiu is a 17-year-old Maori teenager (*rangitahi*) who lives with his mother and older brother in a large city. His parents were divorced some years ago and his mother never remarried. Matiu has two elder sisters who are both married and live in another city. Matiu is in his last year of secondary school. His major interests in life are football, which he plays very well, and socialising with his many friends. He has been 'going steady' with Te Ara for the last three years. Matiu's ambition is to be an 'All Black'. His older brother Manu is doing well at university and has just returned from a year's study overseas, on a scholarship.

Manu takes up the story, explaining that about nine months ago Matiu began to withdraw into himself—staying in his bedroom, giving up football, breaking up with his girlfriend and refusing to speak to anyone. He was suspicious of everyone, including his mother, sisters and his football coach. He thought everyone was against him. When Manu came home from overseas, Matiu told him that he was hearing voices talking about him; arguing about him and telling him he was no good; that he was a 'queer'; and that his girlfriend had given him up for someone else. The voices were telling him that he may as well kill himself. Sometimes Matiu thought it was the neighbours outside his window, but he was never able to catch them, and the same voices were giving him the same messages through his CDs, so he had stopped listening as it was all so distressing.

His mother adds that Matiu has also practically stopped eating, and on and off for weeks he has been pacing the floor most nights, mumbling to himself. She says he is a very good boy and has never acted like this before.

Until this stage in the proceedings you have just been encouraging the family to tell their story and listening. Direct questioning to Matiu elicits no response, other than to look away. At one stage during the telling of the story he mutters something unintelligible, looking sharply upwards, and the older man who has been introduced as his grandfather puts an arm on his shoulder, soothing him. You ask if anyone else in the family has had difficulty like this. Auntie responds that a distant cousin was in a psychiatric hospital years ago, but no one knows what was wrong with her. She has passed away now.

Matiu's family are positive that there is no drug involvement. For one thing he has been at home with no visitors, and also Manu has been around to see his friends, who are also friends of his.

The diagnosis is psychosis, quite obviously, but the questions are: is this functional— that is, schizophreniform psychosis; or organic—that is, drug induced psychosis; or affective—that is, depression, with mood congruent hallucinations and delusions; and what significance do cultural beliefs have in this presentation?

THE MANAGEMENT OF MENTAL HEALTH PROBLEMS AMONG INDIGENOUS PEOPLE

The DSM-IV[15] provides an outline for cultural formulation by acknowledging that there may be difficulties in applying DSM-IV criteria across cultures, and that cultural context is relevant to clinical care. It is suggested the GP describe the patient's cultural identity. Table 6.1 lists each aspect of the DSM-IV formulation and the specific factors that should be covered for Aboriginal people and Maori for each aspect of cultural identity.

IDENTIFY THE PATIENT'S CULTURAL IDENTITY

It is very important to ascertain the cultural identity of a patient from the outset. Cultural and ethnic identity is self-defined. The GP must allow the patient to state how they identify culturally. The GP cannot determine cultural identity from the appearance of the patient.

TABLE 6.1 Factors in facilitating the therapeutic relationship

KEY FACTORS IN THE CLINICAL ENCOUNTER	SUGGESTED CLINICAL APPROACH
Patient's cultural identity and language competencies	During the course of the consultation, you ask the patient (or in the case of Matiu, the family) their ethnicity or cultural identity; this has to be self-defined. Determine their preferred language; an interpreter or cultural consultant may be needed. Is their first language an indigenous form of English—for example, Aboriginal English?
Patient's explanation of the illness	Ask the patient what they think the problem is. How does *whanau*/family view the problem? How does the indigenous health worker (if present) view the problems?
Does the patient have support systems within their cultural group?	Support includes family, extended family, kinship, tribal/*iwi* groups, Aboriginal or Maori health service or organisation, other sources of support, such as church or sports group
Identify sociocultural stressors contributing to illness	Deaths of family members, poverty, unemployment, racism, marginalisation; *mate* Maori—that is, transgression of cultural rules/boundaries
Impact of culture on the therapeutic relationship	Power inequity; 'getting to know each other'; involvement of family/*whanau*, cultural consultant, health worker, practitioner of indigenous medicine in the relationship between GP and patient
Impact of culture on overall outcome	This depends on how well each of the above aspects is managed. Good outcomes can be expected when the GP develops a good relationship with the patient and *whanau*, and respects and accommodates the views of the patient and family/*whanau*/cultural consultant

Ellen, for example, has olive skin, and lives in a comfortable house in a middle class European area of her town; her Aboriginality is not obvious. And yet she identifies strongly as Aboriginal, has strong ties to her community and holds beliefs about wellbeing and illness passed down in her family over many generations. Further, Ellen seems to speak English fluently; however, she actually speaks Aboriginal English, a separate language with its own grammatical rules and lexicon. Misunderstandings can occur between the GP and the patient. In Ellen's case, this is one of the reasons she was initially hesitant in answering questions—for example, she did not understand what the GP meant by 'anxiety'. Later in the interview, the way in which Ellen described her experiences of seeing and hearing her father, and her experiences of seeing him and the ancestors in the bush, add to the GP's difficulty in determining the nature of these experiences. Ellen's sister, on the other hand, is a trained teacher and fluent in both standard English and Aboriginal English, and actually did a lot of interpreting for Ellen, which may not have been obvious to the GP at the time.

Matiu looks Maori; he is brown-skinned and dressed in the 'uniform' of young urban Maori (hooded tracksuit top, baggy trousers and Nike shoes). His *whanau* definitely identify as Maori. They speak Te Reo Maori (the Maori language) and conduct *karakia* prior to the commencement of the consultation. But how does Matiu identify? Is he fluent in Te Reo Maori? Matiu is almost silent during the consultation; however, he should be asked how he identifies culturally. Given he has come to the consultation without apparent coercion, accompanied by *whanau*, it is highly likely that he does identify as Maori, but this cannot be assumed, nor can his fluency in Te Reo Maori (see 'Identify the impact of culture on the therapeutic relationship' on page 82).

IDENTIFY THE PATIENT'S EXPLANATION FOR THE ILLNESS

Aboriginal people and Maori have views of wellbeing and illness that differ from those of Western medicine. Indigenous patients may seek help from an indigenous healer and at the same time consult a Western practitioner. The views of cultural consultants and family members, in addition to those of the patient, on matters pertaining to the nature and cause of the illness, use of indigenous therapies and practitioners can be invaluable for diagnosis, management and treatment compliance. The following questions should not necessarily be asked in a direct manner. The patient and family have come to the GP as the expert, and will lose confidence if the GP appears to be uncertain. However, these questions should be kept in mind and, where necessary, can be brought into the interview to gain an understanding of how the patient and the family/*whanau* view the illness:

- What do you think is wrong?
- Is there is a name for it?
- What may have caused it?
- What do you think should be done now?
- What do you think will be the outcome?

In the case of Ellen, the fact that her sister acted as both a family member and a cultural consultant helped to clarify the experiences Ellen described. She clearly stated that they were not considered to be indicative of illness, but were normal, especially in grief, and especially among people who been taught about Aboriginal medicine and 'the old ways'. This knowledge, and the fact that Ellen's sister was able to take care of her, allowed the GP to let Ellen go home, and to see her regularly over the next few days to rule out medical causes of her symptoms and confirm the diagnosis of depression consequent to unresolved grief.

In Matiu's case, the *whanau* (family) will definitely have an opinion about the problem. In Maori *whanau*, it will often be the senior man who speaks about how the illness is viewed by the *whanau*. It is important to know if the *whanau* believes the illness to be a Maori illness (*mate* Maori) caused by a malignant force (Makutu)[11, 16] or by an infringement of a *tapu* (or sacred lore) by Matiu,[11, 16] or is the manifestation in Matiu of an infringement of *tapu*, committed by ancestors from generations ago. If this is indeed the belief of the *whanau*, they will already have consulted, and may still be visiting, a *Tohunga* (Maori traditional healer). Aboriginal people also often seek help from Western and Aboriginal practitioners at the same time.

Cultural beliefs and experiences, especially those pertaining to spirituality and events surrounding death, can be misinterpreted as psychopathology (Ellen's experiences were regarded as delusional by her local doctor). However, the fact that Ellen's sister did not regard such experiences as unusual, but as aspects of spirituality often experienced by other members of their home community, suggest that such experiences are not psychotic but in fact culturally appropriate experiences during grief.

On the other hand, Matiu clearly has delusional symptoms. His *whanau* do not hold similar beliefs and have in fact brought him to you for treatment. In Matiu's case more information is required, together with a period of observation in a safe environment to determine the exact nature of his illness, particularly as the voices are telling him to kill himself, and the family no longer understands his behaviour. *Mate* Maori and psychosis may co-exist, and both will require appropriate treatment.

IDENTIFY THE SUPPORT AVAILABLE

Ellen and Matiu both have obvious support from the family/*whanau*. Ellen's sister played a vital role in Ellen's successful treatment. She was an interpreter for Ellen and the doctor; she undertook to look after Ellen at home; and it is likely she undertook to intervene in the stalemate between Ellen and her husband, resulting in them getting back together. Where an indigenous patient presents to the consultation alone, it is important to ask about their social supports. The patient may be visiting from another region and have no support from local indigenous groups. GPs, especially those working in rural and remote regions, or where there are large indigenous populations, should make themselves familiar with the local Aboriginal medical service or the local Maori health service provider, respectively. Such organisations are usually able to provide support for visitors. They can also provide cultural consultants or interpreters. Indigenous patients should be asked if they would like to have another indigenous person present at the interview. Family/*whanau* and cultural consultants not only support the patient but can also help the GP and the patient understand each other, as did Ellen's sister and Matiu's *whanau*.

IDENTIFY THE SOCIAL STRESSORS

Sociocultural factors—such as experiences of colonisation, poverty, racism and adverse environmental factors—can increase the risk of mental illness, especially depression and post-traumatic stress disorder, for indigenous people (see Table 6.1 and the 'Introduction' to this chapter).

IDENTIFY THE IMPACT OF CULTURE ON THE THERAPEUTIC RELATIONSHIP

The impact of differences in cultures on the clinical encounter often remains unacknowledged. The failure to acknowledge and understand such differences can lead to misunderstandings, which have a negative impact on the encounter between the indigenous patient and the Western clinician. Ellen's local doctor misinterpreted her symptoms. He did not seek advice from family members or a local cultural consultant. As a result, he misdiagnosed Ellen as psychotic and inappropriately tried to have her admitted to an acute psychiatric hospital. Ellen refused treatment, and would not have sought further treatment had not her sister intervened and taken Ellen to her own GP. Ellen's depression was of mild to moderate severity; however, had she remained untreated there could have been a number of undesirable consequences, including the condition becoming chronic, and the split between Ellen and her husband of thirty years remaining unresolved.

In order to establish a relationship with another person, Aboriginal people, Maori and indeed most indigenous peoples need to 'get to know' the other person. It is important to know who the person is, where they come from and who their family is. On meeting for the first time, Aboriginal people will quickly establish these facts and continue to relate in the knowledge of where each stands with respect to the other. With the help of Ellen's sister, Ellen's doctor in the city was able to feel confident that Ellen was safe, and not psychotic. This in turn allowed him to take the time to get to know Ellen, and let her get to know him. During that time he was able to establish that she was physically healthy, and to diagnose and treat her depression.

Maori speaking at meetings or gatherings where people from different backgrounds are gathered will always place themselves in context by naming the *Waka* (canoe) in which their *iwi* (tribe) travelled to Aotearoa/New Zealand; their *Maunga* (mountain) to which that *iwi* has affiliation; their *awa* (body of water); their *iwi* (tribe); *hapu* (sub-tribe); *marae* (*whanau/hapu* or meeting house), *whanau* (usually just parents); and, finally, their *ingoa* (first name).[16] In this way everyone at the meeting knows who the person is and how they relate to that person and their ancestors. This knowing is of great importance to all indigenous peoples as it is essential for ensuring that proper socially sanctioned interactions occur between people.

In the clinical consultation, getting an understanding of what the patient and/or the family believe is happening is vital, and it will take time. With increasing pressure on all GPs to be time efficient, setting aside such time is difficult; however, it can be the difference between a positive outcome and treatment failure. The GP should feel comfortable about what they reveal about themselves—there is no need to tell their life story—but a preliminary 'chat' before getting straight into the presenting problem is helpful. It is also important that the patient is given time to tell their story in their own time. The patient may even ask a family member to tell part of the story, as did both Ellen and Matiu. The authors find it is often of benefit to see the patient twice within the first week before making decisions on diagnosis and management (this will of course depend on the severity of the disorder and being able to ensure the patient remains safe). Such an approach also allows the GP, the patient and the patient's family to get to know each other, which in turn facilitates understanding and enables issues pertaining to language use and views of wellbeing and illness to be addressed.

LANGUAGE It is important that the GP, the patient and the patient's family have a common understanding of what is being said in the consultations. In Australia and New Zealand, most Aboriginal people and Maori speak English as their first language.

However, Aboriginal English and Maori English are languages in their own right, with their own grammatical rules and lexicons. It cannot be taken for granted that words and expressions in English mean the same thing for both GP and patient. In most clinical encounters between a Western GP and an indigenous patient, the likelihood that misunderstandings will occur because of different language use is high. Some ways to avoid such misunderstanding include:

- having a cultural consultant interpreter present at meetings;
- facilitating the development of a therapeutic relationship in which the patient feels comfortable enough to ask the GP what they mean—for example, in Ellen's case: 'What does anxious mean?';
- being a good listener; and
- always being respectful and not only listening carefully but also explaining your understanding of the problem and your management plan clearly.

CONCLUSION

Indigenous peoples have maintained their identities as the first peoples of their lands. However, their cultures have not remained static, and since colonisation, elements of Western culture and knowledge have been incorporated; in some cases aspects of indigenous cultures have been adopted by Western peoples.

The case studies in this chapter describe two of the most common mental health problems experienced by Aboriginal people and Maori. It is essential to the establishment of a therapeutic relationship between the GP and the indigenous patient with a mental health problem that the GP is aware of the history and current circumstances of indigenous peoples, cultural differences (including linguistic) between the GP and the patient, and that the patient may have a different view of the illness to the Western view.

Indigenous knowledge about mental health can be brought into the clinical encounter by the following:

- facilitating the involvement of family/*whanau* members of the patient;
- involving a cultural consultant—for example, an Aboriginal health worker or a Maori cultural consultant (most mainstream and indigenous health services in Australia and New Zealand employ cultural consultants);
- involving elders—Aboriginal elders or Maori *kaumatua* and *kuia*; and
- jointly managing the patient with an expert in Aboriginal medicine (*Ngangkarri*) or in Maori medicine (*Tohunga*).

Once the GP has conducted a culturally appropriate interview and has very likely forged a strong therapeutic alliance with the family, it is likely that the patient will come again with any concerns they have. This was demonstrated clearly in Ellen's case when her husband, who had previously refused to talk about his son, felt able to attend a consultation with Ellen and her GP. If a person is to be admitted to hospital (as would be the likely outcome in Matiu's case), a strong therapeutic alliance will assist in follow-up and post-discharge management.

The quote at the beginning of this chapter, '*Te whare e kitea, te kokonga ngakau e kore e kitea*' is a Maori proverb. Literally translated, it means that we can see the corners of a house, but the corners of the heart are not visible, thus things are not always as they seem at first glance. We hope that this chapter goes some way towards illustrating the relevance of this proverb to the practice of psychiatry among indigenous peoples, and of how to avoid misunderstanding and misinterpretation and achieve a positive outcome for the patient, the family and the GP.

REFERENCES

1. McKendrick JH. Patterns of psychological distress and implications for mental health service delivery in an urban Aboriginal general practice population. PhD thesis. Melbourne, Victoria: University of Melbourne, 1993.
2. National Inquiry into the Separation of Aboriginal and Torres Strait Islander Children from their Families. Bringing them home. Sydney: Human Rights and Equal Opportunity Commission (Sir Ronald Wilson, president), 1997.
3. McKendrick JH, Charles S. The Report of the Rumbalara Mental Health Project. Melbourne: The Rumbalara Aboriginal Cooperative and Department of Psychiatry, University of Melbourne, 2001.
4. Mason K, Ryan E, Bennett HR. Psychiatric Report 1988. Wellington: Ministry of Health, 1988.
5. Mantell C, Bennett P, Richards D, McKendrick JH. *Kimihia nga mea kua Ngaro*. Auckland: Faculty of Medical and Health Sciences, University of Auckland and Pukaki Ki Te Akitai, 2005.
6. Smith L. Decolonising Methodologies: Research and Indigenous Peoples. London: Zed Books, 1999.
7. McKendrick J, Cutter T, McKenzie A, Chiu E. The pattern of psychiatric morbidity amongst Victorian urban Aboriginal people. Australian and New Zealand Journal of Psychiatry 1992;26(1):40–7.
8. McKendrick JH, Thorpe M. The Victorian Aboriginal Mental Health Network: Developing a Model of Mental Health Care for Aboriginal Communities. Australasian Psychiatry 1994;2(5):219–21.
9. Hunter E. Australian Aboriginal People and suicide: Mental Health Issues. In: Proceedings of the Advanced Study Institute, The Mental Health of Aboriginal Peoples: Transformations of Identity and Community. Montreal: Department of Transcultural Psychiatry, Faculty of Medicine, McGill University, 2000.
10. Durie M. Mauri Ora. Auckland: Oxford University Press, 2001.
11. Bennett P, McKendrick J, Mantell C. Why are Maori over represented in psychiatric hospitals? Part One. Auckland: Health Research Council, 2005.
12. Dyall L, Bridgman G. *Nga Ia o Te Oranga Maori*—Trends in Maori Mental Health 1984–93. Wellington: Te Puni Kokiri, 1996.
13. Swan P, Raphael B. Ways Forward. National Consultancy Report on Aboriginal and Torres Strait Islander Mental Health Care. Canberra: Australian Government Publishing Service, 1995.
14. Kirmayer LJ, Brass G, Tait C. The Mental Health of Aboriginal Peoples: Transformations of Identity and Community. Canadian Journal of Psychology 2000;45(7):607–16.
15. American Psychiatric Association. Diagnostic and Statistical Manual of Mental Disorders. 4th edn. Washington: American Psychiatric Association, 2000.
16. Mead H. Tikanga Maori. Wellington: Huia Press, 2004.

CHAPTER 7

PSYCHIATRIC ASSESSMENT FOR GPs

F Judd, G Hodgins and G Blashki

...more is missed in medicine by not looking than not knowing.

SIR WILLIAM JENNER, *1815–1898*

CASE STUDY 1

Mark, a 40-year-old man who has been recently separated from his wife, presents to your surgery seeking something to help him sleep. He admits he's been drinking more than usual to help his sleep problem. Work has been stressful; he's been irritable and this has caused problems with his workmates.

KEY FACTS

■ Initial psychiatric assessment will generally focus on the detection of psychiatric illness and factors contributing to this.

■ Detection of a possible case by screening needs to be followed up by further assessment to confirm or exclude the presence of a mental disorder, identify the particular disorder, quantify its severity and develop a treatment plan.

■ History taking aims to identify the main complaints and to obtain a biographical understanding of the patient as a person.

■ Identifying personality difficulties is essential:

— A current mental disorder may worsen personality problems and, vice versa, personality problems may worsen a coexisting mental disorder.
— There is a worse prognosis for patients with comorbid mental disorder and personality disorder.

KEY FACTS *continued*

- The severity of a disorder is determined by history, mental state signs and level of functional impairment or disability.

- Psychiatric assessment should always include an assessment of risk.

- Psychiatric assessment, as part of chronic disease management, should focus on:

  — monitoring the level of symptoms (including early warning signs for relapse) and functional impairment or disability;
  — monitoring the level of adherence to treatment and the identification of emerging side effects or other problems; and
  — detecting any emerging comorbid problems.

INTRODUCTION

Psychiatric assessment may occur as the first step in the care of a patient with an acute illness, as a prelude to the treatment of an emergency presentation or as part of continuing care and preventive interventions. The purpose and focus of the assessment may vary according to whether the patient is being seen for the first time, or whether the assessment is part of the ongoing management of a patient with a chronic psychiatric disorder. Furthermore, psychiatric assessment in general practice differs from that undertaken in specialist settings. Important differences may include the patient's perspective of the assessment, the severity of the presenting psychiatric illness and the comprehensiveness of the assessment undertaken. The time constraints and competing demands of general practice generally result in general practitioners (GPs) undertaking targeted assessments. This strategy is not without risk, but it reflects the probabilistic decision-making approach that GPs use in all areas of medicine. Alternatively, a more comprehensive assessment may be undertaken over several consultations.

However, in general, the assessment seeks to determine:

- whether a psychiatric disorder (or disorders) is present;
- whether there are any medical comorbidities;
- whether there is an organic factor contributing to, or possibly causing, the psychiatric disturbance;
- whether there are any significant personality problems and coping difficulties involved in the genesis of the problem;
- what predisposing, precipitating, perpetuating and protective factors are present;
- the severity of the illness and whether the patient poses a risk to self or others; and
- what treatments are currently being provided or what treatments are required.

In summary, the assessment aims to answer these questions:

- What is wrong?
- Why is it wrong?
- What needs to be done to address the current problems?

Assessment will generally involve some, or all, of the following:

- the use of screening methods;
- psychiatric history taking;
- mental state examination;
- physical examination;
- use of special diagnostic tests;
- the use of symptom severity/outcome-monitoring tools; and
- consultation with specialist mental health providers.

Of course, not all the elements listed above will be necessary or appropriate at every assessment; however, it is important to be familiar with these components and to understand when they should be undertaken. For example, in the mental state examination, we detail aspects of the assessment of thought form and content, which are particularly relevant if psychosis is suspected (see Chapter 12), as well as the cognitive assessment, which is particularly important when assessing an elderly person presenting with psychiatric problems (see Chapter 16). The last step in any assessment is a plan for further management.

SCREENING METHODS

Screening can be a useful aid in the detection of illness. A variety of screening methods can be used to detect a possible case (see Chapter 21). Screening methods generally fall into two groups: the use of key questions at some point in the interview, or administration of screening questionnaires. The purpose of these screening methods is to help the GP identify patients who require more detailed assessment in order to confirm the suspicion that they may have a mental disorder. Figure 7.1 lists sample key interview questions used to screen for mental disorders.

FIGURE 7.1 Sample key interview questions for screening for mental disorders

- Have you found you've lost interest or pleasure in doing things?
- Have you been feeling down or depressed?
- Have you been feeling more nervous or anxious than usual?
- Are you worrying a lot about different things?
- Have you been having anxiety attacks or feelings of panic?
- Have you thought you've been drinking too much or that you should cut down on your drinking?
- Has anyone else thought you were drinking too much?
- Have you been worrying about your weight, worrying that you're too fat, trying to lose weight?
- Have you been trying to deliberately lose weight—exercising excessively, vomiting, purging and so on?
- Has your eating been out of control? Do you binge eat?

A variety of questionnaires or scales are used for screening. For example, the Kessler Psychological Distress Scale (K-10) is a simple patient rated scale, widely used to screen for psychological distress. Questions on the K-10 focus on anxiety and depression. The maximum score on the scale is 50, indicating severe distress, and the minimum score is 10, indicating no distress. People who score 16–30 have three times the population risk of having a current anxiety or depressive disorder, while those scoring 30–50 have ten times the population risk of meeting the criteria for an anxiety or depressive disorder.[1]

Detection of a possible case by one of these screening methods then needs to be followed up by further assessment—that is, a history and mental state examination—in order to confirm or exclude the presence of a mental disorder(s), identify the particular disorder, quantify its severity and develop a treatment plan.

PSYCHIATRIC HISTORY TAKING

History taking has two main aims:

■ to detail the main complaints, factors that may have caused the illness and factors that may influence the management and prognosis of the illness; and
■ to obtain a biographical understanding of the patient as a person.

The following section describes important components of history taking. Many GPs may already know much of this information about their patients, particularly if they have been long-standing patients of the practice; however, it is important not to assume the presence or absence of specific information (for example, use of illicit drugs) and to ask specific questions if you are unsure. Sometimes you can be surprised by the answer!

PRESENTING COMPLAINT

It is important to obtain a brief description of the principal complaint and the time frame of the problem. The specific information required includes answers to the following questions:

■ What is the nature of the problem?
■ What specific symptoms are present and what is their duration?
■ What, if any, events led to the current presentation?
■ Why and how has the individual presented at this time?
■ Are the symptoms of recent onset or chronic in nature?
■ What factors increase or decrease the severity of symptoms?
■ Is this an acute episode of illness or does the presentation represent relapse, or recurrence of a chronic illness?
■ If this is a chronic or recurrent illness, what treatment has previously been given and what was the person's response to this treatment?

Where possible, it is always useful to obtain information from corroborative sources such as a partner, parent, employer or the police.

THE PERSONAL (DEVELOPMENTAL) HISTORY

The development of a person's character is strongly influenced by their childhood experiences, environment, and family and peer relationships. In eliciting details of their developmental history, look for: problems in the early post-natal period, such as cerebral trauma, infection or other insults that may have resulted in brain damage; separation or loss from parent figures in early childhood; risk-taking behaviours, substance use or difficulties with social and interpersonal functioning during adolescence; and work and relationship difficulties. If you do not already have information about the following, it should be sought:

- Infancy—drug treatment during pregnancy; emotions and temperament; level of activity; and general development
- Childhood and adolescence—emotional adjustment; relationship with peers, siblings and parents; physical illness; loss or trauma in the family; physical or sexual abuse; peer relationships; and progress at school
- Work history—jobs held; reasons for changing jobs; level of satisfaction with employment; ambitions
- Social history—friendships; peer relationships; recreational interests and activities
- Relationship history—long-term relationships (duration, quality, reasons for break up of relationships)
- Forensic history—history of aggression and/or violence; any contact with the police; and reasons for this

FAMILY HISTORY

GPs are often familiar with the patient's family history but if they are not, it is important to obtain a picture of the patient's family—that is, partner, children, parents and siblings. This information should include each person's age, health, occupation and contact with and quality of relationship with the person. In addition, as many disorders have a familial influence, it is important to obtain information about any psychiatric illness in family members.

PAST PSYCHIATRIC HISTORY

Many mental disorders are chronic or relapsing. Thus it is important to know whether the current presentation has developed de novo, is part of an ongoing problem or an exacerbation of a pre-existing problem.

Where the person has a chronic or recurring illness, it is important to obtain information regarding past episodes of illness, any treatment given for this as well as the response to such treatment. It is also important to identify any untoward reactions, such as allergies or unwanted side effects, to previous treatments.

PAST MEDICAL HISTORY

While it is likely that the patient's medical history is well known to their treating GP, it is important to review this at the time of presentation of any psychiatric illness, and to carefully consider whether medical problems could be contributing to the current presentation (for example, thyroid problems may contribute to the onset of anxiety or depression). Importantly, there may be interactions between currently prescribed medical treatments (including over the counter preparations), complementary medicines and planned psychiatric treatments.

CASE STUDY 2

Dave, a retired engineer in his early fifties, presents frequently to your surgery for blood pressure checks. He has tried several antihypertensive drugs but has experienced side effects with them all. He has become preoccupied with his health and is vigilant about the development of new symptoms. He has sleep problems, is constantly tired, and admits he feels depressed, and at times that life is not worth living. Prescribing an antidepressant will be difficult; in addition to his somatic focus and worries regarding side effects, he has a past history of congestive cardiac failure.

DRUG AND ALCOHOL HISTORY

The use of illicit drugs may precipitate various psychiatric syndromes. In addition, alcohol is commonly used as self-treatment for a variety of psychiatric conditions, particularly anxiety and depression. It is essential to obtain a comprehensive drug and alcohol history, and to examine the possible contribution of substance use to the presenting complaint, current level of functioning and any social, marital or employment difficulties.

CASE STUDY 3

Max, a 56-year-old businessman, attends your practice regularly for management of his peptic ulcer. He mentions he's been depressed, and that his wife feels he should take some medication to help his mood. On checking his history, you note he admits to drinking a bottle of wine each night, and his recent repeat liver function tests were abnormal. Max reluctantly tells you he's recently had his driving licence cancelled for drink driving. Following further exploration, it seems his mood problems are probably secondary to his alcohol use, perhaps exacerbated by the drink driving charge and the problems flowing from this.

PREMORBID PERSONALITY

Understanding the patient's personality is important for a variety of reasons. A current mental disorder such as depression may worsen personality problems and, vice versa, personality problems may worsen a coexisting mental disorder. In addition, patients with both personality difficulties and a mental disorder have a worse prognosis than those without significant personality problems.

The patient should be asked: 'Can you tell me what sort of person you were before you became ill?', but this information should be supplemented by information obtained from the family and other informants. In addition, information obtained from the personal (developmental) history will assist in the assessment of premorbid personality.

When patients present describing chronic symptoms, it is important to consider whether the symptoms may be a feature of a personality disorder rather than a current episode of acute illness. Often this arises when considering a diagnosis of chronic depression. A key feature of personality disorder is a stable pattern of long duration (see Figure 7.2). Thus, the onset can be traced back to adolescence or early adulthood. One should be alerted to the possibility of personality problems rather than a depressive illness when the history starts with: 'I've been depressed for as long as I can remember.'

FIGURE 7.2 Personality disorders

Personality can be defined as a relatively stable and enduring set of characteristic behavioural and emotional traits. Over time, the person will interact with others in a reasonably predictable way. In assessing patients, we need to determine whether there may be evidence of 'personality pathology' or evidence that the individual has a personality disorder. The latter is a variant or an extreme set of characteristics that go beyond the range found in most people. The key features of personality disorders are that patterns of emotions and behaviour:

- are deeply ingrained and of an inflexible nature;
- are maladaptive, especially in interpersonal circumstances;
- are relatively stable over time;
- significantly impair the ability of the person to function;
- distress those close to the person; and
- are ego-syntonic—that is, the behaviours do not distress the person directly.

CURRENT SOCIAL SITUATION

It is always important to look carefully at the individual's current social situation, and in particular to identify factors that may act as a risk for illness or that are resilience factors. These include the patient's social network, family relationships, home situation, occupation (including type of work, job security, job satisfaction) and financial situation.

THE MENTAL STATE EXAMINATION

The mental state examination is a description of what is observed at the time of the interview. This includes observed behaviour, cognitive abilities and inner experiences expressed during the interview. It is important to note that this cross-sectional assessment has limitations. The patient's mental state may fluctuate, and many patients are able to disguise significant problems during a psychiatric interview.

Although a comprehensive mental state examination is undertaken as part of a full psychiatric assessment, GPs will tend to focus on individual components as guided by the clinical situation. For example, in cases of suspected psychosis, the focus will be on affect, thinking and perception, whereas for suspected dementia, cognitive assessment is an important focus.

Usually, the mental state examination complements details obtained in history taking; however, at times the mental state examination may appear unremarkable in contrast to the information obtained during history taking. Where this is the case, findings should not be accepted without further exploration, particularly seeking information from others who know the patient.

The mental state examination should begin as soon as the patient enters the room; observation will reveal important information such as grooming, hygiene, behaviour, gait, and level of interest in and interaction with surroundings. The nine key components of the mental state examination are outlined below.

APPEARANCE, BEHAVIOUR AND RAPPORT

This component includes a description of the individual's physical appearance, their reaction to the present situation and the interviewer, and their motor behaviour. It is important to note the rapport developed—that is, how well you and the patient relate to each other, as revealed by the how the patient interacts during the interview.

SPEECH

The physical aspects of speech can be described in terms of rate, quantity of information (for example, slow, rapid, monotonous, loud, quiet, slurred, whispered) and whether there are any problems with articulation (dysarthrias) or dysphasias (or aphasias). Important characteristics seen in particular psychiatric disorders are shown in Table 7.1.

MOOD AND AFFECT

Mood is the internal feeling or emotion that often influences behaviour and the individual's perception of the world. The mood state is generally fairly constant over significant periods of time, although patients may describe fluctuations—for example, 'my mood has been up and down'. Common descriptions of mood include depressed, euphoric, labile, hostile and anxious.

Affect is the person's external emotional response—that is, what you observe at interview. During the interview, you may observe multiple affects. In describing the individual's affect, it is important to note whether the emotional response is appropriate to the subject matter being discussed. Important variations of affect are shown in Table 7.1.

DISORDERS OF THOUGHT

Disorders of thought include disorders of content of thought and disorders of thought process.

THOUGHT CONTENT Thought content refers to what patients talk about in the substance of the interview. Thought content is considered abnormal if it contains any of the following elements: delusions, overvalued ideas, suicidal or homicidal thoughts, preoccupation with various themes, obsessions, compulsions or phobias.

DISORDERS OF THOUGHT PROCESS Disorders of thought process can be further categorised into disorders of form of thought, stream of thought and possession of thought:

DISORDERS OF FORM OF THOUGHT The term 'formal thought disorder' refers to disorders of conceptual or abstract thinking—that is, the way in which ideas are produced and organised. These types of disorder often occur in schizophrenia and in organic brain disorders. They are described in various ways but commonly used terms include 'loosening of associations' (derailment) and 'tangentiality' (see Table 7.1).

DISORDERS OF STREAM OF THOUGHT This category includes disorders of tempo (flight of ideas, inhibition or retardation of thinking, circumstantiality) and disorders of continuity of thinking (perseveration, thought blocking). (Again, see Table 7.1.)

DISORDERS OF POSSESSION OF THOUGHT Normally, individuals experience their thinking as being their own, and they feel they are in control of their thinking. In some psychiatric disorders, patients experience a sense of losing control of their thinking. This occurs in two major forms—obsessions and thought alienation (seen in individuals with schizophrenia).

PERCEPTION

Perception is the process of experiencing the environment and recognising or making sense of the stimuli received. Disorders of perception include false associations (illusions) or the de novo arrival of a percept without a stimulus (hallucination). (See Figure 7.3.)

Auditory hallucinations are the most common type of hallucination. They most commonly occur in people with a psychotic illness. They are also commonly seen in people with an acute organic brain syndrome (delirium). The presence of visual hallucinations suggests an organic mental disorder.

Illusions can occur as part of a psychotic disorder, mood disorder, anxiety disorder and also as part of an organic disorder. Like hallucinations, illusions may occur in any sensory modality. Other perceptual disturbances include de-realisation, de-personalisation and dissociation.

CASE STUDY 4

Jim, a 17-year-old boy, is brought in by his mother for a 'check-up'. The story quickly unfolds that the young man has been staying in his room most of the day for the last three months, spending most of his time downloading music onto his iPOD. He is dressed in black, leaves his headphones on during the consultation, and has very poor eye contact. Suspecting he may be psychotic, you focus your initial assessment on eliciting any unusual ideas or abnormal thought content and any perceptual disturbance, and assessing his affect and thought processes. In addition, you seek a history of illicit drug use, and re-check to see whether there is a family history of psychosis.

COGNITION

Cognition refers to information processing and draws on both thinking and memory. Important components of cognitive function include the following:

- **Orientation** This is generally tested with respect to the categories of time, place and person.
- **Attention and concentration** Attention refers to the ability to focus and direct cognitive processes, while concentration refers to the ability to focus and sustain attention for a period of time.
- **Memory** Three categories of memory should be tested: immediate, short-term and long-term memory. Immediate memory refers to registration or the capacity for immediate recall of new learning. It lasts for only a few seconds. Short-term memory refers to temporary memory, lasting for a few seconds to a few minutes. Long-term memory remains stable over time and is the type of memory most affected by forms

of amnesia. Long-term memory has two sub-types—declarative and procedural. Procedural memory involves remembering how to perform a set of skills—for example, driving. This form of memory evolves after many trials and often remains largely intact in various forms of amnesia. Declarative memory involves data or facts that can be verbal or non-verbal. This type of memory can be acquired in a short time and is the form most impaired in amnesia.

- **Visuospatial ability** The ability to perform visuospatial functions is an essential part of performing daily activities and affects the ability to navigate, use machinery and perceive the environment.
- **Abstract thinking** This involves the ability to deal with concepts, extract common characteristics from groups of objects, juggle more than one idea at a time and interpret information.

It is often useful to include a standardised test as part of screening for cognitive problems. The most widely used is the Mini Mental State Examination (MMSE) (see Chapter 16).[2] This is a clinician administered tool that is not suitable for making a diagnosis but can be used to indicate the presence of cognitive impairment, such as when dementia or head injury are suspected. The MMSE provides measures of orientation, registration, immediate memory (but not long-term memory) as well as visuospatial and language functioning (see Chapter 16).

INTELLIGENCE

It is important to make an assessment of intelligence. The level of psychosocial functioning and vocabulary are generally used to estimate whether the individual is of average or above IQ. Persons with mental retardation (intellectual disability) have IQ scores of less than 70, combined with significant adaptive deficits that have developed during the developmental period (up to 18 years of age). The vast majority of persons with an intellectual disability fall into the mild category and live in the community with little utilisation of disability services. Detecting individuals with an intellectual disability is important, as the level of comorbid psychiatric and physical disorders among this group is very high.

JUDGMENT

Judgment involves weighing and comparing the relative values of different aspects of an issue. Determining whether a particular judgment is sound is situation dependent. It is important to be clear about judgment, as this may influence any decisions made about the management of the patient.

INSIGHT

Insight refers to the individual's awareness of their situation or illness. Overall, insight includes whether the person understands they are ill, why the illness may have developed and what appropriate treatments are available for the illness.

TABLE 7.1 Key mental state features and disorders associated with these

MENTAL STATE FEATURE	DESCRIPTION	ASSOCIATED DISORDER
Poverty of speech	Restricted amount of spontaneous speech; answers to questions are brief and monosyllabic	Dementia, depression
Pressure of speech	Speech is rapid, difficult to interrupt, loud and hard to understand	Mania
Restricted affect	Limited or decreased range of affect	Depression, anxiety
Blunted affect	Externally expressed emotion is present but much diminished in intensity	Psychosis
Flat affect	No emotional expression—an extreme form of blunted affect	Psychosis
Flight of ideas	Thoughts follow each other rapidly; there is no general direction of thinking; connections between successive thoughts are due to chance (albeit understandable) factors	Mania
Thought blocking	There is a sudden arrest of the train of thoughts, leading to a blank, and an entirely new thought begins	Psychosis, anxiety
Loosening of associations (derailment)	Disorder of the logical progression of thought; unrelated and unconnected (or loosely connected) ideas shift from one subject to another. There is no meaningful connection between the ideas that are being expressed	Psychosis
Tangentiality	Thoughts are logically connected but context shifts from the original topic to one or more different topic areas without ever returning to the original idea—a less severe disruption to organisation of thought than loosening of associations	Psychosis

FIGURE 7.3 Phenomenology—key definitions

DELUSION A false, unshakeable belief out of keeping with the patient's social, cultural and religious background. The content of delusions is influenced by social and cultural background. Common delusions include delusions of persecution, delusions of jealousy, delusions of love, grandiose delusions, delusions of ill health and delusions of guilt.

OVERVALUED IDEA Because of the associated feeling tone, a thought that takes precedence over all other ideas, preoccuping the patient's thinking and affecting their behaviour.

FIGURE 7.3 *continued*

OBSESSION The essential feature of an obsession is that it appears against a person's will but is recognised as part of their own thought. Individuals may experience obsessional mental images, ideas, fears or impulses that are distressing to them.

THOUGHT ALIENATION In thought alienation, the person believes that their thoughts are under the control of an outside agency or that others are participating in their thinking. This category may include thought insertion, thought withdrawal and thought broadcasting.

HALLUCINATION An hallucination is a false sensory perception in which the individual sees, hears, smells, tastes or feels something that other people do not see, hear, smell, taste or feel.

ILLUSIONS These are perceptual distortions. The essential difference between an illusion and a hallucination is that in an illusion there is an object present but what is perceived by the patient is distorted.

FIGURE 7.4 Methods of cognitive testing

ATTENTION This is tested by digit span forwards and backwards (most adults have a digit span of 5–7 numbers forwards and 4–6 numbers backwards without errors).

CONCENTRATION You can assess this by asking the individual to subtract serial 7s from 100. (*Note*: This can be disrupted by performance anxiety, mood disturbance, alteration of consciousness or poor educational level). An alternative is to spell WORLD backwards or to subtract serial 3s, starting from 20.

IMMEDIATE MEMORY This is readily tested by asking the individual to repeat four items—for example, dog, shoe, blue, apple.

SHORT-TERM MEMORY Test a patient's short-term memory by asking the individual to repeat the four items (dog, shoe, blue, apple) after three minutes. If the patient does not recall a word, prompt them with a semantic cue—for example, animal (dog), piece of clothing (shoe), colour (blue), fruit (apple).

LONG-TERM DECLARATIVE MEMORY In order to test long-term declarative memory, ask questions about episodic memory, which is time-tagged, personalised (or autobiographical) and experiential knowledge—for example, the date of the patient's wedding. Semantic memory, which refers to recall of general information a person could reasonably be expected to have learnt, can be tested by asking for information, such as the year World War II started.

VISUOSPATIAL ABILITY This is most readily tested by assessing constructional ability. For example, the patient can be asked to draw a 3D figure, such as a cube, or draw a clock face showing a specified time.

ABSTRACT THINKING This is commonly assessed by asking the individual to interpret the meaning of common proverbs, or by the similarities test—for example, ask patients to compare two objects, such as a desk and chair, and list as many common qualities and differences as they can.

PHYSICAL EXAMINATION

Physical examination is a necessary part of the psychiatric assessment. Organic factors need to be excluded as a cause of symptoms or as contributing to them. In addition, comorbid medical illnesses that affect presentation and management or impede development of judgment, insight and compliance must be identified and, where appropriate, strategies should be put in place to deal with these. The physical examination should include a systems examination, with particular focus on the neurological system. Acute and chronic physical effects of illicit drug taking and alcohol use, including associated infections, must always be sought, even if the patient denies the use of such agents.

THE USE OF SPECIAL INVESTIGATIONS AND DIAGNOSTIC TESTS

When a patient presents for the first time, apart from the general physical examination, the GP should order a full blood examination; tests for renal, liver and thyroid function; and calcium and phosphate estimation. Computerised tomography (CT) scan, magnetic resonance imaging (MRI), functional imaging and electroencephalogram (EEG), to name a few, may form part of the psychiatric assessment, especially where organic cerebral pathology is suspected. Cerebral CT scanning, folate and B12 and syphilis serology should be performed as a routine in older patients, especially if cognitive deficits are present. In younger patients, where there is a history of drug abuse (either known or suspected), testing for hepatitis B, hepatitis C and HIV (with informed consent) may be required. It is important to remember that the comorbid rate of substance abuse and unprotected sexual practice is high in both mania and schizophrenia.

CASE STUDY 5

John, a 47-year-old man, presents at your surgery, describing problems with his memory. He has also experienced difficulty organising tasks at work, something that has never bothered him before. He tells you he's feeling pretty miserable and is just not coping. The cognitive complaints prompt you to check his memory and do some simple tests, and to your surprise he does poorly on the MMSE. Physical examination reveals left-sided weakness, and an urgent CT scan shows a glioma.

USE OF SYMPTOM SEVERITY AND OUTCOME-MONITORING TOOLS

A variety of symptom severity measures may be of assistance in the assessment and subsequent planning of treatment of patients. Table 7.2 provides a list of commonly used symptom severity measures (outcome tools). These should be used to assess symptom severity once a diagnosis has been made, and then later to monitor the effects of treatment. Details of outcome-monitoring tools and their use are provided in Chapter 21.

TABLE 7.2 Commonly used symptom severity measures (outcome tools)

PSYCHIATRIC DISORDER	NAME OF SCALE
Depression	Centre for Epidemiological Studies Depression rating scale (CES-D)[3]
Generalised anxiety disorder	Hospital Anxiety and Depression rating Scale (HADS)[4]
Post-natal depression	Edinburgh Postnatal Depression Scale (EPDS)[5]
Psychosis	Brief Psychiatric Rating Scale (BPRS)[6]
Harmful alcohol use	Alcohol Use Disorders Identification Test (AUDIT)[7]
Organic disorders	Mini Mental State Examination (MMSE)[8] Delirium Rating Scale (DRS)[9]
Overall level of functioning or disability	Medical Outcome Study Short Form Health Survey-12 (SF-12)[10] Global Assessment of Functioning (GAF)[11]

CONSULTATION WITH SPECIALIST MENTAL HEALTH PROVIDERS

Assessment may be aided by consultation with specialist mental health providers. This may involve the specialist seeing the patient for assessment (primary consultation) and providing advice, or the GP discussing the case with the specialist, who does not see the patient (secondary consultation). The timing of such a consultation will vary according to whether advice is needed for immediate crisis management, to assist with differential diagnosis or to plan ongoing treatment. Access to specialist care varies widely across different geographical settings but knowledge of local services is essential for successful referrals (see Chapter 22).

SUMMARY, DIAGNOSIS AND FORMULATION
SUMMARY

Information obtained from history, mental state examination, physical examination and other sources must be collected in a summary that informs the diagnosis and differential diagnosis. In essence, the summary will include information about who the person is, what their problems are and what effects these problems are having on the person (physical, psychological, social, vocational, financial).

DIAGNOSIS/DIFFERENTIAL DIAGNOSIS

Making a diagnosis and considering important differential diagnoses is as important in psychiatry as in general medicine. Murtagh[12] has described a simple and practical approach to diagnosis. This model suggests that five key questions should be considered. They are:

- What is the probability diagnosis?
- What serious disorders must not be missed?
- What conditions are often missed (the pitfalls)?
- Could this patient have one of the masquerades in medical practice?
- Is this patient trying to tell me something else?

These questions are just as applicable to making a psychiatric assessment as to making a general medical assessment.

FORMULATION

Formulation draws the relevant facts together and discusses them from the point of view of aetiology, diagnosis, further investigations, treatment and prognosis. It describes how and why the problems arose in terms of predisposing, precipitating and maintaining (and protective) factors. These factors need to be considered from the biological, psychological and sociocultural perspective. For example, genetic factors may predispose an individual to the development of an illness, while drug use may be a precipitant. An individual's personality strengths or vulnerabilities can predispose to, or protect against, the development of a mental illness. Stressors are often precipitants for the development of illness, while strong social supports may be protective. Using the biopsychosocial approach, Table 7.3 presents a summary of factors that often contribute to the development of disorder.

The formulation is the explanatory conduit between assessment and treatment. A formulation should be able to describe the answer to the question: 'Why is this person ill in this way at this time?' As such, it lays the framework for the planning of treatment and, in particular, the decision to use medication, psychological or social interventions, or a combination of these.

A useful way to acknowledge the relevance and potential interaction of biological, psychological and sociocultural factors is to use the multi-axial approach to diagnosis. As outlined in Chapter 1, the most commonly used system of this type is described in DSM-IV.[13] This approach categorises psychological factors on Axes 1 and II, biological factors on Axis III and sociocultural factors on Axes IV and V, as follows:

- **Axis 1** This axis is used to record mental disorders:
  — organic and cognitive disorders
  — mood disorders
  — anxiety disorders
  — psychotic disorders
  — somatoform disorders
  — eating disorders
  — substance use disorders
- **Axis II** Personality disorders, prominent maladaptive personality features and intellectual disability are recorded on this axis. A common approach to classifying personality disorders is that used in DSM-IV, which puts personality disorders phenomenologically into similar clusters:
  — Cluster A: odd or eccentric—paranoid, schizoid, schizotypal

TABLE 7.3 Factors determining illness

PERSPECTIVE	PREDISPOSING FACTORS	PRECIPITATING FACTORS	MAINTAINING FACTORS	PROTECTIVE FACTORS
Biological	Family history of medical and psychiatric illness	Physical illness Medication side effects Alcohol/drug use	Physical illness Medication side effects Alcohol/drug use	Treatment of illness
Psychological	Personality traits Defence/coping mechanisms Past psychiatric history	Life events Stressors	Stressors Personality traits	Personality traits Defence/coping mechanisms Treatment of illness
Sociocultural	Family environment Early relationships	Social circumstances Occupational circumstances	Relationship problems Occupational problems Financial problems	Supportive environment Faith

Source: Adapted from Bloch S, Singh BS. [14]

— Cluster B: dramatic, emotional or erratic—antisocial, borderline, histrionic, narcissistic

— Cluster C: anxious or fearful—avoidant, dependent, obsessive-compulsive

■ **Axis III** Recorded here are general medical conditions, including any medical conditions that are potentially relevant to the understanding or management of the individual's mental disorder.

■ **Axis IV** Psychosocial and environmental problems that may affect the diagnosis, treatment and prognosis of any mental disorders are recorded here.

■ **Axis V** This axis is used to record the assessment of the individual's overall level of functioning.

An important part of the assessment that flows from such a multi-axial approach is an understanding of the severity of the disorder, and an assessment of risk. The severity of the disorder is determined by history, mental state signs and level of functional impairment or disability. In addition, severity can be quantified using a disorder specific symptom-rating scale (see Table 7.2). Assessment of risk should always be included in the psychiatric assessment. Such an assessment should include a consideration of risk to both self and others, and encompass a range of areas, including:

■ self-harm risk;
■ suicide risk;
■ danger to others;
■ likelihood of substance abuse;
■ vulnerability to exploitation by others;
■ likelihood of deterioration of mental state;
■ non-compliance with treatment;
■ homelessness; and
■ risk of self-neglect.

Figure 7.5 lists factors known to be associated with an increased risk of suicide, and Figure 7.6 describes the key areas of enquiry that should be pursued when a patient admits or describes self-harm or suicidal ideation.

FIGURE 7.5 Factors associated with increased risk of suicide

■ Age—rate rises steadily with age
■ Sex—male > female (particularly high rate for males aged 15 to 30, especially in rural areas)
■ Marital status—single, widow(er)
■ Socioeconomic status—rate increased for lower socioeconomic class
■ Unemployment—rate increased for unemployed
■ Physical illness—especially chronic and/or painful conditions
■ Psychiatric illness—especially depression, schizophrenia
■ Alcohol or drug abuse/dependence
■ Distressing life events

FIGURE 7.6 Assessing suicide risk at interview

In addition to the general risk factors, assessment of risk in patients who report suicidal ideation requires consideration of:

- Level of wish or intent to die
- Level of wish or intent to live
- Wish to die versus wish to escape situation or feelings
- Fixed versus ambivalent suicidal ideation
- Preparation for attempt—for example, collecting tablets, buying a gun
- Final acts in anticipation of death—for example, making a will, sorting out insurance
- Presence of a plan
- Lethality of chosen means for self-harm
- Access to and knowledge of how to use those means
- Presence or absence of supports
- Presence or absence of 'protective' individual factors
- Presence of deterrents or reasons to stay alive—for example, family, religion
- Purpose or reason for attempt

ASSESSMENT OF PATIENTS WITH RECURRENT OR CHRONIC MENTAL ILLNESS

Ongoing psychiatric assessment is required as part of chronic disease management for many individuals with mental disorders. The focus of such assessment will be informed by the nature of the chronic illness (for example, see Figure 7.7 for a description of 'phases' of illness), any comorbid conditions and factors identified as having an important role in precipitating episodes of illness, and those factors that protect against relapse. Thus, continuing assessment should focus on:

- monitoring the level of symptoms and functional impairment or disability;
- determining the level of adherence to treatment and identification of any emerging side effects or problems with treatments (for example, weight gain and altered lipid profile and blood glucose levels with antipsychotic medications);
- regular review of the psychosocial factors that represent a high risk for relapse;
- regular review and enhancement of the operative protective factors that may buffer against any propensity to relapse;
- regular assessment to identify any emerging comorbid problems—individuals with chronic psychiatric illness have an increased risk of physical morbidity and mortality; and
- a patient's unique relapse 'signature',[15] —that is, a sequential emergence of symptoms and signs that herald impending relapse. Ongoing assessment as part of chronic disease management should include a review with patients of their typical sequence of warning signs, so that they can better understand their significance and develop a plan to deal with them when they arise.

FIGURE 7.7 Phases of illness

In affective disorders, it is usual to talk of an acute episode, remission and recovery phases (see Figure 7.8).

- The acute episode refers to the experience of pervasive and persistent depressed mood together with the characteristic biological and psychological symptoms of depression.
- Remission refers to a sustained period of time in which improvement occurs so the individual is asymptomatic. During remission, relapse can still occur—that is, there can be a return of symptoms that are still ongoing but symptomatically suppressed in this episode.
- Recovery refers to a prolonged remission. If symptoms now occur, they are assessed as representing an entirely new episode.[16]

Similarly, four phases of psychosis have been described: prodrome, acute phase, early recovery and late recovery phases. These generally refer to individuals experiencing first episode psychosis, with the term 'chronic schizophrenia' being reserved to describe recurrent episodes of acute psychosis and, for some patients, ongoing positive and/or negative symptoms that do not resolve.

FIGURE 7.8 Depression—phases of illness

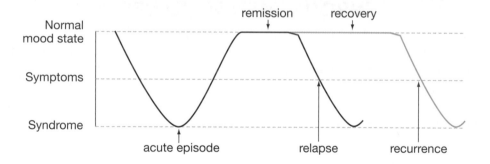

TREATMENT PLANNING

The final phase of psychiatric assessment is developing an appropriate management plan. This may involve:

- further assessment by the GP;
- referral to others for further assessment and/or treatment; and
- initiation of treatment on the basis of the assessment to date.

Important considerations should always include: whether there are indications for immediate referral for management of a psychiatric crisis or high level of risk; whether there are indications for referral to a psychiatrist, psychologist or specialist mental health service (see Figure 7.9); or whether there is a need for inpatient treatment (see Figure 7.10). It is also critical to assess the patient and their family's attitude to referral, and how practical issues such as cost and possible travel will be addressed.

WHO SHOULD PROVIDE TREATMENT?

As mentioned above, it is always important to consider whether referral to a specialist is appropriate. In addition to the factors listed in Figure 7.9, the stepped collaborative care model provides a useful framework for guiding any decision to refer a patient. As discussed in Chapter 1, this model defines different types of intervention based on patient need. It advocates the treatment of patients with mild disorders by GPs as well as the provision of opportunities for referral to specialist services for patients with complex presentations or who do not respond to usual care (see Figure 7.11). When referral is made to a specialist (psychiatrist, clinical psychologist or other allied health professional), it is important to be clear about the nature and extent of the collaboration required (see Chapter 22).

FIGURE 7.9 Are there indications for referral?

Referral should be considered when:

- There is diagnostic uncertainty.
- The patient has an acute illness and fails to respond to usual treatment.
- The severity or presentation of illness entails treatment beyond one's competency.
- Other factors such as concomitant medical problems complicate treatment.
- Troublesome side effects complicate treatment.
- Hospitalisation is indicated.

FIGURE 7.10 Does the patient need inpatient treatment?

Inpatient treatment should be considered in the following circumstances:

- Because of illness, the patient poses a threat to self or others.
- Because of illness, the patient's behaviour is intolerable in their own environment.
- Outpatient treatment has been unsuccessful.
- Treatment is best initiated in hospital.
- The complexity or intensity of treatment requires the resources of an inpatient unit.
- Further necessary diagnostic assessment is not possible while the individual is an outpatient.
- Treatment is facilitated by removing the patient from their environment.
- Withdrawal from alcohol or drugs is, or will, complicate further assessment and treatment.

WHICH TREATMENTS?

The diagnosis—together with identification of the predisposing, precipitating, maintaining and protective factors—lays the framework for planning treatment, which may include the use of medication, a psychological intervention or both. Additional factors that may influence the decision to choose a particular treatment include:

- the severity of the presenting problems;
- patient preference and motivation for a particular treatment;
- any previous treatment and response to this;

- treatment goals (symptom reduction or more enduring change);
- patterns of behaviour that may suggest that psychological intervention would be useful;
- suitability of the patient to a particular approach;
- skill level and training of the practitioner;
- context in which the patient is being seen;
- cultural considerations; and
- resource issues.

FIGURE 7.11 Stepped collaborative care model

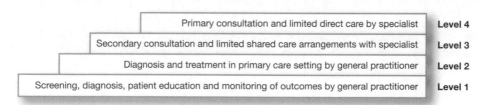

Primary consultation and limited direct care by specialist	**Level 4**
Secondary consultation and limited shared care arrangements with specialist	**Level 3**
Diagnosis and treatment in primary care setting by general practitioner	**Level 2**
Screening, diagnosis, patient education and monitoring of outcomes by general practitioner	**Level 1**

CONCLUSION

As with other areas of medicine, psychiatric assessment requires a thorough history and examination (that is, mental state and physical exam) and appropriate investigations in order to generate a diagnosis and differential diagnosis. In addition, a formulation using the biopsychosocial approach is needed. This lays the framework for planning treatment, and includes consideration of which interventions, who should be involved in treatment and where treatment should occur.

REFERENCES

1. Andrews G, Slade T. Interpreting scores on the Kessler Psychological Distress Scale (K-10). Australian and New Zealand Journal of Public Health 2001;25:494–7.
2. Folstein MF, Folstein SE, McHugh PR. Mini Mental State: a practical method for grading the cognitive state for the clinician. Journal of Psychiatric Research 1975;12:189–98.
3. Radloff LS. The CES-D Scale: A self-report depression scale for research in the general population. Applied Psychological Measurement 1977;1:385–401.
4. Zigmond AS, Snaith RP. The Hospital Anxiety and Depression Scale. Acta Psychiatrica Scandinavica 1983;67:361–70.
5. Cox JL, Holden JM, Sagovsky R. Detection of postnatal depression. Development of the 10-item Edinburgh Postnatal Depression Scale. British Journal of Psychiatry 1987;150:782–6.
6. Overall JE, Graham DR. The Brief Psychiatric Rating Scale (BPRS): recent developments in ascertainment and scaling. Psychopharmacology Bulletin 1988;24:97–9.
7. Saunders JB, Aasland OG, Babor TF, De La Fuente JR, Grant M. Development of the alcohol use disorders identification test (AUDIT): WHO collaborative project on early detection of persons with harmful alcohol consumption. Addiction 1993;88:791–804.
8. Folstein MF, Folstein SE, McHugh PR. 'Mini-mental state': a practical method for grading the cognitive state of patients for the clinician. Journal of Psychiatric Research 1975;12:189–98.
9. Trzepacz PT, Baker RW, Greenhouse I. A symptom rating scale for delirium. Psychiatry Research 1988;23:89–97.

10. Ware JE, Kosinski M, Keller SD. SF-12: How to Scale the SF-12 Physical and Mental Health Summary Scales. Boston: Health Institute, New England Medical Centre, 1995.

11. Endicott J, Spitzer RL, Fleiss JL, Cohen J. The Global Assessment Scale: A procedure for measuring overall severity of psychiatric dysfunction. Archives of General Psychiatry 1976;33:766–71.

12. Murtagh J. General Practice. Sydney: McGraw Hill Book Company Australia Pty Ltd, 1994.

13. American Psychiatric Association. Diagnostic and Statistical Manual of Mental Disorders. 4th edn. Washington DC: American Psychiatric Association, 1994.

14. Bloch S, Singh BS. Foundations of Clinical Psychiatry. Melbourne: Melbourne University Press, 1994.

15. Birchwood M, MacMillan F, Smith J. Early intervention. In: Birchwood M, Tarrier N, eds. Innovations in the Psychological Management of Schizophrenia. Assessment, Treatment and Services. Chichester: John Wiley & Sons, 1992;115–45.

16. Frank E, Prien RF, Jarrett RB, Keller MB, Kupfer DJ, Lavori PW, Rush AJ, Weissman MM. Conceptualisation and rationale for consensus definition of terms in major depressive disorder: remission, recovery, relapse and recurrence. Archives of General Psychiatry 1991;48:851–855.

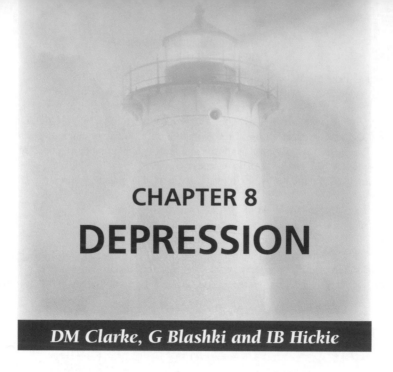

CHAPTER 8

DEPRESSION

DM Clarke, G Blashki and IB Hickie

Depression is a disorder of mood, so mysteriously painful and elusive in the way it becomes known to the self...as to verge close to being beyond description. It thus remains nearly incomprehensible to those who have not experienced it in its extreme mode, although the gloom, the 'blues' which people go through occasionally and associate with the general hassle of everyday existence are of such prevalence that they do give many individuals a hint of the illness in its catastrophic form.

WILLIAM STYRON, 1991[1]

CASE STUDY

Marlene is a 52-year-old woman who has worked in private child care for seven years. She presents with her 26-year-old daughter, who is concerned that her mother is 'losing it' and going to have a 'nervous breakdown'. Marlene expresses feelings of frustration, short-temperedness and a lack of motivation and purpose in life. She describes herself as a hard worker who has overcome many obstacles in her life. Due to family circumstances, she left school early and took a job. She got along well with her brothers and sisters, and they all tolerated the strict family environment created by their father. She married in her early twenties. Her husband was difficult to live with, had problems with gambling and alcohol, and was verbally and emotionally abusive to her. Ten years ago she decided to leave her husband; 'It was either that or kill myself,' she says.

At her consultation with the general practitioner (GP) she looks shrunken and afraid, and tears come easily as she speaks. She describes how, following the separation from her husband, she struggled to keep going. She was successful in getting employment and worked hard to look after the children. Although she still has contact with the children, since they have left home she has felt increasingly lonely, being often at home alone in the

---

evenings. She has lost enthusiasm for a life that seems more and more pointless; at times she feels like giving up. She has no definite plan of suicide, and states that she would never take her own life, but feels 'so helpless'.

The GP arranges two long appointments with her to gain a fuller understanding of the problem and arrange investigations. She feels that Marlene is indeed depressed, and spends time discussing the meaning of this diagnosis and postulating reasons for the depression as well as things that might be of help. The GP suggests a number of lifestyle changes—gentle exercise, planning regular activities—and some tips for improving her sleep. They discuss treatment options such as psychological approaches to depression and the use of antidepressants, and Marlene decides she will talk to her daughter before embarking on such treatment.

KEY FACTS

■ Depression is distinguished from normal sadness and grief by its persistence and its pervasiveness into all areas of life and the often accompanying pessimism, guilt and self-deprecating thoughts.

■ Depressive disorders often coexist with anxiety disorders, somatisation, substance abuse disorders and physical illness.

■ Depression needs to be understood within the context of the patient's current life situation. Exploring the life context of a depressive disorder may give both patient and doctor a sense of understanding and control, and lead naturally to a psychological intervention that explores interpersonal issues and the origins of guilt or shame.

■ The most 'depressogenic' life circumstances are those that are chronically stressful, such as chronic marital difficulties, caring for a demented relative, prolonged unemployment or having a chronically painful physical illness. By contrast, acute losses tend to give rise to short lived bereavement responses.

■ Depression in mid-life often follows earlier experiences of anxiety and may frequently commence, but not simply be explained by, other triggering factors, such as physical illness, loss of a job or a marital separation.

■ Depression often has a relapsing course, and predisposing factors and life stressors relevant to the first episode of depression may persist.

■ Depression is associated with increased risk of suicide, so assessment of risk of self-harm is essential.

■ The chances of suicide or accidental death are greatly increased in men, particularly among those who abuse alcohol and other substances and/or live alone.

■ Any episode of depression may in fact be a presentation of bipolar disorder. Such a diagnosis has specific treatment implications. It is therefore important to enquire into a personal or family history of mania or hypomania.

■ Depression during pregnancy and/or after delivery of a child is often not immediately recognised for what it is, yet has important implications for the mother, the child and the family.

continued overleaf

KEY FACTS *continued*

■ Antidepressant medication is recommended for moderate and severe or persistent depression, with selection guided by the presence of comorbidities (anxiety, substance use, physical diseases), potential side effects, past treatment responsiveness and doctor preference.

INTRODUCTION

Every day thousands of patients with stories like Marlene's present to GPs. Although each has their own personal story, they all present with the same essential characteristics of an illness that we diagnose as a depressive disorder. As in Marlene's case, the depressive themes and symptoms will be embedded within the narrative of their lives. Sensitive discussion and negotiation is usually required to identify the cardinal features of depression that differentiate it from the other common psychological disorders and normal distress.

Patients generally are aware of the stressors they face, although frequently underestimate their importance or severity; but they are often unfamiliar with other relevant risk factors for depression, such as family history (genetic liability), medical disorders (cerebrovascular disease, recent infectious illness), medications (for example, steroids) or other psychological disorders (premorbid anxiety). The patient's narrative may contain key psychosocial stressors while omitting some of these other factors. But the patient's story is not the whole story. Depression needs to be diagnosed on its own terms—on the presence of depressive symptoms and signs. Many people in difficult or traumatic circumstances do not have a depressive disorder, while others with depression are unable to provide a contextual explanation for their distress. The GP and the patient need to embark together on an exploration that leads to a shared understanding of the problem and what needs to be done.

In this chapter, we provide an overview of depression, the different classification systems, the way it presents in general practice, its epidemiology and aetiology as well as management approaches based on current best practice principles of psychological and pharmacological treatments. We also discuss the special conditions of bipolar disorder—an important differential diagnosis of unipolar depression—and perinatal depression.

DEFINITIONS

The essential features of a depressive disorder are lowering of mood and a pervasive loss of interest and pleasure in normal activities (see Figure 8.1). There are a variety of words and expressions that people use to describe this condition—depressed, down, sad, flat, blue, unhappy, black, miserable, full of dread, dead inside, unable to feel anything, disturbed, preoccupied—and yet, as the opening quote from William Styron reminds us, there are frequently no words to describe the experience. Hence the importance of doctors being able to correctly empathise with the feeling and help the patient find the words.

The loss of the ability to experience pleasure (anhedonia), as distinct from the more normative concept of sadness, is central to the depressive experience and important in distinguishing a clinical depression from normal mood reactivity. This is not just the loss of pleasure in one situation (for example, at work) but a pervasive anhedonia. It is not situational. Anhedonia is evident because of the patient's lack of reactivity of mood, even in usually pleasurable circumstances.

Classically, depression affects thinking. A depressed person will tend to be negative about their past, their present and their future. They may feel pessimistic and hopeless that things will ever be different, losing hope that anything, perhaps even God, could save them. Depressed people commonly feel bad about themselves; they have a low sense of self-value, feeling self-critical and worthless. These negative thoughts can quite easily become so far removed from reality that we consider them delusional. Delusions of worthlessness, guilt, of the need for punishment or feeling that one is being punished are not uncommon. Such thoughts may be intermittent or may occupy the whole of the person's waking hours, even keeping sufferers awake at night. Thoughts of giving up, that life is not worth living or that one would rather be dead can easily arise from feelings of hopelessness, unworthiness, guilt or a desire for relief from the torment.

Depression has marked physical and biological effects. Particularly characteristic is the altered circadian rhythm, evidenced by early morning waking and a worsening of the mood in the morning as seen in melancholic depression. Loss of appetite with accompanying loss of weight, and loss of sexual interest probably represent further neuroendocrine disturbances. Most common in depression are fatigue or tiredness and lack of energy. Psychomotor retardation is demonstrated by slowing or poverty of thinking and slowing or poverty of movement. Of course, some people experiencing depression will be agitated and this will be evident in increased psychomotor activity, rumination and restlessness.

The combination of anhedonia, negativity and pessimism, together with loss of drive and a feeling that life is of no value, leads to withdrawal from people and activities, lack of self-care and neglect of responsibilities.

FIGURE 8.1 Summary of depressive symptomatology

MOOD DISTURBANCE

■ Depressed or lowered mood (feeling sad, blue)

ANHEDONIA

■ Loss of ability to experience pleasure or joy
■ Reduced reactivity of mood in pleasurable circumstances

DEPRESSIVE THOUGHT

■ Brooding
■ Pessimism
■ Low self-worth, self-loathing
■ Guilt, shame
■ Hopelessness
■ Thoughts of death and suicide

continued overleaf

FIGURE 8.1 *continued*

PHYSICAL AND BIOLOGICAL CHANGES

- Sleep disturbance
- Diurnal variation of mood and accompanying symptoms
- Appetite change and accompanying weight change
- Fatigue, tiredness, loss of energy
- Psychomotor change—slowing of thought, impaired concentration, poverty of movement, rumination, agitation
- Loss of sexual drive

SOCIAL WITHDRAWAL

- Withdrawal from people
- Neglect of responsibilities and self-care

CLASSIFICATION

The categories of depression, as described in the two commonly used psychiatric classifications DSM-IV[2] and ICD-10[3], are listed in Table 8.1. Important criteria on which classifications are based include:

- severity (major depression being more severe than adjustment disorder);
- specific symptom sub-types (for example, melancholic depression characterised by anhedonia and psychomotor retardation);
- duration (dysthymia being a chronic form of depression);
- course (adjustment disorder being expected to resolve once the stressful situation resolves); and
- whether it is secondary to a physical or other psychiatric condition.

SEVERITY OF DEPRESSION

Severity of depression is conventionally categorised as mild, moderate or severe according to the severity and numbers of symptoms. This is a little arbitrary, and a chronic and persistent depression may in fact cause more impairment of functioning and more impact on life and family than a briefer but more severe depression. Factors the clinician can consider and implicitly combine into a measure of severity include: the number of symptoms, the severity of symptoms, the duration of symptoms, the level of hopelessness and the degree of functional impairment. The following need to be considered:

- severity of depressed mood—this is probably the most important and is measured empathically; how depressed do you feel the person is?
- constancy of depression—is the depression present all day every day or does it vary?
- pervasiveness of the depression—is the inability to enjoy life pervasive through all activities and all situations and times?
- degree of depressed content in thought—particularly hopelessness, feelings toward the self, such as self-deprecation and guilt, and the will to live or die;

TABLE 8.1 Current major classifications of mood disorders

DSM-IV MOOD DISORDERS	ICD-10 MOOD (AFFECTIVE) DISORDERS
MAJOR DEPRESSIVE DISORDER	**DEPRESSIVE EPISODE**
■ Mild	■ Mild
■ Moderate	■ Moderate
■ Severe	■ Severe
■ With melancholic features	■ With somatic symptoms
■ With psychotic features	■ With psychotic features
■ Single episode	■ Recurrent depressive disorder
■ Recurrent	
Bipolar disorder	*Bipolar affective disorder*
■ Most recent episode depressed, manic or mixed	■ Current episode depression, manic or mixed
Dysthymic disorder (chronic depression)	*Dysthymic disorder*
Cyclothymic disorder	*Cyclothymic disorder*
Adjustment disorder	*Adjustment disorders*
■ With depressed mood	■ Brief depressive reaction
■ With mixed anxiety and depressed mood	■ Prolonged depressive reaction
	■ Mixed anxiety and depression
Mood disorder due to [specify general medical condition]	*Organic mood (affective) disorder*

- presence of neurovegetative symptoms—sleep disturbance, fatigue, psychomotor activity; and
- impairment of functioning—inability to concentrate, work and care for oneself; level of withdrawal from people and activities.

A schema for thinking about severity is presented in Table 8.2.[4] There is a number of rating scales that can assist in the assessment of severity—for example, the CES-D (see Chapter 21).

SUB-TYPES OF DEPRESSION

MELANCHOLIA Melancholia is an important sub-type of depression. It is a marker for more severe depression, and is characterised by depressed mood as well as:

- loss of ability to experience pleasure or joy when pleasurable things happen (anhedonia);
- loss of reactivity of mood (not being able to be cheered up);
- a distinct quality to the mood—the person identifies that it is not the normal (albeit severe) sadness that one might experience after a bereavement;
- early morning waking (about two hours earlier than usual);
- diurnal variation—the depression is worse in the morning;

TABLE 8.2 Classification of severity of depressive illness, based on clinical features

SYMPTOM CLUSTER	MILD	MODERATE	SEVERE
Mood	■ Lowered mood ■ Reduced joy ■ Crying ■ Anxiety ■ Irritability	■ Reduced interest in things ■ Reduced pleasure in things ■ Reduced reactivity	■ No interest in things ■ No pleasure in things ■ No reactivity
Depressive thought	■ Loss of confidence	■ Pessimistic about the future ■ Feeling worthless or a failure ■ Paranoid ideas	■ Hopeless, see no future, self-reproach, guilt, shame ■ Consider illness a punishment ■ Paranoid or nihilistic delusions
Cognition	■ Minor forgetfulness or lack of concentration	■ Indecisiveness ■ Forgetfulness	■ Unable to make decisions ■ Slowed mentation, seems cognitively impaired (pseudodementia)
Somatic	■ Low drive ■ Loss of interest in food ■ Lowered libido ■ Mild initial insomnia; wake 1–2 times a night	■ Low energy, drive ■ Eat with encouragement; mild weight loss ■ Loss of libido ■ Initial insomnia; wake several times a night	■ No energy, drive ■ Unable to eat; severe weight loss ■ No libido ■ Psychomotor retardation or agitation ■ Sleep only a few hours
Social	■ Mild social withdrawal	■ Apathy and social withdrawal ■ Work impairment	■ Apathy and social withdrawal ■ Marked work impairment ■ Poor self-care
Suicidality	■ Life not enjoyable, not worth living	■ Thoughts of death or suicide	■ Plans or attempts suicide

- observable psychomotor retardation or agitation ;
- significant loss of appetite and weight; and
- excessive guilt.

The first two characteristics are persistent (occurring every day for two weeks or more) and pervasive (occuring in all situations, not just while at work, for instance).

A melancholic picture of depression is probably associated with a range of neurochemical disturbances (as demonstrated by an abnormal Dexamethasone Suppression Test) and a good response to physical treatment, either antidepressant medication or electroconvulsive therapy.

ADJUSTMENT DISORDERS Adjustment disorder describes brief depressive symptoms in response to a life crisis in someone who is usually well and who can expect a good recovery. It is considered a mild form of depression, although if the stresses continue, the depression may continue and lead to significant ongoing distress and impairment.

DEMORALISATION When the stress is severe and experienced as threatening one's life or integrity (for example, with the diagnosis of cancer, chronic disability or a degenerative disease), the depression can be understood in terms of demoralisation. This occurs when there is overwhelming helplessness. If help is not available, hopelessness, impaired self-esteem, a feeling of aloneness and finally despair and thoughts of suicide can ensue. Demoralisation is a severe form of 'adjustment disorder' which, although situational, can lead to a person wanting to end their life.[5]

SECONDARY DEPRESSION Depression may occur secondarily to medication (organic mood disorder). It frequently occurs with physical illness, and in this situation may be biologically mediated (for example, a reaction to inflammatory cytokines), or be a psychological response (as in demoralization) which is more commonly the case. Health practitioners often ignore even severe depressive disorders that occur in association with medical conditions because they seem 'understandable'. Such depressions do result in ongoing morbidity, disability and poor physical health outcomes, however, and therefore require treatment in the usual way.

Sometimes depression is the first presentation of an occult malignancy, and this possibility should be considered when depression occurs for the first time in an older person. Depression may also occur as part of, or subsequent to, another psychiatric illness (for example, post-psychotic depression) or as secondary to substance abuse (most often alcohol abuse). One of the most common comorbidities in older persons is cerebrovascular disease, including subcortical small vessel disease (typically undetected neurologically) as well as larger strokes. Such disorders tend to result in significant neuropsychological impairment and place the older person at high risk of requiring institutional care (see Chapter 16).

DYSTHYMIC DISORDER Another criterion on which to classify depression is the time course of illness. Dysthymic disorder is a chronic, fluctuating depression lasting at least several years. The depression may fluctuate apparently spontaneously or in response to everyday stresses. Although it is not as acutely severe as major depressive disorder, dysthymic disorder is very disabling because of its chronicity and unpredictability, and it is often accompanied by significant impairment in interpersonal and work related functioning. Its chronicity makes it difficult to distinguish dysthymia from a depressive personality or disposition.

EPIDEMIOLOGY

Depression is common in the community, contributes significantly to the worldwide burden of disease and presents commonly to general practice in the first instance. The World Health Organization has identified unipolar depression as the fourth leading cause of disability, and has predicted that by 2020 depression will contribute the second largest burden of disease worldwide.[6] In the Australian community, depression has been estimated to be prevalent in approximately 5% of the community in any one year.[7] Indeed, presentation to a GP for management of depression is estimated to be the fourth most frequent reason for a GP consultation.[8] Furthermore, depressed patients are equally likely to present to GPs with non-specific physical symptoms such as tiredness, headaches and chronic pain as they are with more overt psychological disturbances.[9]

AETIOLOGY

The risk factors for depression are multiple and in any individual will reflect interactions between their innate characteristics (genetics, biochemistry, developmental experiences) and their current environment, the latter providing potential stress (for example, marital distress, unemployment) as well as protection (family, social network, employment). Each person will have greater or lesser vulnerability on the basis of heritable characteristics, developmental history and social supports. This will be evidenced by a past personal history or family history of depression, or by a depressive, anxious or obsessional personality. Important predisposing, precipitating and perpetuating factors are listed in Table 8.3.

TABLE 8.3 Aetiological factors for depression			
CAUSE	**PREDISPOSING**	**PRECIPITATING**	**PERPETUATING**
Biological	■ Hereditary factors ■ Temperament	■ Medication ■ Other drugs ■ Physical illness	■ Medication ■ Other drugs ■ Physical illness
Psychosocial	■ Early loss of parent ■ Difficult early life ■ Parent with mental illness, alcoholism or chronic illness ■ Abuse ■ Neglect ■ Chronic illness	■ Divorce or bereavement ■ Redundancy or retirement ■ Empty nest ■ Physical illness ■ Mental illness	■ Repeated losses ■ Chronic illness and incapacity ■ Social isolation

In general, people who have 'good genes' (that is, no family history of mental illness) and an emotionally secure upbringing will be more resilient than those without these factors. The specific genetic contributions to common forms of anxiety and depression have recently been more clearly delineated, with particular focus on the increased vulnerability to life stress conferred by polymorphisms of the serotonin transporter gene.[10]

Losses, such as a parent leaving or dying, are stressors at any age and may predispose to, or precipitate, depression. Certain stages in life—such as adolescence, first time motherhood or retirement—provide unique stresses associated with role transition and changes in social networks and responsibilities. With increasing age, physical illness, incapacity, cumulative loss and relative social isolation often combine to produce a potent depressogenic cocktail. For other people, some of these stresses just present challenges to be overcome. Old age can bring a sense of satisfaction and completion as a person enjoys the fruits of a rich life lived to the full. For a person who is depressed, understanding their unique story and the meaning of events for them will help make sense of the depression and give a degree of control that facilitates recovery and aids management planning. This is the purpose of the 'formulation'—making sense of the unique story of the patient to understand the interacting biological, psychological and social determinants (see Chapter 7 for a fuller discussion of the formulation).

COURSE OF ILLNESS

Major depressive episode (MDE) is an episodic illness, and it is customary to think of it in three phases—acute episode, remission and recovery.

- **Acute episode** The patient currently experiences persistently depressed mood and/ or pervasive anhedonia, together with the characteristic biological and psychological symptoms of depression.
- **Remission** A recent acute episode is followed by a sustained period of improvement, during which relapse can still occur—that is, there can be a return of symptoms of a still ongoing, but symptomatically suppressed episode.
- **Recovery** There is a prolonged remission; if symptoms then recur they are considered as representing an entirely new episode.

The risk of relapse increases with each episode experienced by a patient. Between 50% and 60% of patients who have one depressive episode will have a second; 70% of those who have two episodes will have a third; and 90% of those who have had three episodes will have a fourth. Put another way, over five years, 80–90% of patients do recover at some time but of these, 70–80% subsequently relapse. Over ten years, only 25% of patients have a single episode of major depression. Furthermore, 10–20% of depressed patients continue to experience persistent symptoms of fluctuating severity.

Bipolar disorder is generally characterised by recovery and relapse. Patients may experience repeated episodes of depression with few manic episodes, frequent manic episodes and few depressive episodes, or alternate between the two. Episodes tend to become less frequent with increasing age. As with unipolar depression, some patients with bipolar disorder do not experience full remission of symptoms between acute episodes.

DIAGNOSIS OF DEPRESSION IN GENERAL PRACTICE

Despite the substantial burden of depressive disorders on communities, and on individuals and their families, studies around the world consistently report that about half the depressed patients who present to GPs remain undiagnosed. There are complex reasons for this underdiagnosis that relate to the way patients present, to GP attitudes to managing depression and to our system of health care.

A patient's attitude to depression clearly influences whether they choose to disclose depressive symptoms to their GP. There is still much stigma associated with having depression, and it is often regarded as a sign of weakness or something that people should 'just get over'. In addition, depressed patients frequently attend the GP complaining of somatic symptoms or non-specific presentations, such as tiredness or vague aches and pains, often making the diagnosis difficult.

Furthermore, some GPs are less inclined than others to make the diagnosis of depression, and this relates to their own attitudes or lack of knowledge about the condition. Studies show that a GP's consulting style influences detection rates significantly: patients are more likely to disclose emotional symptoms when the GP asks more open-ended questions, listens attentively and enquires about psychosocial issues during the consultation.[11] Whether GPs have enough time to adequately explore psychological issues also influences GP behaviour and the rate of diagnosis of depression.

Beyond patient and doctor characteristics, both the physical layout of the general practice and the practical extent to which the general practice team is organised to address these issues have major impacts on diagnosis rates and the quality of treatment provided.[9] Practices that emphasise time spent with a patient, routine use of case detection or 'screening tools', additional mental health training for the practitioner and continuity of care with specific patients will achieve the best results.

DIFFERENTIAL DIAGNOSIS

When a patient presents describing depressed mood, this may be due to a depressive illness (such as those listed in Figure 8.1); however, a variety of other explanations also need to be considered. Figure 8.2 shows a simple flow chart summarising the assessment and diagnostic decisions of a patient with depressive symptoms.

NORMAL MOOD RESPONSE TO A STRESSFUL SITUATION

This diagnosis is a judgment made by assessment of the level (number and severity) of symptoms, their persistence, the degree of distress and impairment caused, and the degree to which this is considered appropriate to the circumstances. A normal grief reaction may involve quite severe disturbance of mood (pangs of grief, pining) and moderate impairment of functioning (see Chapter 19). But it does not involve feelings of worthlessness or guilt and does not go on forever. Similarly, with adaptation to a diagnosis of serious physical illness, the acute shock and stress might be severe, as might feelings of helplessness, but there should be movement (adaptation), anhedonia should not be pervasive (there will be joy in some areas of life) and there should be no self-deprecation.

FIGURE 8.2 Depressive symptoms

Are **depressive symptoms** a change from the usual way of feeling and thinking, and do they represent a discrete depressive episode (consider symptom number, severity, persistence and duration)?

No **Depressive personality** or **Dysthymia**

Yes

Is there a history of manic symptoms? *Yes* **Bipolar disorder**

No

Is depression secondary to bereavement or other psychosocial stressor, such as illness? *Yes* **Grief, adjustment disorder** or **demoralisation**

No

Is depression due to an 'organic' cause, such as medical illness, medication or substance? *Yes* **Depression secondary** to:
• substance use
• medication
• physical illness

No

Is depression a secondary part of another psychiatric disorder? *Yes* **Depression secondary** to other psychiatric illness (e.g. psychosis, obsessive-compulsive or other anxiety disorder)

No

Is melancholia present?

Yes **MDD with melancholic features**

No

Are delusions or hallucinations present?

Yes **MDD with psychotic features**

No

Major depressive disorder (MDD)

COMORBID ANXIETY DISORDER

Patients with a mixture of anxiety and depressive symptoms are frequently seen in general practice settings. Such patients could be given a diagnosis of depression (as in major depressive disorder, perhaps an agitated depression) or any anxiety disorder (for example, panic disorder with secondary depression), or one of mixed anxiety and depressive disorder. Management is generally determined by the most prominent symptoms. As antidepressants also have an anxiolytic effect, where medication is deemed appropriate an antidepressant rather than an anxiolytic (for example, benzodiazepine) will usually be the drug of choice. Cognitive therapy for depression and anxiety symptoms, behavioural management for avoidance behaviour, sleep–wake cycle regulation, reduction of alcohol and other harmful substance use, and pleasant events scheduling are all examples of how therapy will help both anxiety and depression (see Chapter 17 for more details about these therapeutic techniques).

PERSONALITY

Despite its non-recognition in current diagnostic manuals, the depressive personality has a long theoretical and clinical tradition. Emil Kraepelin described the depressive temperament as being characterised by 'a permanent gloomy emotional stress in all experiences of life'. He emphasised persistent gloominess and joylessness, and a predominantly depressed, despondent and despairing mood.[12] Depression in these people has an early onset (perhaps it is always present) and is stable, durable and resistant to change across situations and time. Although the distinction between depressive personality and dysthymic disorder is at times difficult to make, it is important to do so, as the latter may respond to treatments such as cognitive behavioural treatment (CBT), interpersonal therapy (IPT) and antidepressants, while patients with depressive personality may be best helped with longer term psychotherapies and supportive care (see Chapter 17).

ORGANIC MOOD DISORDER

As it is potentially remedial, organic mood disorder is an important diagnosis to make. The GP should consider it if depression occurs for the first time after mid-life, if there is any indication of physical illness or newly commenced drug therapy, or if there is any change in cognitive capacity suggesting intracranial pathology. Table 8.4 lists the common potential organic causes of depression.

BIPOLAR DISORDER

A patient with depression may in fact be presenting with their first episode of a bipolar illness. People with bipolar disorder have episodes of both major depressive disorder and mania or hypomania. In its most acute phase, bipolar disorder presents with florid psychosis that can be difficult to distinguish from other forms of psychosis, such as schizophrenia and drug induced psychoses (see Chapter 12). During a manic episode, a patient will typically have what is termed an elevated or expansive mood combined with grandiosity, hyperactivity (racing thoughts, pressure of speech, increased goal directed activity and reduced sleep) and impaired judgment (overconfidence, excessive engagement in pleasurable activities, often with risk). Delusions in bipolar disorder

TABLE 8.4 Organic causes of depression	
Neurological and intracerebral disease	Small and large vessel cerebrovascular disease, Parkinson's disease, Huntington's disease, tumours, SLE (lupus), multiple sclerosis, cerebral infections, stroke, arteriovenous (A-V) malformation
Occult neoplasms	Especially abdominal, such as pancreatic carcinoma
Medications	Antihypertensives, beta blockers, corticosteroids, interferon, oral contraceptives
Infections	Particularly viral; HIV, infectious mononucleosis
Endocrine disorders	Addison's, Cushing's and thyroid disease

are usually mood congruent, in contrast to the often non-mood congruent or bizarre delusions of schizophrenia. Hypomanic episodes are more subtle versions of mania. A history of a previous manic or hypomanic episode should be sought, either in depressed patients to exclude or confirm a diagnosis of bipolar disorder, or in their family history to suggest a provisional diagnosis of bipolar disorder. Other features that may suggest a diagnosis of bipolar disorder include poor response to antidepressant therapies, significant alcohol or substance abuse, severe sleep–wake cycle disturbance, periods of sustained irritability or highly unstable interpersonal relationships. The significance of this diagnosis is that more care will need to be given to the use of antidepressants, with the mainstay of treatment being mood stabilisers (see Chapter 20).

PERINATAL DEPRESSION

This used to be called postnatal depression, but the term 'perinatal' reflects the fact that some women are already very anxious or depressed at the time they become pregnant or during the pregnancy. Only a subset becomes depressed for the first time after delivery. Depression is common during and after pregnancy, and in most respects is like any other depression. What is important is that it is frequently not recognised. This is because it may be considered normal or just part of the 'baby blues', or alternatively is so associated with a lack of confidence in mothering that women are ashamed to admit their difficulties and fail to present for help. It is important here to recognise the attendant risks for the developing infant and family if the depression is not recognised and treated—problems of neglect, impaired mother–child bonding, family stress, suicide or infanticide. As a result there is a considerable argument for routinely screening women for depression after they have given birth (for example, using the Edinburgh Postnatal Depression Scale).[13] (See Chapter 21.) Remember also that women with a past history of depression, as with women with a past history of bipolar disorder or schizophrenia, are particularly vulnerable to a recurrence or relapse in the perinatal period, so they should be observed carefully, and serious consideration should be given to pharmaceutical protection, either during pregnancy or in the immediate postnatal period.

Treatment of depression in the perinatal period is effective. The commonly used antidepressants are relatively safe in pregnancy, although recent guidelines for the use of medicines in pregnancy should be consulted before prescribing. In particular, concerns have been raised about the use of selective serotonin reuptake inhibitors (SSRIs) during pregnancy (see Chapter 20), and the potential for withdrawal symptoms in a neonate whose mother has been treated with SSRIs and venlafaxine. Similarly, in the post-partum period, medication is relatively safe, with only low levels of most drugs being excreted into breast milk, but again, specific advice from therapeutic guidelines should be sought.

INVESTIGATIONS

A diagnosis of major depression is made on the basis of the history and mental state examination. As part of the GP assessment, baseline investigations should be performed to exclude organic causes of depression, particularly when the presentation is atypical or when the first episode of depression occurs in an older person. These investigations can also form part of good preventive care—remember that depression increases the risk for a range of physical illnesses, including heart disease. A balance is needed to ensure that appropriate physical investigations are undertaken but unnecessary overinvestigation is avoided. The latter is particularly important when patients present with prominent somatic symptoms where multiple investigations can reinforce inappropriate somatic concerns. A commonsense approach will be guided by the presence of comorbid illnesses and the clinical presentation, which may direct the GP to particular investigations—for example, for cardiovascular problems, malignancy or abnormalities related to substance abuse.

Baseline blood tests recommended for patients with a depressive disorder include: a full blood examination, urea and electrolytes, thyroid tests, random glucose and lipid profile. Additional tests may be warranted, according to the clinical setting, but tests worth considering include an electrocardiogram (ECG) where patients are experiencing palpitations, a computerised tomography (CT) or magnetic resonance imaging (MRI) brain scan where neurological disease is thought a possibility, and urine microscopy and culture to detect urinary infection.

MANAGEMENT
INFORMATION AND EDUCATION

It is important to give patients information about depression and to use the consultation to help patients understand the nature of stress and how they cope with it (psychoeducation). If a patient is experiencing physical symptoms or sleep disturbance, explaining that these are physiological responses to stress or arousal will take away some of the mystery of the experience. Giving both the patient and their family or carers high quality pamphlets, books or websites about depression is likely to be particularly helpful (see Chapter 3).

PSYCHOLOGICAL AND BEHAVIOURAL INTERVENTIONS

Psychological and behavioural interventions are an important and effective approach to managing depressive disorders, either alone or in combination with antidepressant medications, and need to be considered by the GP. A range of approaches suitable for general practice are described in detail in Chapter 17. The purpose of this section is to highlight how the GP may use these various techniques to specifically assist the depressed patient.

First we stress the importance of a committed and trusting relationship with the patient. There should be a therapeutic alliance between the GP and the patient; where there are specific personal or cultural barriers that prevent this, it is better to refer the patient to another provider (see Chapters 5 and 6). In addition, not all GPs have the time, inclination and/or training to enter into psychological treatment with the patient, and here again, the patient's interests may be best served by management by another GP with specific psychological interests or by referral to another mental health specialist (see Chapter 22).

Simple behavioural interventions—such as education about the principles of sleep (sleep–wake cycle management), relaxation (using progressive muscle relaxation or imagery) and planning mastery and pleasurable events (activity scheduling)—are very helpful and within the repertoire of every GP. These are the first steps to be considered.

Following that, choosing a psychological approach that will most likely assist the patient depends on a number of things, in particular the nature and severity of the depression and the predisposing and precipitating factors that have been identified in the assessment and formulation (see Chapter 7). The psychological approaches we describe fall into five categories: empathic attunement, stress management, problem-solving, interpersonal therapy and cognitive behavioural strategies (see Chapter 17).

Empathic attunement is often overlooked in discussions of psychological therapies on the assumption that its importance is assumed. But it is the most important skill and needs to be made explicit. If a doctor can genuinely empathise with a patient, they will be telling the patient that they are not alone, their experience is not so strange and that they can be understood. They will also be saying to the patient that they are worthy of being listened to. For very depressed patients, these things can be empowering and life giving. Empathic attunement is not a passive thing: it involves actively listening, trying to understand the patient's experience, getting 'into their shoes', and reflecting back so that the patient appreciates that the doctor really understands their experience.

Following empathic understanding, stress reduction (see Chapter 17) and pleasant event scheduling (see Chapter 17) are perhaps the techniques that GPs most commonly use with a depressed patient. Through lack of confidence and energy, depressed patients invariably withdraw from pleasurable activities and activities that give them a sense of accomplishment. Identifying these activities with them and using a simple activity-scheduling strategy can help patients to rediscover some enjoyment and mastery. Both these activities (stress reduction and pleasant event scheduling) are not time consuming; they are activities the patient learns to do themselves. These activities help with the current depression, and give the patient both a sense of competence in the present time and a skill learnt for life in future time. Similarly, structured problem solving (see Chapter 17) helps solve the current dilemma (and hence perhaps the depression and anxiety), and gives the patient a new skill and competence. All these therapies are easily delivered by GPs. In the context of these behavioural interventions, consideration should be given to social supports and how these may be strengthened and mobilised.

Other techniques derived from more formal counselling and psychotherapy can be learnt by enthusiastic GPs, although they take more time to both learn and deliver. We have already noted that most depression, especially first episode depression, usually occurs in the context of some stressful life occurrence that has significance of an interpersonal nature—for instance, grief, job redundancy, retirement and interpersonal disputes. Interpersonal counselling (see Chapter 17) addresses these by exploring with patients their life and relationships, and providing understanding of their current life events in the context of their hopes and expectations for their relationships. This type of approach requires up to six sessions of 30 minutes duration each. Utilising cognitive strategies, focusing on the recognition of cognitive distortions and challenging negative automatic thoughts (see Chapter 17), is also an effective way to approach therapy for a depressed patient, particularly where there are obvious cognitive distortions. However, this also takes training and delivery time. More formal cognitive and interpersonal therapies are available in some primary care settings, usually by referral to psychologists or psychiatrists.

PHARMACOLOGICAL INTERVENTIONS

Antidepressants are useful for the treatment of the more severe forms of depression, but not so much for mild depression. Simple psychological therapies, 'watchful waiting' and the giving of information (bibliotherapy or psychoeducation) are therefore particularly important first line measures in all cases of depression. Not all patients will require antidepressants. However, for the more severe depression, and persistent depression, there are now a range of drugs and a range of classes of antidepressants available that, on the whole, have similar effectiveness.[14] Each class of antidepressants has a different side effect profile, although these are not highly predictable in individual patients. The choice of antidepressants is therefore usually based on minimising side effects and other drug interactions, as well as on the GP's familiarity with particular drugs. Detailed information about the various antidepressants, their mode of action and common side effects is described in Chapter 20 and is not repeated here.

Recent guidelines[15] generally recommend an SSRI as the first line of treatment. When selecting an SSRI, factors to consider are potential drug interactions (cytochrome P-450 enzyme systems), severity of withdrawal syndromes and tendency to cause initial agitation. SSRIs may be associated with worsening sleep patterns in the first few weeks of therapy, during which time a night sedative will be helpful. SSRIs are effective for anxiety, including panic, and are therefore useful for treating mixed depression and anxiety.

If there is no or inadequate improvement using the maximum dose of SSRI for a period of 6–8 weeks, the GP needs to go to a second line treatment, using another agent such as venlafaxine or a tricyclic antidepressant—that is, not an SSRI. At this stage, if there is uncertainty about progress, the GP should seek a specialist opinion. Psychiatrists sometimes use combinations of drugs and mood stabilisers, although there is little hard evidence apart from clinical experience of the value of these treatments. Of course, if the clinical situation demands more urgency, speedy referral to specialist care ought to be obtained.

Patients with melancholic or severe depression may do less well with SSRIs, and therefore benefit from commencing therapy with selective norepinephrine reuptake inhibitors (SNRIs) or tricyclic antidepressants.[16] It is important to note that the widespread use of antidepressant medications, in association with greater provision of other therapies, has been associated with falls in suicide rates in Australia.[17]

REFERRAL TO A SPECIALIST OR FOR HOSPITALISATION

When they feel out of their depth or need advice, GPs will refer patients to a specialist. Sometimes GPs complain that it is hard to find a specialist, but it is important that they identify appropriate referral pathways and consider the type of relationship they might have with the specialist. For example, do they want to work in a shared care relationship or are they seeking to transfer clinical responsibility?[18] Referral to a psychiatrist for either opinion or management is advised if the patient is not getting better after several months of treatment. Referral is also indicated if the depression is severe, evidenced perhaps by mental and physical slowing, if the patient has delusions (often of worthlessness or guilt) or if there are strong suicidal ideas. Electroconvulsive therapy (ECT) is indicated if the gravity of the clinical situation demands a quick effective treatment, for treatment of resistant cases and where psychotic phenomena are present.

The drug treatment of patients with bipolar disorder is usually managed in association with a specialist psychiatrist (see Chapter 20). The mainstay here is mood-stabilising drugs, with lithium carbonate having the greatest efficacy. Although they have the potential to cause mood swings, antipsychotics and antidepressants have their place in treating cycles of mania and depression.

One thing that is very clear in the drug treatment of depression is that there is a high incidence of relapse upon cessation of medication. It is therefore important to offer information about depression and encourage compliance. It is currently recommended that patients continue antidepressant medication for a year after they have achieved remission from the first episode of depression, and for two years following repeated episodes. The outcomes are better if psychological and behavioural therapies are combined with drug therapies.

CONCLUSION

Depression is now so common in the population that all GPs will encounter it. Research has given us a good understanding about the aetiology of, and treatments for, depression. Much of this treatment, of course, occurs in general practice, although GPs are wise to establish good relationships with specialist psychiatrists and psychologists who can assist in delivering the best pharmacological and psychological care for these patients. Depression is intimately related to a person's general physical health and functioning and so, even with specialist involvement, the GP's role will remain central.

REFERENCES

1. Styron W. Darkness Visible: A Memoir of Madness. London: Jonathan Cape, 1991;7.
2. American Psychiatric Association. Diagnostic and Statistical Manual of Mental Disorders. 4th edn. Washington DC: American Psychiatric Association, 1994.
3. World Health Organization. The ICO-10 Classification of Mental and Behavioural Disorders. Geneva: WHO, 1992.
4. Judd FK, Mijch AM. Psychiatric disturbances and HIV infection. In: Crowe S, Hoy J, Mills J, eds. Management of the HIV-infected Patient. Cambridge: Cambridge University Press, 1996;125–41.
5. Clarke DM, Kissane DW. Demoralisation: its phenomenology and importance. Australian and New Zealand Journal of Psychiatry 2002;36:733–42.

6. Murray CJL, Lopez AD. Alternative projections of mortality and disability by cause 1990–2020: Global Burden of Disease Study. Lancet 1997;349:1498–504.

7. Andrews G, Hall W, Teesson M, Henderson H. The Mental Health of Australians. Canberra: Mental Health Branch, Commonwealth Department of Health and Aged Care, April 1999.

8. Britt H, Miller GC, Knox S, Charles J, Valenti L, Pan Y, Henderson J, O'Halloran J, Ng A. General practice activity in Australia 2003–04. AIHW Cat. No. GEP 16. Canberra: Australian Institute of Health and Welfare, General Practice Series No. 16, 2004.

9. Hickie IB, Davenport TA, Scott EM, Hadzi-Pavlovic D, Naismith SL, Koschera A. Unmet need for recognition of common mental disorders in Australian general practice. Medical Journal of Australia 2001;175(Suppl.)16:S18–24.

10. Caspi A, Sugden K, Moffitt TE, Taylor A, Craig IW, Harrington H, McClay J, Mill J, Martin J, Braithwaite A, Poulton R.. Influence of life stress on depression: moderation by a polymorphism in the 5-HTT gene. Science 2003;301:386–9.

11. Goldberg DP, Jenkins L, Millar T, Faragher EB. The ability of trainee general practitioners to identify psychological distress among their patients. Psychological Medicine 1993;23:185–93.

12. Sass H, Jünemann K. Affective disorders, personality and personality disorders. Acta Psychiatrica Scandinavica 2003;108(Suppl. 418):34–40.

13. Cox JL, Holden JM, Sagovsky R. Detection of postnatal depression. Development of the 10-item Edinburgh Postnatal Depression Scale. British Journal of Psychiatry 1987;150:782–6.

14. Boerner RJ, Moller HJ. The importance of new antidepressants in the treatment of anxiety/depressive disorders. Pharmacopsychiatry 1999;32:119–26.

15. Ellis PM, Smith DAR. Treating depression: the beyondblue guidelines for treating depression in primary care. Medical Journal of Australia 2002;176:S77–83.

16. Boyce P, Judd F. The place for the tricyclic antidepressants in the treatment of depression. Australian and New Zealand Journal of Psychiatry 1999;33:323–7.

17. Hall WD, Mant A, Mitchell PB, Rendle VA, Hickie IB, McManus P. Association between antidepressant prescribing and suicide in Australia, 1991–2000: trend analysis. British Medical Journal 2003; 326:1008–13.

18. Blashki G, Selzer R, Judd F, Hodgins G, Ciechomski L. Primary care psychiatry: taking consultation liaison psychiatry to the community. Australasian Psychiatry 2005;13:302–6.

CHAPTER 9
ANXIETY DISORDERS

F Judd and H Malcolm

We are, perhaps, uniquely among earth's creatures, the worrying animal. We worry away our lives, fearing the future, discontent with the present, unable to take in the idea of dying, unable to sit still.

LEWIS THOMAS, *1913–1993*

CASE STUDY

Sandra, a 33-year-old woman, first presented requesting a repeat prescription for paroxetine. She said this had been prescribed for depression and panic but that the problems were now 'under control'. She returns some weeks later with worsening anxiety, feeling on edge, panicky and hopeless. She describes lifelong anxiety, but has only been receiving treatment for the past four years or so.

KEY FACTS

- Anxiety disorders are the most common group of psychiatric illnesses in the general population.

- The most common presentations in primary care are generalised anxiety and panic disorder with or without agoraphobia.

- Anxiety disorders are frequently under-diagnosed and under-treated.

- Comorbidity is the rule—there may be another anxiety disorder, depression, alcohol abuse or drug abuse (particularly benzodiazepines).

- While there is overlap in symptoms and treatment, making a specific diagnosis provides the best management outcomes.

continued overleaf

■ 'Organic' causes of anxiety—such as thyroid disease, substance intoxication and/or withdrawal—are common and should be excluded.

■ Anxiety disorders usually have an early age of onset and precede the development of other disorders (particularly mood disorders).

■ Anxiety disorders are characterised by a chronic course, albeit often with relapse and remission.

■ Cognitive behavioural therapies, either alone or in combination with medication, are effective for the treatment of anxiety disorders.

■ Lifestyle may have a major impact on these disorders—for example, even small amounts of alcohol and caffeine may cause a significant exacerbation of symptoms.

INTRODUCTION

Anxiety is a normal emotion frequently experienced in mild and self-limited forms. Characteristic features of anxiety include fearful mood, increased arousal, restless behaviour and avoidance of situations. Mild levels of anxiety may enhance performance, but excessive anxiety has a detrimental effect. Anxiety may be an adaptive behaviour: when faced with a threat or trauma, physiological arousal experienced as the 'fight or flight response' facilitates action.

Anxiety disorders are a group of conditions characterised by tension, worry, fear, dread or arousal that is excessive or prolonged, that appears unrelated to any current threat, and that results in distress or significant impairment in functioning. This generally includes academic and occupational functioning as well as in relationships with family and friends. Consequently, the financial cost of these disorders can be substantial, involving both indirect costs (that is, affecting social and occupational functioning) as well as the direct costs of medical treatment.[1]

CLASSIFICATION

The anxiety disorders can be separated into a number of discrete conditions. However, there is significant comorbidity between the different anxiety disorders and with mood disorders. The two main classifications of anxiety disorders (DSM-IV[2] and ICD-10[3]) are shown in Table 9.1.

EPIDEMIOLOGY

Anxiety disorders are the most common of all psychiatric illnesses; the twelve-month prevalence rate is almost 10%.[4] They often have an early onset (in the teens and twenties) and follow a chronic course. Generalised anxiety disorder (GAD) and obsessive-compulsive disorder (OCD) tend to be chronic conditions where the symptoms wax and wane, often worsening at times of stress. Social phobic (SP) symptoms tend to be continuous and disabling. Panic disorder with agoraphobia (PDA) is often an episodic

TABLE 9.1 Current major classifications of anxiety disorder

DSM-IV: ANXIETY DISORDERS	ICD-10: NEUROTIC, STRESS RELATED AND SOMATOFORM DISORDERS
■ Panic disorder (with/without agoraphobia)	■ Phobic anxiety disorders
■ Agoraphobia without history of panic disorder	— Agoraphobia (with/without panic disorder)
■ Specific phobia	— Social phobia
■ Social phobia	— Specific phobias
■ Obsessive-compulsive disorder	■ Other anxiety disorders
■ Post-traumatic stress disorder	— Panic disorder
■ Acute stress disorder	— Generalised anxiety disorder
■ Generalised anxiety disorder	— Mixed anxiety and depressive disorder
■ Anxiety disorder due to general medical condition	■ Obsessive-compulsive disorder
■ Substance induced anxiety disorder	■ Reaction to severe stress, and adjustment disorders
■ Adjustment disorder with anxiety	■ Acute stress reaction
■ Adjustment disorder with mixed anxiety and depressed mood	■ Post-traumatic stress disorder
	■ Adjustment disorders—mixed anxiety and depressive reaction

TABLE 9.2 Anxiety disorders: epidemiology

ANXIETY DISORDER	MALE TO FEMALE RATIO	AGE OF ONSET	LIFETIME PREVALENCE (%)
Panic disorder with or without agoraphobia	1:2	Late adolescence to mid-thirties	3.5[1,5]
Social phobia	F>M	Mid-teens	13.3[5]
Specific phobia	1:3	Childhood	11.3[5]
Generalised anxiety disorder	1:2	Childhood to adolescence	5.1[5]
Obsessive-compulsive disorder	F>M	Childhood to young adulthood	2.5[6]

condition, varying from having years of remission between attacks to one of chronic severe symptoms. Those disorders, which begin in childhood and adolescence, are more likely to be associated with significant comorbidity and chronicity. (See Table 7.2.)

AETIOLOGY

The current understanding of the aetiology of anxiety disorders is based broadly on the stress–diathesis model,[7] where vulnerability and stress combine to result in an anxiety disorder. According to this model, anxiety is likely to develop in individuals who have a vulnerability (diathesis) to the disorder when they find themselves in a high-risk situation. A variety of biological, psychological and social factors have been identified as important to the development of anxiety disorders (see Figure 9.1). Some of these (for example, genetic factors, personality style) are regarded as vulnerability factors. Others (for example, stressful life events or work or family stress) are precipitants to the development of the disorder or act to maintain or cause an exacerbation of symptoms. In addition, there may be a 'weakening effect' when supports or resources (protective factors) are temporarily removed or unavailable.

FIGURE 9.1 Aetiological factors of anxiety disorders

- Early family background; child–parent relationships[8]
- Parental loss or threat of such loss in childhood[9]
- Cognitive style—schemata, information processing, inferences[10, 11]
- Personality—trait anxiety, neuroticism[12, 13]
- Genetic factors—significant heritability demonstrated for PD, SP (generalised type) and OCD[14]
- Neurobiology—abnormalities of noradrenergic function (PD), serotonergic function (PD, OCD, GAD) and γ–amino butyric acid (GABA)—benzodiazepine complex (GAD)[15–19]
- Cardiovascular function—decreased heart rate variability in PD[20]
- Life events—threat, loss, adversity[21]

CLINICAL FEATURES

Anxiety disorders are characterised by excessive and recurring fears and anxiety that do not dissipate with reassurance and that are accompanied by somatic symptoms, subjective feelings of foreboding and thoughts or actions that seem excessive. These symptoms occur in the context of a perceived threat and are disproportionate to the triggering situation.

All anxiety disorders share three common symptom components—physiological, behavioural and cognitive;[22] these constitute the anxiety triad (see Figure 9.2). The physiological component is autonomic hyperarousal, which occurs when the individual faces perceived danger. Physical changes arise from the physiological response to threat and cause the somatic symptoms of acute anxiety, seen most clearly during a panic attack. These somatic manifestations are shown in Table 9.3. Prolonged anxiety results in additional symptoms, such as those listed in Figure 9.3.

The behavioural component involves strategies for dealing with the threatening situation. The most common behavioural strategy is avoidance of the anxiety-provoking situations. Other behaviours include frequent safety checks or seeking constant support and reassurance from others.

The cognitive component is that when anxious, an individual's thoughts become focused on the perceived threat and other contextual information is excluded. Often the individual believes they are unable to cope with the situation. Thoughts may include specific fears or non-specific foreboding, thoughts that something bad is about to happen. Content varies between the different anxiety disorders as described below.

FIGURE 9.2 The anxiety triad

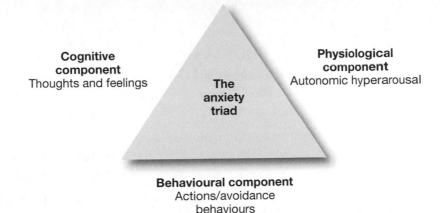

Cognitive component
Thoughts and feelings

Physiological component
Autonomic hyperarousal

The anxiety triad

Behavioural component
Actions/avoidance behaviours

TABLE 9.3 Somatic manifestations of acute anxiety

SYSTEM	SYMPTOMS
Cardiovascular	Palpitations, chest pain, faintness, flushing, sweating
Respiratory	Shortness of breath, hyperventilation, dyspnoea
Gastrointestinal	Choking, lump in throat, dry mouth, nausea, vomiting, diarrhoea
Neurological	Dizziness, headache, paraesthesia, vertigo
Musculoskeletal	Muscle ache, muscle tension, tremor, restlessness

FIGURE 9.3 Somatic manifestations of prolonged anxiety

- Tiredness
- Being easily startled
- Irritability
- Difficulty concentrating
- Constipation or diarrhoea
- Frequent urination
- Difficulty falling asleep or staying asleep
- Feeling keyed-up or on edge
- Feeling depressed

PANIC DISORDER

The key features of panic disorder (PD) are the experience of recurrent panic attacks—that is, abrupt, unexpected and unpredictable attacks of fear or discomfort, reaching peak intensity within minutes and accompanied by the physiological symptoms of the 'fight or flight response' as well as a range of characteristic cognitive symptoms, including fear of dying, fear of going crazy and fear of losing control. Typically, anxiety levels build up as the individual expects further attacks (anticipatory anxiety), and phobic avoidance behaviours develop in an attempt to stay away from anxiety-provoking situations. Most often, this leads to the development of agoraphobia, less often to avoidance of only social situations.

PHOBIAS

The key feature of phobic disorders is a fear that is excessive or unreasonable and that leads to avoidance of events or situations. There are three distinct varieties of phobic disorders: agoraphobia, social phobia and specific phobia.

AGORAPHOBIA Agoraphobia is the fear and avoidance of a variety of situations (crowds, public places, trains, trams, being home alone) from which the individual may not be able to escape, or where help may not be available should they experience a panic attack.

SOCIAL PHOBIA Social phobia is the fear and avoidance of scrutiny or of being the focus of attention in social situations in case one acts in a way that results in humiliation or embarrassment (this may include having a panic attack).

SPECIFIC PHOBIA Specific phobia is the excessive and unreasonable fear and avoidance of specific objects and situations. These include: insects and animals; natural events or objects such as storms, heights or water; specific situations such as tunnels, bridges, elevators or enclosed spaces; and seeing blood or an injury, or receiving an injection or other invasive medical procedure.

OBSESSIVE-COMPULSIVE DISORDER

The key feature of obsessive-compulsive disorder (OCD) is the presence of obsessions and/or compulsions. Obsessions are recurrent intrusive thoughts that cannot be ignored, resisted or reasoned away. Compulsions are repetitive actions that are performed in a stereotyped way and that are excessive and inappropriate (for example, repetitive checking, cleaning, counting, repeating words and imagining the opposite). Compulsive acts temporarily reduce the anxiety caused by the obsessions. Notably, individuals with OCD often also exhibit marked avoidance of objects or situations that may trigger the obsessional thoughts.

GENERALISED ANXIETY DISORDER

The key feature of generalised anxiety disorder (GAD) is persistent tension, anxiety and worry over everyday events and problems accompanied by somatic symptoms of anxiety. The worry is typically described as 'uncontrollable' and this is the main characteristic that differentiates pathological worry from normal worry.

POST-TRAUMATIC STRESS DISORDER

The key feature of post-traumatic stress disorder (PTSD) is the experience of recurrent intrusive recollections and re-experiencing of a traumatic event together with high levels of arousal and distress. Typical symptoms include nightmares, flashbacks and avoidance of cues that remind the individual of the traumatic event. These are experienced against a background of a sense of numbness and emotional blunting and detachment from other people.

MIXED ANXIETY AND DEPRESSION

This diagnosis is used when symptoms of both anxiety and depression are present but neither set of symptoms considered separately is sufficiently severe to justify a diagnosis. This mixture of comparatively mild symptoms is frequently seen in primary care settings.

ANXIETY DUE TO A GENERAL MEDICAL CONDITION

This diagnosis refers to situations in which significant anxiety (either in the form of panic attacks or generalised anxiety) is a direct physiological effect of a specific medical condition. As shown in Figures 9.4 and 9.5, many medical conditions as well as a variety of drugs can cause anxiety symptoms.

FIGURE 9.4 Medical conditions that may cause anxiety

- Anxiety is the most common ictal manifestation of temporal lobe epilepsy.
- Cardiac arrhythmias (of varying aetiology) may produce symptoms mistaken for anxiety.
- Recurring pulmonary emboli may present with repeated episodes of acute anxiety associated with hyperventilation and dyspnoea.
- Phaeochromocytoma is a rare condition that may produce acute or chronic symptoms of anxiety. Hypertension is usually present during acute episodes.
- Hypoglycaemia may produce panic attacks associated with hunger.
- Anxiety is a common symptom of hyperthyroidism.

FIGURE 9.5 Drugs that may cause anxiety

- Use of, or intoxication with, a variety of substances—for example, caffeine, amphetamine, cannabis or cocaine.
- Withdrawal from a variety of substances—for example, narcotics, alcohol or benzodiazepines.
- A variety of medications and over the counter preparations—for example, bronchodilators, theophylline, calcium channel blockers, pseudoephedrine.

ASSESSMENT

Individuals with anxiety may present with a variety of complaints. Patients rarely present specifically stating that they are over-anxious. The most common presenting problem is of somatic complaints, which may occur as part of any of the anxiety disorders. Other common presentations may be with secondary features of the anxiety—for example, difficulty concentrating, feeling stressed and less capable at work, troubles at home managing the children, conflict with spouse, loss of confidence. A third common presentation is with symptoms relating to comorbid disorders. Substance abuse problems are particularly common, especially where patients are self-medicating (for example, with alcohol) to cope with their anxiety. Another important presentation is with symptoms of depression, which frequently develops as a secondary feature in those with an anxiety disorder.

History taking should focus on the delineation of the cognitive, behavioural and physiological aspects of the problem. This should identify any known triggers and any avoidance behaviours. Identifying the cognitions associated with the experience of anxiety symptoms is important in differentiating between anxiety disorders. For example, fear of having a heart attack is often seen in PD, while fear of embarrassing oneself in front of others is a key feature of SP. Six key questions can be of use in determining which anxiety disorder(s) is present. These are:

- Is there a history of panic attacks?
- If so, are the panic attacks spontaneous (as in PD) or cued (as in phobic disorders)?
- Is there a history of phobic avoidance?
- Are there obsessions and/or compulsions present?
- Is there a traumatic cause as the precipitant?
- Is the patient generally tense, anxious or worried?

The use of symptom checklists or rating scales is often useful in characterising and quantifying symptoms and in monitoring response to treatment (see Table 9.4). A description of these scales can be found in Chapter 21.

The next task is to check for symptoms suggestive of any comorbid disorder—that is, the presence of more than one anxiety disorder or a comorbid depressive illness or substance abuse or dependence.

In addition to identifying the symptoms of the disorder, assessment should focus on the circumstances that led to the current presentation, and any factors that are linked to exacerbation, remission or relapse of symptoms. It is always important to identify protective factors (for example, supportive family network), and to be clear how available these are currently to the patient. Finally, it is important to assess the level of impairment experienced by the patient as a result of their anxiety symptoms and any suicidal thoughts or behaviour. The symptom rating scales listed in Table 9.4 can assist here.

In all patients, it is essential to be clear whether the individual is suffering from a primary anxiety disorder, or whether there is an organic cause for the symptoms. It is important to note that medical disorders may present as—that is, mimic—anxiety, cause anxiety or exacerbate anxiety disorders. It is important to do enough to confidently exclude possible organic disease but not to overdo it, particularly in the situation where the patient is preoccupied with concerns of organic disease. Figure 9.6 shows a simple assessment checklist that may be of assistance.

REVISITING THE CASE STUDY

With the deterioration in Sandra's symptoms, she is seen for a more detailed assessment. She describes that she has been anxious for as long as she can remember, although she has only been on treatment for the past four years. Her symptoms have been worse since recontacting her father, whom she had not seen for many years. Her parents' marriage broke up when she was aged 2, and she subsequently lived with her father, who was very strict and 'never there' emotionally for her. She was sent to boarding school and describes that as 'hell'. She says she was raped when she was in Year 10 and felt that her father had abandoned her at that time. At the time of assessment, she is working in an office job and in a supportive relationship with her partner of nine years. She describes having few interests outside the home. She is rather socially isolated,

TABLE 9.4 Assessment of anxiety

DISORDER	DISORDER SPECIFIC FEATURES	AIDS TO ASSESSMENT
PDA	■ Panic attacks—spontaneous or cued ■ Anticipatory anxiety ■ Phobic avoidance—wide variety of situations ■ Somatic focus/hypochondriacal preoccupation ■ Fear of physical collapse or loss of control	■ Panic attack diary ■ Body Sensations Questionnaire (BSQ)[23] ■ Fear Questionnaire (FQ)[24] ■ Mobility inventory (MI)[25]
SP	■ Panic attacks—cued ■ Anticipatory anxiety ■ Phobic avoidance—social or performance situations ■ Fear of negative evaluation and shame	■ Fear Questionnaire (FQ)[24] ■ Liebowitz Social Anxiety Scale—Self-Report (SR)[26]
Specific phobia	■ Panic attacks—cued ■ Phobic avoidance—specific object or situation	■ Fear Questionnaire (FQ)[24]
OCD	■ Obsessions—thoughts, impulses, images ■ Compulsions ■ Avoidance of triggers for obsessions ■ Fear of harm to self or others	■ Yale-Brown Obsessive Compulsive Scale—Self-Report (Y-BOCS-SR)[27]
PTSD	■ Re-experiencing the traumatic event—recollections (images, thoughts, perceptions), dreams, flashbacks ■ Avoidance of stimuli associated with the trauma ■ Persistent symptoms of increased arousal	■ Post-Traumatic Stress Disorder Checklist (PTSD-C)[28]
GAD	■ Worry—pervasive and 'uncontrollable' ■ Symptoms of motor tension, autonomic over-activity and hyperarousal	■ Hospital Anxiety and Depression Scale (HADS)[29]

FIGURE 9.6 Assessment checklist

1 HISTORY

(a) Is the story consistent and/or typical? Can a positive diagnosis be made?

(b) Is this person 'at risk' for one of the medical conditions that may cause anxiety? (See Figure 9.4.)

(c) Substance use and/or withdrawal checklist:
  (i) Caffeine
  (ii) Alcohol
  (iii) Illicit drugs

(d) Prescribed drugs review
  (i) Dose change?
  (ii) New drug?

(e) Over the counter preparations

2 PHYSICAL EXAMINATION

(a) Extent and focus of physical examination should be guided by the clinical presentation

(b) General health, cardiovascular system, thyroid status

(c) Signs of substance use/withdrawal

(d) Blood pressure, pulse

3 INVESTIGATIONS

(a) Consider thyroid function, blood sugar, electrocardiogram (ECG), drug screen.

(b) Conduct special investigations according to index of suspicion.

---

feeling out of place in social situations and mentions that even visiting friends is anxiety provoking for her.

When questioned about specific symptoms, she describes panic attacks (which have been of such severity that she was hospitalised two years previously), high levels of general tension and anxiety, and intermittent feelings of depression.

At the time of her assessment, she describes feelings of hopelessness and suicidal thoughts, and feels that she can't see the light at the end of the tunnel.

Previous treatments include sertraline, paroxetine and moclobemide. Sandra has previously seen a psychiatrist for assessment and been treated as an inpatient in a private psychiatric hospital.

She describes a family history of psychiatric disorder, with her grandmother and aunt being treated with antidepressants, and she feels her mother suffered from anxiety and/or depression although this was not acknowledged or treated.

Mental state examination shows her to be a young woman who appears anxious and on edge, wringing her hands during the interview. Her mood is sad, angry and frustrated; her affect is anxious and depressed. There is no abnormality of form or content of thought and no perceptual disturbance, and cognitive testing is normal.

To assist assessment and management planning, she is given the CES-D scale, scoring 43 (for information on the CES-D scale, see Chapter 21). Given her description of feeling out of place in social situations, she is given the Leibowitz Social Anxiety Scale to more specifically assess for symptoms of social phobia. Her responses to this show that, while she expresses some anxiety in social situations—that is, going to a party, and being the centre of attention—her symptoms are not sufficiently severe or pervasive to suggest that she has social phobia. Exploring this further, it appears that her discomfort in social situations is related more to low self-esteem, poor self-confidence and high levels of interpersonal sensitivity.

MANAGEMENT

The several discrete anxiety disorders described above have many things in common as well as clear differences. With respect to management, there are some strategies that apply to all the anxiety disorders (although these need to be tailored differently for each) and some treatments that are specific to only one disorder.

The essential first part of management is comprehensive assessment. The key steps necessary for guiding the management of a patient include:

- establishing that the individual does have an anxiety disorder;
- determining which anxiety disorder is present (see the six key questions described in 'Assessment' and the symptom scales in Table 9.4);
- determining the severity of the disorder, including the resulting degree of functional impairment;
- excluding/treating any possible biological factors causing or exacerbating the anxiety;
- excluding/treating any possible psychosocial factors causing or exacerbating the anxiety (for example, relationship problems);
- identifying any secondary complications of the disorder (for example, depression, alcohol or drug abuse, social, marital and employment problems); these all need to be considered in the treatment plan;
- always assessing and being aware of the risk of suicide both in the presence and absence of depression; and
- excluding/changing any lifestyle factors causing or exacerbating the anxiety (for example, alcohol use, as even small amounts may cause significant symptom exacerbation; excessive caffeine intake; excessive work; inadequate sleep).

The next step is to provide information to the patient. The GP should include a description of what the problem is, always stating what the problem is not—that is, dispel any fears or myths the patient may have—and what can be done to help. Information should be provided verbally and in written form.

All patients with anxiety disorders should be encouraged to participate in some form of relaxation therapy. This may include meditation, yoga, tai-chi or relaxation training provided by a therapist (further information about these strategies is provided in Chapter 17).

A variety of other stress management approaches should be discussed and encouraged. These may include specific strategies, such as structured problem solving, or non-specific approaches, including activity scheduling, modifying lifestyle factors—such as improving sleep habits, increasing exercise, avoiding self-medication—and problem focused counselling (for example, financial counselling).

Supportive psychotherapy can be used to facilitate each treatment approach. Components of this therapy include reassurance, explanation, guidance, suggestion, encouragement and assistance in effecting changes in the patient's environment.[30]

PANIC DISORDER

Specific management strategies for PD must target two key areas—control of panic attacks and overcoming phobic avoidance. Three key strategies are important in the control of panic attacks:

- **Control of hyperventilation** This is usually present as part of panic. Breathing retraining is used to address it. This includes educating the patient about the bodily effects of hyperventilation, demonstrating that they do hyperventilate and teaching the slow breathing technique.
- **Cognitive therapy** The cognitive model of PD proposes that panic results from the catastrophic misinterpretation of normal bodily sensations.[31] Cognitive therapy focuses on the reinterpretation and decatastrophising of bodily sensations associated with hyperventilation.
- **Pharmacotherapy** Medication may be required for patients with more severe forms of PD and for those who do not achieve sufficient control using psychological techniques alone. Several medications have been shown to be effective for the treatment of panic. These include tricyclic antidepressants (TCAs), monoamine oxidase inhibitors (MAOIs), selective serotonin reuptake inhibitors (SSRIs) and high-potency benzodiazepines.[32] These medications are of equal efficacy, blocking panic attacks in about 70% of cases. TCAs, MAOIs and SSRIs have a delayed onset of action of 2–4 weeks. It should be noted that SSRIs and, to a lesser extent, TCAs may exacerbate anxiety before producing an antipanic effect. Benzodiazepines have an immediate action and thus are often preferred by patients. The risk of developing dependence and/or abuse with benzodiazepines should be noted. This is particularly a problem with short-acting medications such as alprazolam or oxazepam.

Once panic attacks are controlled, specific therapy (graduated in vivo exposure therapy) is required to help the patient overcome phobic avoidance.

SOCIAL PHOBIA

Key components in the management of SP are:

- control of hyperventilation and other measures to deal with panic attacks;
- cognitive therapy to identify and challenge distortions or errors in cognitive processing that produce anxiety;
- assertiveness and social skills training;
- graduated in vivo exposure therapy to overcome avoidance behaviour; and
- possibly medication for those with more severe forms of social phobia.[33] SSRIs are generally regarded as first line pharmacotherapy for social phobia. MAOIs have well established efficacy but are less commonly used because of the risk of hypertensive reactions and the requirement for dietary restrictions. Beta blockers may be useful for people with prominent symptoms of autonomic arousal.

SPECIFIC PHOBIAS

Graduated exposure therapy is the mainstay of treatment for specific phobias. This may be done in imagination or in vivo.

OBSESSIVE-COMPULSIVE DISORDER

There are two key approaches to the treatment of OCD: cognitive behavioural therapy and pharmacotherapy.

COGNITIVE BEHAVIOURAL THERAPY Cognitive behavioural therapy relies on two key elements: exposure to the cues or triggers that cause discomfort or anxiety (these may be external cues or internal cues such as thoughts, images, feelings or impulses); and prevention of rituals in which the patient engages in order to reduce discomfort or anxiety.[34]

PHARMACOTHERAPY For those with more severe forms of the disorder, medication is frequently needed in addition to cognitive behavioural therapy. Medications that have an effect on the serotonergic system have been shown to be effective. These include the serotonergic TCA clomipramine, and the SSRIs.[35] These medications have a prolonged delay in onset of action of up to twelve weeks before anti-obsessional effects are evident. Often higher doses of medication are required—for example, clomipramine at 300 mg per day or fluoxetine at 60–80 mg per day. There is a high relapse rate following discontinuation of medication, with symptoms recurring over weeks to months following medication cessation.

POST-TRAUMATIC STRESS DISORDER

The treatment focus for PTSD is on three key components:

- damping down arousal, for which medication can be useful. Recommended drugs include the SSRIs or the MAOIs. Anticonvulsants such as sodium valproate and atypical antipsychotics can be helpful in dealing with extreme irritability and flashbacks; [36]
- dealing with the meaning of the traumatic event, for which a variety of psychotherapeutic approaches have been used;
- using exposure techniques to desensitise the traumatic memories and teach coping skills. Exposure treatments for PTSD involve repeated reliving of the trauma with the aim of facilitating the processing of the trauma, which is thought to be impaired in those who suffer from chronic PTSD. This may include in vivo and imaginal exposure;[37] and
- importantly, addressing comorbidity, as pure post-traumatic stress disorder is the exception and comorbidity the rule.

GENERALISED ANXIETY DISORDER

The two major approaches to treatment of GAD are cognitive therapy and the use of medication.[38] The cognitive model of anxiety proposes that bias at various levels of information processing influences an individual's response. Patients with GAD overestimate the likelihood of negative events and underestimate their ability to cope with difficult or stressful situations. Cognitive therapy uses various methods of cognitive restructuring to target the faulty appraisal system and change thinking so that it is more realistic and logical.

Medication is required for the treatment of comorbid depression (one of the antidepressants) or when non-drug treatments are insufficient to reduce anxiety and disability to a manageable level. Several classes of medication have been shown to be effective.[39] These include:

- TCAs, effective in low dose (for example, 75 mg nocte) for the treatment of GAD;
- venlafaxine, again in low doses (up to 75 mg per day);
- SSRIs, generally used at doses similar to that used in depression;
- benzodiazepines (athough they are effective, patients may become dependent on and/or abuse the medication so they should be prescribed with caution and careful monitoring); and
- buspirone (a 5HT1A drug), effective in doses of 15–30 mg per day. It has a gradual, relatively slow, onset of action and, for many patients, response occurs only after several weeks.

Note that the uncontrollable nature of the worry means that reassurance is rarely effective.

TREATMENT OF COMMONLY CO-OCCURRING MENTAL DISORDERS

Where there is comorbid alcohol abuse or dependence, the alcohol abuse must be addressed first. Regardless of whether the alcohol problems are primary or secondary, they assume an independent course that can seriously impair the patient's ability to benefit from therapy for their anxiety disorder.

Where symptoms of both anxiety and depression are present, priority should be given to treatment of the depression, particularly if it is severe. Once the depressive symptoms have improved, the need for further specific treatment for the anxiety disorder can be assessed and initiated as appropriate. Comorbid major depression leads to more psychological and social impairment, increased risk of suicide and a greater likelihood of relapse, recurrence and chronicity than in those with an anxiety disorder alone.[40–1]

WHEN TO REFER

Referral to a psychiatrist, psychologist or specialist mental health service should occur when:

- there is diagnostic uncertainty;
- the patient fails to respond to usual treatment;
- other factors—for example, concomitant medical problems—complicate treatment;
- troublesome side effects complicate treatment; or
- hospitalisation is indicated.

LONG-TERM MANAGEMENT

Anxiety disorders tend to be chronic conditions, albeit often accompanied by relapse and remission. Thus any treatment plan must include a long-term management strategy that includes consideration of the need for continuation of treatment and the development of a relapse prevention plan. Maintenance therapy is often required and will be particularly indicated where significant psychosocial stressors contribute to symptom exacerbation or where the individual has a history of previous relapse following cessation of treatment or incomplete symptom resolution. When maintenance treatment includes medication, this should be subject to regular review. There should also be continuing discussion about psychological strategies for controlling anxiety, and any known factors that contribute to the exacerbation or maintenance of symptoms should be addressed.

REVISITING THE CASE STUDY

Comprehensive assessment of Sandra led to the following conclusions:

- Sandra has a long-standing anxiety disorder, specifically PD.
- Previous assessment had excluded any biological factors contributing to the anxiety.
- Unresolved issues with respect to recurrent losses during her earlier life as well as unresolved aspects of her relationship with her father were identified as factors contributing to her anxiety.
- She was noted to have a moderately severe depression as a secondary complication to her anxiety disorder.
- Sandra displayed significant impairment in social functioning but less so with respect to occupational functioning.
- She was noted to have expressed suicidal ideas and ideas of hopelessness. An important protective factor identified was the supportive relationship with her partner.

While there were symptoms of both PD and depression, the depression was of moderate severity and thus priority was given to treating this. To this end, paroxetine was continued and cognitive strategies were used to address the negative biases in Sandra's thinking. Behavioural strategies, particularly activity scheduling, were also used to address her depression. To assist with control of her anxiety, Sandra attended a stress management course and was taught structured problem solving. In order to address the underlying vulnerability factors, she was encouraged to talk about aspects of her earlier life that had been difficult for her and, in particular, her relationship with her father, as her unresolved feelings towards him were clearly a source of distress for her. Breathing retraining was used as a specific strategy to help her control her panicky feelings.

CONCLUSION

Anxiety disorders are common, and frequently coexist with other disorders. Comprehensive assessment is required to identify both the disorder(s) present and the factors that contribute to the onset or maintenance of symptoms. Effective treatment must address the anxiety disorder, its causes and its consequences.

REFERENCES

1. Leon AC, Portera L, Weissman MM. The social costs of anxiety disorders. British Journal of Psychiatry 1995;166(Suppl. 27):19–22.
2. American Psychiatric Association. Diagnostic and Statistical Manual of Mental Disorders. 4th edn. Washington DC: American Psychiatric Association, 1994.
3. World Health Organization. The ICD-10 Classification of Mental and Behavioural Disorders. Geneva: WHO, 1992.
4. Andrews G, Hall W, Teesson M, Henderson H. The Mental Health of Australians. Canberra: Mental Health Branch, Commonwealth Department of Health and Aged Care, April 1999.
5. Kessler RC, McGonagle KA, Zhao S, Nelson C, Hughes M, Eshelman S, Wittchen HV, Kendler KS. Lifetime and 12-month prevalence of DSM-IIIR psychiatric disorders in the United States: results from the National Comorbidity Survey. Archives of General Psychiatry 1994;51:8–19.
6. Robins LN, Helzer JE, Weissman MM, Orraschel H, Gruenberg E, Burke JD, Repier DA. Lifetime prevalence of specific psychiatric disorders in three sites. Archives of General Psychiatry 1984;41:949–58.
7. Zubin J, Spring B. Vulnerability—a new view of schizophrenia. Journal of Abnormal Psychology 1997;86:103–26.
8. Judd FK, Norman TR, Burrows GD. Theories on the aetiology of anxiety disorders. In: DenBoer JA, Sitsen JMA, eds. Handbook of Depression and Anxiety: A Biological Approach. New York: Marcel Decker, 1994;225–46.
9. Silove D. Perceived parental characteristics and reports of early parental deprivation in agoraphobic patients. Australian and New Zealand Journal of Psychiatry 1986;20:365–9.
10. Beck AT. Cognitive Therapy and Emotional Disorders. New York: International Universities Press, 1976.
11. Beck AT, Emery G. Anxiety Disorders and Phobias: A Cognitive Perspective. New York: Basic Books, 1985.
12. Andrews G, Stewart G, Morris-Yates A, Holt P, Henderson S. Evidence for a general neurotic syndrome. British Journal of Psychiatry 1990;157:6–12.
13. Tyrer P, Casey P, Gall J. Relationship between neurosis and personality disorder. British Journal of Psychiatry 1983;142:404–8.
14. Marks IM. Genetics of fear and anxiety disorders. British Journal of Psychiatry 1986;149:406–18.
15. Connor KM, Davidson JRT. Generalised anxiety disorder: Neurobiological and pharmacotherapeutic perspectives. Biological Psychiatry 1998;44:1286–94.
16. Pigott TA. OCD: where the serotonin selectivity story begins. Journal of Clinical Psychiatry 1996;57(Suppl. 6):11–20.
17. Charney DS, Krystal JH, Southwick SM, Delgardo PL. The role of noradrenergic function in human anxiety and depression. In: DenBoer JA, Sitsen JMH, eds. Handbook of Depression and Anxiety: A Biological Approach. New York: Marcel Decker, 1994;497–514.
18. Haefley W. Benzodiazepines, benzodiazepine receptors, and endogenous ligands. In: DenBoer JA, Sitsen JMH, eds. Handbook of Depression and Anxiety: A Biological Approach. New York: Marcel Decker, 1994;573–608.
19. Westenberg HGM, DenBoer JA. The neuropharmacology of anxiety: a review on the role of serotonin. In: DenBoer JA, Sitsen JMH, eds. Handbook of Depression and Anxiety: A Biological Approach. New York: Marcel Decker, 1994;405–46.
20. Kawachi I, Sparrow D, Vokonas PS, Weiss ST. Decreased heart rate variability in men with phobic anxiety (data from the Normative Aging Study). American Journal of Cardiology 1995;75:882–5.
21. Andrews G. Stressful life events and anxiety. In: Burrows G, Noyes R, Ross M, eds. Handbook of Anxiety. Vol 2: Classification, Aetiological Factors and Associated Disorders. Amsterdam: Elsevier, 1988;163–74.
22. Beck AT, Rush AJ, Shaw BF, Emery G. Cognitive Therapy of Depression. New York: Guilford Press, 1979.
23. Chambless DL, Caputo GC, Bright P, Gallagher R. Assessment of fear in agoraphobics: The Body

Sensations Questionnaire and the Agoraphobic Cognitions Questionnaire. Journal of Consulting and Clinical Psychology 1994;52:1090–7.

24. Marks IM, Matthews AM. Brief standard rating scale for phobic patients. Behaviour Research and Therapy 1979;17:263–7.

25. Chambless DL, Caputo GC, Jasin SE, Gracely EJ, Williams C. The mobility inventory for agoraphobia. Behaviour Research and Therapy 1985;23:35–44.

26. Fresco DM, Coles ME, Heimberg RG, Liebowitz MR, Hami S, Stein MB, Goetz D. The Liebowitz Social Anxiety Scale: a comparison of the psychometric properties of self report and clinician administered formats. Psychological Medicine 2001;31:1025–35.

27. Goodman WK, Price LH, Rasmussen SA, Mazur C, Fleischmann RL, Hill CL, Heninger GR, Charney DS. The Yale-Brown Obsessive Compulsive Scale. Archives of General Psychiatry 1989;46:1006–11.

28. Weathers FW, Litz BT, Herman DS, Houska JA, Kene TM. The PTSD Checklist (PCL): Reliability, Validity and Diagnostic Utility. Boston, MA: National Centre for PTSD, 1991.

29. Zigmond AS, Snaith RP. The Hospital Anxiety and Depression Scale. Acta Psychiatrica Scandinavica 1983;67:361–70.

30. Bloch S. Supportive psychotherapy. In: Bloch S, ed. An Introduction to the Psychotherapies. 2nd edn. Oxford: Oxford University Press, 1986;252–78.

31. Clark DM. A cognitive approach to panic. Behaviour Research and Therapy 1986;24:461–70.

32. Royal Australian and New Zealand College of Psychiatrists Clinical Practice Guidelines Team for Panic Disorder and Agoraphobia. Australian and New Zealand Clinical Practice Guidelines for the Treatment of Panic Disorder and Agoraphobia. Australian and New Zealand Journal of Psychiatry 2003;37:641–6.

33. Blanco C, Raza MZ, Schneier FR, Liebowitz MR. The evidence-based pharmacological treatment of social anxiety disorder. International Journal of Neuropsychopharmacology 2003;6:427–42.

34. Salkovskis PM. Understanding and treating obsessive compulsive disorder. Behaviour Research and Therapy 1999;37(Suppl. 1).S29–52.

35. Zohar J, Sasson Y, Chopra M, Amital D, Iancu I. Pharmacological treatment of obsessive compulsive disorder: a review. In: Maj M, Sartorius N, Okasha A, Zohar J, eds. Obsessive Compulsive Disorder. 2nd edn. Chichester: John Wiley & Sons, 2002;43–61.

36. Schoenfeld FB, Marmar CR, Neylan TC. Current concepts in pharmacotherapy for posttraumatic stress disorder. Psychiatric Services 2004;55:519–31.

37. Foa EB, Steketee G, Rothbaum B. Behavioural/cognitive conceptualisations of posttraumatic stress disorder. Behaviour Therapy 1989;20:155–76.

38. Gould RA, Otto MW, Pollack MH, Yap L. Cognitive behavioural and pharmacological treatment of Generalised Anxiety Disorder: a preliminary meta-analysis. Behaviour Therapy 1997;28:285–305.

39. Gale C, Oakley Browne M. Anxiety disorder. British Medical Journal 2000;321:1204-7.

40. Hollifield M, Caton W, Skipper B, Chapman T, Ballenger JC, Mannuzza S, Fyer AJ. Panic disorder and quality of life: variables predictive of functional impairment. American Journal of Psychiatry 1997;154:766–72.

41. Judd FK, Burrows GD. Anxiety disorders and their relationship to depression. In: Paykel ES, ed. Handbook of Affective Disorders. Edinburgh: Churchill Livingstone, 1992;77–87.

CHAPTER 10

ALCOHOL AND OTHER DRUG MISUSE

B Monheit and A Gijsbers

If we could sniff or swallow something that would, for five or six hours each day, abolish our solitude as individuals, atone us with our fellows in a growing exaltation of affection and make life in all its aspects seem not only worth living, but divinely beautiful and significant, and if this heavenly world-transfiguring drug were of such a kind that we could wake up each morning with a clear head and an undamaged constitution—then it seems to me all our problems (and not merely the one small problem of discovering a novel pleasure) would be wholly solved and earth would become paradise.

ALDOUS HUXLEY, *Brave New World, 1949*

CASE STUDY 1

Harry, 58 years old, presents to you on a Monday morning, claiming to feel a bit crook with indigestion and lethargy. He looks quite unwell and requests a certificate to take two days off work to recover. On examination his blood pressure is 150/96 and he has some epigastric tenderness. There are no stigmata of chronic liver disease and the rest of his examination is normal.

When you ask about his drinking alcohol, he says he had 'a few' over the weekend and agrees he may have given it 'a bit of a nudge'. More specific questioning reveals that he had three alcohol-free days a week, but drank a total of sixty standard drinks in an average week.

- General practitioners (GPs) are key practitioners in dealing with substance misuse issues in the community.

- Controlled studies show that GP management of patients with substance misuse issues can be effective.

- The majority of patients expect their doctor to know their substance use history and do not regard questions in this area as an intrusion.

- The legal drugs, tobacco and alcohol, are the substances most commonly misused in the community; illicit drug use is comparatively rare.

- A third of the community has tried cannabis. Designer drugs are often used recreationally and the hardcore illegal drugs such as heroin, amphetamine and cocaine are only tried by a small minority of the population.

- The GP's attitude is crucial to the success of a management program. The therapeutic relationship is the cornerstone to recovery.

- The GP needs to show empathy and engagement, but there is a fine line between acceptance of the patient and indulgence towards their unacceptable behaviour.

- An adequate assessment determines where the patient is in relationship to the stages of change.

- GPs can be most helpful if they are familiar with their local drug and alcohol inpatient and outpatient services.

INTRODUCTION

GPs are increasingly being asked by their patients, government and public health authorities to become more involved in the diagnosis and management of drug and alcohol problems. Many GPs resist taking on that role, and this may stem from lack of confidence and skills in this area as well as a belief that intervention is doomed to failure. Yet the results of interventions by GPs can be very significant. Brief interventions for alcohol abuse, smoking cessation and opiate pharmacotherapies for heroin addiction are common examples of effective GP initiated treatments that have been proven by multiple studies in Australia and overseas.

The high incidence of coexisting mental health problems with substance abuse disorders creates an additional challenge for GPs, who should become familiar with this serious health problem.

GENERAL PRINCIPLES

Substance misuse issues differ from other psychiatric conditions in that there are significant moral and legal responses to drug problems in a community.[1] This intimate conjunction of social and medical issues makes drug treatment a fascinating area of medicine.

CLASSIFICATION OF PSYCHOACTIVE SUBSTANCES

The most common psychoactive substances that are abused can be divided into three groups:[2]

- psychodepressants—for example, alcohol, sedatives, hypnotics, cannabis, volatile solvents and opioids;
- psychostimulants—for example, amphetamines, ecstasy, cocaine and nicotine; and
- hallucinogens—for example, LSD (lysergic acid diethylamide), designer drugs such as GHB (gamma hydroxybutyrate), cannabis, ecstasy.

Note: Cannabis and ecstasy are found in two separate categories.

HOW DO THESE SUBSTANCES WORK?

Activation of the mesolimbic dopamine pathway by psychoactive drugs mimics basic motivational human responses to hunger, thirst, sexual desire and the presence of danger. The reward pathways in the nucleus accumbens and ventral pallidum are modified by circuits from other centres. Thus the prefrontal cortex and the anterior cingulate gyrus are associated with control, the orbitofrontal cortex is associated with drive and the amygdala and hippocampus are associated with memory. Cravings are thought to arise from the orbitofrontal cortex, and lack of control is thought to occur because of poor connections between the prefrontal cortex and the anterior cingulate gyrus on the one hand and the mesolimbic system on the other. In susceptible people, the brain responds as if the drugs and their associated stimuli are biologically needed. With repeated exposure, the association becomes stronger, evoking a larger behavioural and neurochemical response. These responses are of course also influenced by environmental and genetic factors.[3]

DOMAINS OF SUBSTANCE MISUSE

Below is an outline of the domains of substance misuse: intoxication, withdrawal, dependence, abuse, misuse and damage. Intoxication and overdose are more common causes of death than chronic problems such as dependence and physical damage.

INTOXICATION This is the acute effect of psychoactive substances. They alter a person's perception, mood, behaviour, judgment and functioning. Some may sedate to the point of death. There are degrees of intoxication, from mild to fatal.

WITHDRAWAL Sudden cessation of a psychoactive substance can lead to a withdrawal syndrome characteristic of the drug.

DEPENDENCE Sometimes a distinction is drawn between physiological and psychological dependence. The former is characterised by tolerance and dependence, the latter by the behavioural aspects of substance dependence. This distinction is starting to blur as we understand the neurophysiology of cravings and drives and as we recognise the psychological aspects of tolerance and withdrawal. A summary of DSM-IV[4] criteria for abuse and dependence is found in Figure 10.1.

ABUSE Within the DSM-IV classification, this is a lesser form of problem substance use and would include problems due to intoxication, bingeing and physical damage short of dependence.

MISUSE This is a useful general term to describe all damage, including intoxication, withdrawal, abuse and dependence.

DAMAGE Drug misuse can lead to physical, psychological and social damage without the person being dependent. It is important to recognise these patients, as brief interventions by GPs in this population are highly successful.

FIGURE 10.1 Definition of drug dependence and abuse

DEPENDENCE

A diagnosis of dependence is made if three or more of the criteria below occur together in a twelve-month period. The syndrome is defined by behaviours and physiological changes, not by specific levels of substances consumed, patterns of use or any blood test results.

1   There is tolerance to the effects of the substance.
2   The patient experiences withdrawal symptoms on cessation of the substance.
3   The substance is often taken in larger amounts or over a longer period than was intended.
4   There is a persistent desire or there are unsuccessful efforts to cut down or control substance use.
5   A great deal of time is spent on drug related activities.
6   Important social, occupational or recreational activities are given up or reduced because of substance use.
7   The substance use is continued despite knowledge of it causing persistent or recurrent physical or psychological problems.

ABUSE

If the criteria for dependence are not fulfilled, a diagnosis of abuse can be made if one or more of the following criteria is present.

1   Recurrent substance use results in failure to fulfill social roles.
2   The patient recurrently uses the substance in physically hazardous situations.
3   The patient experiences recurring substance related legal problems.
4   There is continued use despite recurrent social or interpersonal problems.

Source: Summarised from DSM-IV.[4]

SPECIFIC SUBSTANCES

This section outlines four categories of substances: alcohol, cannabis, heroin, and amphetamines and other psychostimulants. These and other substances are listed in Table 10.1, which describes each substance, how it acts, its acute intoxicant effect, complications of intoxication, its withdrawal syndrome and complications of withdrawal. The relative frequency of substances used in Australia in the previous twelve months is recorded in Table 10.2.

TABLE 10.1 Summary of psychoactive substance effects: drugs of dependence—their use

DRUG AND MODE OF ACTION	INTOXICATION	COMPLICATIONS OF ACUTE USE/INTOXICATION
ALCOHOL ■ Increases inhibitory effects of GABA (gamma aminobutyric acid) and decreases excitatory effect of glutamate on dopamine pathways	■ Disinhibition, poor insight and judgment, inco-ordination, disorientation, poor attention, memory loss, ataxic gait. Later hypotension, loss of gag reflex	■ Aspiration pneumonia ■ Coma, death ■ Risky behaviour ■ Violent behaviour ■ Social impact ■ Gastrointenstinal upset/inflammation, haematemesis ■ Alcoholic blackouts ■ Dehydration and glycogen depletion (hangover) *Note*: Synergistic behaviour can occur with opioids and benzodiazepines.
OPIOIDS ■ Activate various opioid receptors such as mu, kappa and delta	■ Sedation ■ Hypotension, slow pulse, pin point pupils, itching, scratching, slurred speech, impaired attention and memory	■ Respiratory depression ■ Unconsciousness ■ Death *Note*: Synergistic effects can occur with alcohol and benzodiazepines

and complications

COMPLICATIONS OF CHRONIC USE	WITHDRAWAL	COMPLICATIONS OF WITHDRAWAL
■ Chronic liver disease ■ Alcohol related brain injury (dysexecutive syndrome): — Cerebellar vermis ataxia — Peripheral neuropathy — Stroke — Alcoholic hallucinosis ■ Chronic pancreatitis ■ Cardiomyopathy ■ Hypertension ■ Trauma ■ Psychosocial deterioration ■ Depression ■ Anxiety ■ Other complications (see, e.g. reference 9)	■ Agitation, restlessness, headaches, sweats, insomnia, nightmares, anxiety, tachycardia, hypertension, hyperthermia ■ Vomiting, diarrhoea ■ Perceptual disturbances ■ Peak symptoms: days 2–4 ■ Duration: 3–7 days	■ Delirium tremens ■ Disturbance of consciousness with confusion, disorientation, hallucinations ■ Seizures ■ Anxiety/depression
■ Financial and legal issues are common ■ Infections by bacteria and by blood borne viruses such as hepatitis C and HIV. ■ Xerostomia and the development of dental caries	■ Sweats, yawning, lacrimation, rhinorrhoea, restlessness, irritability, goose flesh, dilated pupils, nausea, vomiting, abdominal cramps and diarrhoea, muscle aches, dysphoria and sleep disturbance *For heroin:* ■ Peak symptoms: 2–3 days ■ Duration: 5–7 days ■ Insomnia, irritability, mood swings, anxiety and cravings may persist for 6 months	■ Worsening physical and psychiatric disorder *Note:* Risk of overdose is higher if patient recommences use after withdrawal because tolerance is lost, therefore the usual dose may be fatal

continued overleaf

TABLE 10.1 *continued*

DRUG AND MODE OF ACTION	INTOXICATION	COMPLICATIONS OF ACUTE USE/INTOXICATION
BENZODIAZEPINES ■ Facilitate the actions of endogenous inhibitory neurotransmitters, especially GABA	■ Sedation, poor memory, disinhibition, hypotension, slurred speech, drooling, nystagmus, diplopia ■ Can be misinterpreted as alcohol intoxication	■ Unconsciousness, coma, death *Note*: Synergistic effect with alcohol and opioids *Note*: Possible paradoxical reaction with activation, agitation
CANNABIS ■ Activates cannabinoid receptors CB1 and CB2 and increases dopamine activity	■ Disinhibition, talkativeness or withdrawal, altered perception, (especially slowing of time), paranoia, increased appetite, tachycardia, dry mouth, conjunctival injection ■ Psychosis may occur in high doses of purer forms	■ Poor co-ordination and disinhibition may lead to violence in social situations ■ Impairment of co-ordination and driving skills
NICOTINE ■ Stimulates nicotinic receptors ■ Ganglion stimulant and blocker	■ Tachycardia, hypertension, increased myocardial contractility and oxygen demand	■ Multi-organ effects resulting in smoking being the greatest contributor to drug related deaths
AMPHETAMINES, COCAINE ■ Amphetamine increases release of dopamine and inhibits dopamine reuptake	■ Hyperactive, talkative, disinhibited, decreased appetite, nausea, vomiting, tachycardia, hypertension, tremor, dilated pupils and acute psychosis	■ Confusion, seizures, coma, dehydration, hyperthermia, ■ Stroke, ventricular arrhythmias

COMPLICATIONS OF CHRONIC USE	WITHDRAWAL	COMPLICATIONS OF WITHDRAWAL
■ Underlying psychiatric illness may be masked ■ Chronic ataxia and sedation ■ Lowered mood ■ Increased risk of overdose, especially in conjunction with other sedatives	■ Anxiety, agitation, tremor, restlessness, insomnia, nightmares, hyperventilation, sensory disturbances, derealisation, confusion, depersonalisation, tachycardia, hypertension and perceptual disturbances *Note*: It can be difficult to interpret if symptoms are due to withdrawal or to the underlying psychiatric condition resurfacing	■ Withdrawal seizures ■ Anxiety disorder due to drug withdrawal ■ Re-emergence or rebound of the underlying anxiety disorder
■ Smoking related harms such as pharyngeal cancer ■ Precipitation of psychiatric problems (psychosis, schizophrenia) in susceptible individuals ■ 'Amotivational syndrome'	■ Insomnia is usually the biggest symptom ■ Agitation, restlessness, irritability, mood swings, lethargy, cravings *Note*: Some of the symptoms are due to nicotine withdrawal	
■ Chronic obstructive lung disease, lung cancer ■ Cardiovascular disease	■ Anger, anxiety, craving, difficulty concentrating, hunger, impatience and restlessness ■ Peak in 1–2 days, lasts 3–4 weeks ■ Cravings often last much longer	*Note*: Bupropion, used to assist with smoking cessation, may cause anxiety, depression or psychosis
■ Tendency to paranoia, psychosis, weight loss, poor nutrition, poor performance and concentration, xerostomia (therefore prone to dental caries)	■ *Crash*: days 1–3 ■ Lowered mood, anxiety, irritability, insomnia (or hypersomnia), agitation ■ *Withdrawal*: days to weeks Insomnia, vivid dreams, fatigue, irritability, mood fluctuations, anxiety, depression, cravings	■ Prolonged depression (often with suicidal intensity)

continued overleaf

TABLE 10.1 *continued*

DRUG AND MODE OF ACTION	INTOXICATION	COMPLICATIONS OF ACUTE USE/INTOXICATION
ECSTASY (MDMA) ■ Increases dopamine, noradrenaline and serotonin release ■ Blocks dopamine reuptake	■ Euphoria and benevolence towards others, anorexia, teeth grinding, nausea, muscle aches and stiffness, ataxia, sweating, tachycardia, hypertension, paranoia, hallucinations, insomnia	■ Anxiety, hypertension, cardiac rhythm abnormalities, hyperthermia, confusion, collapse, convulsions, rhabdomyolysis, acute renal failure, coma, death (rare). *Note*: These symptoms are more likely if drug use is associated with vigorous exertion and fluid imbalance—for example, at 'rave parties'
LSD ■ Serotonin, glutamate and acetylcholine receptors affected	■ Conflicting perceptual and mood changes, mood lability, visual hallucinations, tachycardia, hypertension, pupillary dilatation, tremor	■ Hyperpyrexia, panic episodes, confusion, tremor, vomiting
VOLATILE SUBSTANCES ■ For example, aerosol sprays, including chrome paints, cleaning fluids, petrol	■ Euphoria, disinhibition, disorientation, visual hallucinations	■ Seizures, coma, ventricular arrhythmias, respiratory depression

COMPLICATIONS OF CHRONIC USE	WITHDRAWAL	COMPLICATIONS OF WITHDRAWAL
■ Weight loss, exhaustion, jaundice, 'flashbacks', irritability, paranioa, depression, psychosis	■ Fatigue and insomnia, dysphoria (especially low mood) commonly reported 3–5 days after an episode of use	■ Ecstasy is a relatively 'young drug' so there are substantial gaps in the knowledge regarding long-term effects of use and of withdrawal in humans
■ Schizophreniform psychosis; derangement of memory function, problem solving and abstract thinking	■ An LSD withdrawal symptom has not been identified	■ None described
■ Chronic cough, tinnitus, red watery eyes, nose bleeds, depression, anxiety, tiredness, weakness, chest pains, angina, indigestion, stomach ulcers, myocardial damage, cerebral oedema, lead poisoning (liver damage, cerebral degeneration, nephropathy and anaemia)	*Hangover effects:* ■ Tremor, headache, nausea, vomiting, loss of appetite, fatigue, muscle cramps, delirium *Withdrawal:* ■ Cravings, lethargy, headaches, nausea, loss of appetite, poor concentration	

Source: Adapted from a table prepared by Turning Point Alcohol and Drug Centre, Fitzroy, Victoria, 1998.

TABLE 10.2 Prevalence of recent drug use in Australia

DRUG	% OF POPULATION AGED 14+ WHO USED DRUG IN PREVIOUS 12 MONTHS
Alcohol	83.6
Tobacco	20.7
Cannabis	11.3
Ecstasy/designer drugs	3.4
Amphetamines	3.2
Analgesics (for non-medical purposes)	3.1
Tranquillisers/sleeping pills for non-medical purposes	1.0
Cocaine	1.0
Hallucinogens	0.7
Inhalants	0.4
Ketamine	0.3
Heroin	0.2
Other opiates/opioids for non-medical purposes	0.2
GHB	0.1
Any illicit drug	15.3

Source: National Drug Strategy Household Survey, 2004.[5]

ALCOHOL

Alcohol's attraction lies in its euphoriant and relaxant properties. Alcohol makes people forget their problems (for a while) and it treats the dysphoria associated with both anxiety and depression. However, alcohol is a depressant in its own right and its withdrawal can be associated with severe anxiety symptoms. Alcohol comes in many forms. Its dosage is calculated according to standard drinks. A standard drink contains 10 g of alcohol (see Table 10.3).

TABLE 10.3 Calculating standard drinks

TYPE OF ALCOHOL	NO. STANDARD DRINKS*
1 glass of standard beer	0.8 to 1.2
1 stubby or 1 can of standard beer	1.5
1 bottle of standard beer	3
1 glass (100 mL) table wine	1
1 bottle table wine	7–8
4 L cask of wine	40
1 nip (30 mL) spirits	1
1 bottle spirits	22

* A standard drink contains 10 g of alcohol.

Note: For further information see the Australian Government website: http://www.alcohol.gov.au/

Like any drug, alcohol has acute and chronic effects. Acute and chronic damage can occur in the absence of dependence. Cohort studies have shown that there is some reduction in cardiovascular risk in those cohorts consuming small amounts of alcohol compared with those who are totally abstinent. However, male cohorts consuming on average more than four standard drinks a day and female cohorts drinking on average more than two standard drinks a day are associated with increased incidence of death due to physical damage. Most of the current literature regards these associations as causal.

CANNABIS

Cannabis use is common in Australia. Most cannabis users smoke it only intermittently or recreationally. The acute effects of cannabis include impaired motor skills and inability to perform complex cognitive functions. It can also affect memory acquisition.

About 5–10% of cannabis users become dependent on it. Current evidence shows that the majority of subjects who take cannabis do not become psychotic and that the majority of psychotic patients have not taken cannabis. However, cannabis can exacerbate psychotic illness and cannabis use can precipitate schizophrenia in people who are vulnerable because of a personal or family history of schizophrenia.[6]

HEROIN

Heroin use in Australia is relatively low, but it is a significant cause of death, injury and illness, particularly for younger people. Public health problems associated with injecting drug use include hepatitis B and C, HIV infection, overdoses (both fatal and non-fatal), and localised and systemic infections, such as abscesses, septiciaemia and endocarditis. In addition, there is considerable public concern about heroin use and crime, safety in public places and potential corruption of public officials.

Natural history studies of heroin use show that many individuals who commence heroin use continue to do so for a relatively brief period (weeks or months). Among individuals who then become dependant, 2–3% become abstinent each year, without any formal treatment. At the end of a ten-year follow up, usually about 40% are abstaining from heroin. The remaining 60% are actively using, imprisoned or dead. Retention in treatment is associated with better outcomes.[7]

AMPHETAMINES AND OTHER PSYCHOSTIMULANTS

Speed is the powder form of amphetamine. It is usually injected or snorted but is sometimes swallowed. Since the mid-1990s, most of the speed sold in Australia is actually methamphetamine. This is manufactured by adding a methyl group to the amphetamine molecule, making the product more potent, with stronger psychoactive effects.

Ecstasy is sold as tablets, particularly at parties and 'raves'. True ecstasy pills contain a methamphetamine derivative called MDMA (methylenedioxymethamphetamine). These pills are generally imported from Europe or Asia because few illicit chemists in Australia have the expertise to make MDMA. Therefore most of the tablets sold as ecstasy here are locally manufactured methamphetamine tablets that are sometimes mixed with other drugs such as ketamine in an attempt to mimic the effects of MDMA.[8]

The extent of amphetamine use in Australia is rising and it now ranks as the second most common illicit drug used after cannabis. According to the 2004 National Drug Strategy Household Survey, 9.1% of the general population aged 14 years and over have used this drug and 3.2% stated using it in the last year. In addition, 3.4% of the household survey population reported using ecstasy in the last twelve months, the majority of users belonging to the 20–29 years age group.

GENERAL PRINCIPLES OF ASSESSMENT AND MANAGEMENT

When should patients be assessed? Figure 10.2 lists the features that should trigger questions about substance misuse. If the GP feels hesitant about a direct approach to taking a substance history, the questions can be embedded within a general lifestyle assessment that includes questions about exercise, diet, coffee and cigarette consumption, before taking an alcohol and other drug history. Some of the general principles of assessment and management of substance misuse include:[9, 10]

- Establish and maintain an empathic relationship with the patient based on respect, interest in their welfare and a non-judgmental attitude regarding their drug use and lifestyle.
- Take a drug and alcohol history. For each drug consumed, ask about quantity used, frequency of use, pattern of use and route of administration. Drugs can be used casually, in a binge fashion and dependently.
- Assess the level of risk associated with that use. Risks include overdose, damage, withdrawal and relapse. Is the patient likely to go through withdrawal, and if so, how severe will that withdrawal be?
- What are the underlying reasons for substance misuse?
- Give feedback to the patient on the current problems and risk.
- Assess the patient's motivation to change and, if appropriate, use brief intervention techniques.
- Discuss the patient's wishes regarding their drug use.
- Depending on the patient's 'readiness for change', offer information and treatment options or commence therapy.

MANAGEMENT ACCORDING TO STAGES OF CHANGE

Fundamental to substance misuse counselling is recognising that patients present at various stages of the natural history of their drug use. Effective substance misuse counselling requires the GP to match their strategies according to the patient's current stage of drug use. According to the DiClemente model[11], patients can be classified into the following categories: precontemplation, contemplation, decision, action, maintenance or relapse.

PRECONTEMPLATION These are the 'happy users' who have not thought about changing their substance use. The reasons for using are much more powerful than the reasons for not using. They present to the medical profession with problems other than their drug use, but that clinical encounter can be used as an opportunity to shift their attitude to the next stage.

CONTEMPLATION These are the ambivalent users who are considering change, but have not yet acted. They are weighing up the pros and cons of using. At this point

---

FIGURE 10.2 Common conditions that should alert the GP to substance misuse

GENERAL

- Poor work or school performance
- Moodiness
- Relationship difficulties

ALCOHOL

- Indigestion
- Hypertension
- Raised liver enzymes, especially gamma-GT
- Depression
- Anxiety
- Unexplained fractures
- Failing memory
- Unexplained falls

TOBACCO

- Chronic bronchitis
- Asthma
- Peripheral vascular disease
- Angina and other coronary chest pains

INTRAVENOUS DRUG USE

- Infections—local and septicaemia
- Blood-borne virus infections—hepatitis, HIV/AIDS
- Psychostimulants
- Anxiety
- Agitation
- Psychosis

---

the disparity between what they would like and their actual stage of use may create a considerable degree of discomfort, but a GP skilled in the art of motivational interviewing may help move the patient to the next stage.

DECISION The patient may decide not to do anything about their drug use and return to the first stage, or they may decide to act.

ACTION At this stage the patient has decided to change and the GP can facilitate that change. However, most addictive behaviour is associated with relapse, and therefore the next phase is crucial in consolidating recovery.

MAINTENANCE At this stage effective relapse prevention strategies will help keep a patient off drugs, but the astute GP will be anticipating relapse and will develop strategies to prevent the next stage.

RELAPSE This is the most common outcome of withdrawal from any drug, but this need not be a disaster if the patient learns why the relapse occurred and how to prevent it happening again. Thus a relapse can actually help consolidate the recovery.

This classification of readiness to change is crucial, as inappropriate prescribing of diazepam for alcohol withdrawal for precontemplators and contemplators can lead to the development of a combined alcohol and benzodiazepine dependence. Likewise the inappropriate prescribing of relapse-preventing agents such as naltrexone and acamprosate to precontemplators and contemplators is unlikely to be successful.

MOTIVATIONAL INTERVIEWING STRATEGIES

The key to management here is to engage the patient in articulating for themselves the positives and negatives about their drug use. Doctors need to walk a fine line between drawing out what a person knows about their drug use and informing the patient about the medical consequences of their drug use. Motivational interviewing is about patients finding their own motivation rather than being told by their doctor what is good for them.[12] It may be useful to work with the patient to develop a motivational matrix to help them move from the precontemplative to the contemplative stage (see Figure 10.3).

FIGURE 10.3 Motivational matrix

Consequences	For substance use	Against substance use
Immediate consequences	Relaxes me Makes me forget Stops withdrawals Helps me socialise Feels good	
Long-term consequences		After-effects the next day Health Relationships Income Work

Counsellors should pay attention to the reasons why a patient continues their substance use. A patient will need to find alternative ways to socialise and relax, and will need to find alternative forms of pleasure, or forego pleasure when they are giving up substances. Good substance misuse counselling will help a patient to find an alternative, much more satisfying lifestyle rather than just simply encourage a person to give up their substance use.

Motivational interviewing assesses how important changing the substance misuse is for the patient, and how empowered they will feel about change. There is a skill in increasing the patient's sense that change is possible and to actually encourage change.

MANAGEMENT OF SPECIFIC SUBSTANCE MISUSE PROBLEMS
ALCOHOL DEPENDENCE

The management of a patient's excessive drinking, such as that foreshadowed in case study 1, should follow these principles:

- Assess the severity of the drinking. Is it recurrent intoxication, damaging drinking or dependent drinking requiring withdrawal therapy (see below)?
- Link the patient's presenting symptoms to their alcohol consumption.
- Encourage the patient to articulate for themselves the advantages and disadvantages of their alcohol consumption.
- Present the patient with the NHMRC criteria for safe drinking: two alcohol-free days a week; for men an average of four standard drinks a day and not more than six standard drinks at any one sitting; and for women an average of two standard drinks a day and not more than four standard drinks at any one sitting. As our case study patient Harry has three alcohol-free days in the week, it is unlikely that he will suffer from withdrawal, and thus the main aim of therapy this time is to try and reduce his alcohol consumption to 'safe' levels, or alternatively to stop.
- The Australian Drug Foundation's *A Guide to Changing Your Drinking Habits* contains a lot of basic information for patients about alcohol as well as a drink diary that a patient can fill in and discuss with their doctor next time they visit.[13]
- A patient's liver function tests (especially the gamma-GT) and full blood examination (especially the mean corpuscular volume, or MCV) can be useful markers for following a person's progress towards safer drinking and abstinence. While their sensitivity can be low (depending on the severity of the disease), their specificity is fairly high in general practice, especially if the patient is not on other medications that can raise the gamma-GT.
- If the patient is unable to control their drinking, they need to consider a period of abstinence, and perhaps permanent cessation.
- A review in 2–3 weeks will give the patient time to test their decision to change, and to discuss the results of blood tests.
- When relapses occur, help the patient to focus on what was successful before planning the next attempt.
- Dispassionately analyse the times of excessive consumption and develop an alternative strategy so that the patient can avoid these problems next time.

RECOGNISING AND MANAGING ALCOHOL WITHDRAWAL

WITHDRAWAL SYNDROME Alcohol withdrawal usually occurs in patients who are drinking daily, who drink to treat the shakes and who start drinking early in the morning. It is notoriously difficult to anticipate how tough a withdrawal will be, but if previous withdrawals have been severe, the next one is also likely to be so. Particular care should be taken for patients with a history of delirium tremens (DTs) and withdrawal fitting. Withdrawal symptoms usually start within 6–24 hours of the last drink of alcohol. Symptoms reach their peak on days 2–3 and subside by days 5–7. Complications of withdrawal, DTs and seizures, usually occur within the first three days of the withdrawal.

Beware of attributing symptoms from concomitant conditions to withdrawal. Thus perspiration could be due to a myocardial infarction or to infection, or restlessness could be due to a space-occupying lesion in the brain; confusion may be due to an infection or to hepatic encephalopathy. While the overwhelming majority of cases are straightforward, a GP needs to continue to assess patients astutely and engage specialist assistance if things are out of the ordinary.

WITHDRAWAL MANAGEMENT The agitation and restlessness of alcohol withdrawal can be controlled with adequate amounts of diazepam, which should be titrated according to clinical response. The dose varies widely, from 5 g–40 mg per day. A higher dose should only be dispensed in an inpatient facility, where higher doses may be necessary in patients with concomitant benzodiazepine dependence. Diazepam may be given as frequently as hourly for the first day. After day 3, the dose should be rapidly tapered so that by days 7–8 the patient should be drug free. Occasionally there may be ongoing insomnia, but even this should be primarily treated expectantly and with reassurance. If there is any doubt that patients will not control their diazepam consumption, the doses can be dispensed daily or every second day. This minimises the risk of diazepam overdose.

Sometimes the patient may need paracetamol for headache, and antinausea and antidiarrhoeal agents, although this tends to occur only in a case of severe withdrawal.

In the days of compromised nutrition, patients were given thiamine, multi-B vitamins and occasionally vitamin C and magnesium. If the patient is nutritionally deficient, these should still be given, but the need for them is not as great as it was in the past. However, if in doubt, thiamine and multi-B vitamins should be given.

WITHDRAWAL SETTING Some drug and alcohol services offer a home-based withdrawal service, where a nurse visits daily to supervise the withdrawal. This is offered for those with a stable home environment whose withdrawal is not severe enough to warrant admission to hospital. Withdrawal nurses will depend on the GP to prescribe appropriate amounts of diazepam and other medications to treat the withdrawal. The GP needs to be careful that they prescribe to patients who are not at risk of complications. The patient should be reviewed regularly, both by trained staff and by the GP, and there should be adequate inpatient backup if there are complications. Inpatient withdrawal facilities are limited, but some private withdrawal facilities are available in Australia for those with private health insurance.

RELAPSE PREVENTION Substance dependence is a chronic relapsing condition, so patients should be prepared for this post-withdrawal. Relapse prevention involves both counselling and pharmacotherapy. Counselling should address the following points:

- Develop alternative wind-down strategies to going out with friends for a drink. This may include exercise, hobbies and relaxation.
- Identify situations where the patient is at a high risk of relapse. These may include going out with friends or being bored at home. Develop specific strategies to either avoid these high risk situations or to work through those that cannot be avoided.
- Develop refusal skills—how should the patient handle being asked out for a drink by friends?

■ Underlying psychiatric issues such as depression and anxiety may need specific therapy—either counselling or medications.

■ Most relationships are tested by alcohol dependence but some relationships may be severely dysfunctional and require specific work. There may be an underlying personality disorder.

■ There is a place for more extended rehabilitation programs; these are designed to teach new coping strategies and skills.

■ Long-term support groups are available. They may either be professionally run through psychiatric clinics and drug and alcohol services, or through the self-help groups such as Alcoholics Anonymous (AA) or the New Life program. These are particularly useful in resocialising patients. AA develops the spiritual dimension of a patient's recovery and lets them work through the hurts of the past and take responsibility for them.

Pharmacology can play a part in controlling the craving for alcohol, often a major cause of relapse. Randomised controlled trials of naltrexone and acamprosate have shown that both drugs increase the duration of abstinence and reduce the size of the relapse.[14, 15] Naltrexone is taken as one 50 mg tablet daily. The first two doses are halved to reduce the incidence of nausea. It is an opioid blocker so that patients need to carry a card stating that, should they present to an emergency needing opioids (for example, for a myocardial infarction or a fracture or an acute abdomen), the opioids will not be effective and alternative analgesia will need to be given. Acamprosate acts at the GABA receptors (NMDA receptors). If the patient is over 60 kg, two 333 mg tablets need to be taken three times a day. If the patient is under 60 kg, the first two doses are reduced to one tablet. Acamprosate has been studied in more trials and for a longer duration, but head to head studies suggest that naltrexone is somewhat superior to acamprosate. Disulfiram (antabuse) has been disappointing in controlled trials but anecdotally there are sometimes useful responses. It works by blocking the aldehyde dehydrogenase enzyme, which is part of the alcohol degradation pathway. Disulfiram leads to the buildup of aldehyde, which causes nausea, flushing, chest pains, diarrhoea and a general sense of unwellness. Thus it deters alcohol consumption. The drug works better if a third party supervises the medication.

Relapses can be quite devastating to the patient, and non-judgmental support from their doctor can go a long way to recovering morale after such an event.

CANNABIS ABUSE OR DEPENDENCE

CASE STUDY 2

Mrs Grant, a patient of yours, comes in one afternoon with her 20-year-old son Jim. Jimmy, she explains, smokes cannabis 'most of the time' and sits at home doing nothing. She seeks your help. You ask to speak to Jim alone and then take a drug and alcohol history.

Jim explains that he has been smoking marijuana for the past four years, but the amount has gradually escalated to 1–2 g per day. He smokes it now in a bong (waterpipe). It provides him with relaxation and enjoyment, and helps to pass the time. His parents separated five years ago. He has had no job since he left school and he has been just coasting along. He gets anxious if he does not smoke, and he cannot sleep without 1–2 bongs at night. He occasionally goes out binge drinking with his friends. He smokes 5–6 cigarettes per day, but uses no other drugs. He denies being depressed and he exhibits no thought disorder or other symptoms suggestive of psychosis.

Jim meets the DSM-IV criteria of dependence. He also abuses alcohol and smokes cigarettes. He may be using much more tobacco than initially indicated, as he may be mixing his cannabis with tobacco. There is no evidence of any comorbid psychiatric illness in Jim's history or presentation. His general indolence has been described as an 'amotivational syndrome', thought to be peculiar to cannabis.

Risk factors for his drug problem require further exploration. He has had difficulties adjusting to his parent's separation, but other issues may emerge. Sometimes no clear risk factors are found.

Jim's management is based on motivational interviewing strategies. If Jim were ready to stop using (this might take a few sessions), simple sedatives such as diazepam during the day and temazepam during the night may help to reduce the agitation and insomnia associated with cannabis withdrawal. Should there be any concern about benzodiazepine abuse, daily pickups from the chemist can be arranged. The principles of relapse prevention are the same as for alcohol use, but there are no specific anticraving drugs directed against cannabis use. While abstinence is the goal, from a practical point of view harm reduction strategies such as the following are often necessary:

- Reduce daily intake—for example, smoke only at night instead of all day.
- Reduce smoking tobacco cigarettes, as the additive amount with cannabis increases the risk of bronchitis, emphysema and cancer.
- Do not drive for 3–4 hours after smoking cannabis, as driving skills are impaired during that time.
- Do not smoke cannabis at all if there is a family history of mental illness, especially schizophrenia.

HEROIN DEPENDENCE

Heroin users visit their doctors for a wide variety of reasons. Ceasing drug use is often not the main reason. Common presentations are requests for scripts to ease opiate withdrawal symptoms such as insomnia or anxiety, or for the management of drug related complications. The management of some of these requests for sedatives is dealt with in Chapter 18.

To manage heroin dependence, the GP needs to apply the principles of the stages of change and motivational interviewing. This acknowledges the chronic relapsing nature of this condition. Quick fixes generally do not work. On the other hand, an empathic harm reduction approach, with the aim of attracting the patient into treatment and keeping them engaged, has been shown to save lives. Without treatment the mortality rate among heroin injectors is thirteen times that of non-heroin using peers.[16]

Comorbidity of medical and psychiatric conditions is common in heroin dependent people. GPs may be asked to treat their skin infections and local abscesses at injection sites as well as drug overdoses, social crises and specific psychiatric conditions. The prevalence of hepatitis C infection among heroin injectors is 75% after five years of drug use (compared with 0.3% in the general Australian population). Australia's HIV prevalence of 2–3% among intravenous drug users is remarkably low compared with other Western countries. This important achievement is attributed to the wide availability of clean needles and syringes and good access to opiate substitution treatment for dependence.[17]

There are three broad treatment strategies for managing heroin dependence: drug withdrawal, maintenance pharmacotherapy and long-term rehabilitation programs.

DRUG WITHDRAWAL Heroin withdrawal symptoms generally start within 6–12 hours of last use, peak at 48–72 hours and last about 5–7 days. In most cases withdrawal can be safely completed at the patient's home if there is sufficient support and supervision. However, withdrawal (or 'detox') success rates are higher if the process is undertaken in a residential drug treatment centre. Withdrawal completion rates vary from 10% to 20% with a home withdrawal to 75% in a residential unit. However, the relapse rate within three months for both groups is over 50%.

Short-term medications often used in Australia for heroin withdrawal are:

- buprenorphine—a 5–7 day reduction regimen; or
- symptomatic treatment, consisting of:
  - analgesic/anti-inflammatory—for example, ibuprofen 400 mg qid, and a sedative if required—for example, diazepam 5 mg tds for three days then tapering off; and
  - clonidine at 100–150 µg tds can ease withdrawal symptoms but it can also cause hypotension, so close monitoring is required.

In some Australian states legislation requires anyone prescribing buprenorphine to be specially trained to prescribe this drug. A permit is required from state authorities for each patient. However, the effectiveness of buprenorphine is considerably better than the other opiate withdrawal regimens described above.

MAINTENANCE PHARMACOTHERAPY Methadone and buprenorphine are long-acting synthetic opiates that have been used successfully around the world to treat heroin dependence. In Australia these opiate maintenance programs are tightly regulated by state health departments, which approve specially trained doctors to prescribe and pharmacists to dispense these opiates. Both methadone and buprenorphine have been demonstrated in multiple trials to reduce heroin use as well as to reduce at risk behaviour such as needle sharing and criminal activity. They lower the mortality rate in opioid dependent persons.

Maintenance opiate pharmacotherapy keeps people engaged in treatment and therefore allows time for lifestyle changes to occur and coexisting mental or social problems to be addressed. Treatment evaluation studies have shown that higher doses and longer duration of treatment with these pharmacotherapies are associated with more favourable outcomes. However, experience indicates that the right dose is the one that stops the heroin use.

The opiate receptor-blocking drug naltrexone has proved to be disappointing in treating heroin dependence. This is mainly due to non-compliance of daily tablet taking. The role of naltrexone implants requires further development and evaluation.

LONG-TERM RESIDENTIAL REHABILITATION PROGRAMS Residential programs offer residential facilities for 3–12 months as part of an intensive rehabilitation program that is usually medication free. The regimented program of daily work activities and group discussions suits certain people, but some of the programs have a high drop out rate, especially in the first month.

PSYCHOSTIMULANT ABUSE

The effects of psychostimulant use depend on dose, route of administration and frequency. Most users only tend to use these drugs casually—for example, at weekend parties— so physical dependence and withdrawal problems are less commonly encountered in general practice than with alcohol or heroin use. However, psychological disturbance such as anxiety, panic attacks and mild psychotic features (for example, perceptual disturbances and paranoia) may lead to help seeking by the patient. As the dose of the psychostimulant increases, its toxicity is associated with aggressive behaviour, hostility and medical complications such as hypertensive and hyperpyrexic crises, both of which require emergency medical treatment.

Treatment of psychostimulant intoxication involves explanation, reassurance and symptomatic treatment. This is also sufficient for withdrawal from most amphetamines and ecstasy. For more severe episodes, sedative medication can be used for 2–3 days to treat the agitation that sometimes follows the 'crash'. Benzodiazepines—for example, diazepam at 10 mg tds—may relieve some of the anxiety and insomnia symptoms. Antidepressants are sometimes also used to help patients with persistent psychomotor retardation and low mood associated with psychostimulant withdrawal.

Drug induced psychosis may occur after regular long-term use as well as after short-term and even single large dose use of psychostimulants. This psychosis has been compared to the presentation of acute schizophrenia, as the clinical picture can be very similar; however, they differ in their etiology and duration of the presenting psychotic disorder.

Drug induced psychosis and withdrawal symptoms will abate within a few days of drug cessation, but the post-withdrawal lethargy and intense drug cravings that are associated with amphetamine cessation often lead to relapse and the return to the drug-seeking merry-go-round. The cravings may persist for a month or more. As yet there is no medication available to reduce these intense cravings. Once again the principles of motivational interviewing and relapse prevention should be applied to the management of these patients.

DUAL DIAGNOSIS

Dual diagnosis denotes the co-occurrence of mental illness and substance use disorders. Substance use disorder is the most common and clinically significant comorbidity among patients with severe mental illness. Clinical perspectives in this field can be confusing. Psychiatrists are mostly concerned with dual diagnosis patients who have schizophrenia, bipolar disorder or severe depression and whose use of illicit drugs—especially cannabis, amphetamine or heroin—complicates their mental illness. These patients are generally treated in the public mental health system in Australia. GPs, on the other hand, are more likely to encounter dual diagnosis problems among clinic patients who have a personality disorder and who also use alcohol or other drugs (see Chapter 18). These patients usually suffer from depression (and high suicide risk), anxiety and social phobia symptoms. Patients may often use illicit substances as a form of self-medication. Correct management of their underlying psychiatric condition is then an important part of their recovery. On the other hand, patients may present to their GP with symptoms of anxiety, phobias, depression and/or a traumatic past history, in which the first step to recovery may well be removing the depressant effects of alcohol or other sedatives or the anxiety-producing effects of recurrent withdrawal symptoms. Patients with borderline personality disorder may be self-medicating their emotional dysregulation, and will need specific counselling and occasional psychiatric pharmacotherapy once their drugs of abuse have been withdrawn.[18, 19]

A clear and ongoing assessment of the patient's underlying psychiatric and psychosocial issues is an important part of the total management of patients with substance misuse problems, but access to acute psychiatric or drug and alcohol services when a GP's patient's mental health deteriorates may be difficult. This is generally due to poor co-ordination, different treatment philosophies and gaps between treatment services for dual diagnosis patients. Better integration across disciplines is needed in our fragmented and overspecialised health care system (see Chapter 22). GPs play a key role in providing primary care, especially for those with mild to moderate comorbid disorders. This patient group represents the majority of people affected by dual disorders. GPs need, and should have access to, expertise from specialist mental health and drug and alcohol services as required. This would enable them to undertake the following tasks:

- early detection of the disorders;
- brief interventions to minimise the harm from excessive drug use;
- care co-ordination with other service providers;
- pharmacotherapy, if required, for both the psychiatric and substance abuse disorder; and
- long-term monitoring and follow up.

It is generally acknowledged, however, that the effectiveness of GP management of dual disorders is relatively unexplored. There is also concern that the GP may be unable to meet the expectations of researchers and special interest groups in managing these issues. Substantially more human resources, training and financial support to cover the extra time required by GPs for case co-ordination and counselling is likely to be needed before GPs can fully take on this challenging task.[20]

CONCLUSION

In this chapter the prevalence of substance abuse, with its associated morbidity and mortality, has been highlighted. Community attitudes vary widely on how to best tackle this serious problem. GPs have a unique role and opportunity in assessing, diagnosing and treating patients with drug problems. The treatment often involves a team approach, as addiction is now best regarded as a chronic relapsing medical condition. Evidence based treatment can work in ameliorating the physical and mental disorders associated with abuse of alcohol and other drugs.

REFERENCES

1. The National Drug Strategy. Australia's integrated framework 2004–2009. Canberra: Commonwealth of Australia, 2004.

2. Pagliaro L, Pagliaro A. Pagliaros' Comprehensive Guide to Drugs and Substances of Abuse 2004. Washington DC: American Pharmacists Association, 2004.

3. World Health Organization. Neuroscience of Psychoactive Substance Use and Dependence: Summary. Geneva: WHO, 2004.

4. American Psychiatric Association. Diagnostic and Statistical Manual of Mental Disorder. 4th edn. Washington, DC: American Psychiatric Association, 1994.

5. Australian Institute of Health and Welfare. National Drug Strategy Household Survey 2004. http://www.aihw.gov.au/publications/phe/ndshs04/ndshs04-c00.pdf

6. Hall W, Degenhardt L, Teeson M. Cannabis use and psychotic disorders: an update. Drug and Alcohol Review 2004;23:433–43.

7. Premiers Drug Advisory Council. Drugs and Our Community: Report of the Premiers Drug Advisory Council. Melbourne: Victorian Government, 1996.

8. McKetin R, McLaren J. The methamphetamine situation in Australia: a review of routine data sources. Monograph Series 1. Sydney: National Drug Law Enforcement Research Fund, 2004.

9. Hulse G, White J, Cape G, eds. Management of Alcohol and Drug Problems. Oxford: Oxford University Press, 2002.

10. National Centre for Education and Training on Addiction (NCETA) Consortium. Resource Kit for GP Trainers on Illicit Drug Issues. Flinders University, Adelaide: Australian Department of Health and Ageing, 2004.

11. Hester R, Miller W, eds. Handbook of Alcoholism Treatment Approaches: Effective Alternatives. 3rd edn. New York: Allyn and Bacon, 2002.

12. Rollnick S, Kinnersley P, Scott N. Methods of helping patients with behaviour change. British Medical Journal 1993;307:188–90.

13. Australian Drug Foundation. A Guide to Changing Your Drinking Habits. Melbourne: Australian Drug Foundation, 2001.

14. Keifer F, Jahn H, Tarnaske T, Helwig H, Briken P, Holzbach R, Kampf P, Stracke R, Bachr M, Naber D, Wiedemann K. Comparing and combining naltrexone and acamprosate in relapse prevention of alcoholism: a double blind, placebo controlled study. Archives of General Psychiatry 2003;60:92–9.

15. Rubio G, Jiménez-Arriero MA, Ponce G, Palomo T. Naltrexone versus acamprosate: one year follow-up of alcohol dependence treatment. Alcohol and Alcoholism 2001;365:419–25.

16. Seivewright N, Iqbal M. Prescribing to drug misusers in practice—often effective, but rarely straightforward. Addiction Biology 2002;7:269–77.

17. Dore G, Pritchard-Jones J, Fisher D, Law M. Who's at risk? Hepatitis C—a management guide for general practitioners. Australian Family Physician 1999;28:S18–13.

18. Hickie I, Koschera A, Davenport T, Naismith L, Scott M. Comorbidity of common mental disorders and alcohol or other substance misuse in Australian general practice. Medical Journal of Australia 2001;175:S31–6.

19. NSW Health Department. The Management of People with a Co-existing Mental Health and Substance Use Disorder: Service Delivery Guidelines. Sydney: NSW Health Department, 2000. Accessed via www.health.nsw.gov.au

20. McCabe D, Holmwood C. Co-morbidity in General Practice: The Provision of Care for People with Coexisting Mental Health Problems and Substance Use by General Practitioners. Flinders University Adelaide: Primary Mental Health Care Australian Resource Centre, Department of General Practice, 2002. www.parc.net.au/comorbidityreportrevised2002.doc

CHAPTER 11
SOMATISATION

DM Clarke and L Piterman

One of the unpardonable sins in the eyes of most people is for a man to go about unlabelled. The world regards such a person as the police do an unmuzzled dog, not under proper control.

THOMAS H HUXLEY, *Evolution and Ethics, 1893*

KEY FACTS

- In general practice up to 30% of common physical symptoms are not explained by physical disease.

- Somatisation is defined as the expression of distress in an idiom of bodily complaints with help seeking from medical or health practitioners.

- Somatisation involves, or may involve, overly sensitive bodily perceptions, a somatic attribution of cause, excessive illness worry and abnormal illness behaviour.

- There is a lack of concordance between the patient's belief that they have a physical illness and the doctor's view that they do not.

- Medically unexplained symptoms are the first clue to somatisation; however, a diagnosis of somatisation also requires the identification of psychological aetiological factors.

- Unexplained somatic symptoms are associated with anxiety and depression; the likelihood of depression and anxiety being present increases with the number of somatoform symptoms or unexplained symptoms present.

- Because of their understanding of biopsychosocial determinants of illness and their provision of long-term continuous care, general practitioners (GPs) are well placed to undertake the management of people with somatoform disorders.

continued overleaf

■ Management involves clarification of the diagnosis, reassurance and re-attribution (moving a person from a somatic conviction to considering psychological contributions).

■ The care of chronic somatisers involves case management with an emphasis on: minimising investigations, physical treatment and polypharmacy; and avoiding abandonment of the patient.

INTRODUCTION

The clinical method is a process used by doctors and aimed at reaching a precise diagnosis that determines management and prognosis. That process involves history taking, clinical examination and investigation, and encompasses science (biomedical and social) as well as craft. Central to the diagnostic process is the consultation, the quality of which is determined by the knowledge, skills, attitudes and beliefs of the doctor, the patient's expression of their symptoms, the patient's knowledge, attitude and beliefs regarding these symptoms, and the nature of the doctor–patient relationship. Culture, context and past experience play a vital role. The rapid growth in scientific knowledge has been followed by a parallel growth in medical nosology. There is an abundance of literature describing the classification and labelling of diseases and syndromes (International Classification of Diseases (ICD), International Classification of Primary Care (ICPC), Diagnostic and Statistical Manual of Mental Disorders (DSM) and so on), all of which aims to introduce precision into diagnostic classification and management (see Chapters 1 and 7). Unlike many branches of medicine, general practice still remains characterised by a 'high level of illness and low level of disease',[1] with uncertainty, complexity and ambiguity often making definitive diagnosis difficult. This has resulted in management strategies based on the exclusion of serious physical illness, the development of a probabilistic diagnostic hypothesis,[2] and a management plan that matches the hypothesis, allowing for review and revision with the passage of time. Probabilistic thinking and management may be improved with the inclusion of two important frameworks—the biopsychosocial and the biopsychosocial-semiotic.[3] In the former, attention is given to all three dimensions—biological, psychological and social—in the causation and diagnosis of disease. The latter adds a patient centred perspective and seeks to gain an understanding of the meaning of the presenting symptoms to the patient.

Despite these developments in systematic approaches to diagnostic conceptualisation, large gaps still exist in achieving definitive diagnoses in many general practice encounters. Somatic symptoms with which patients present do not always fit neatly into the text book descriptions of diseases that GPs studied at medical school; nor do they always match established nosologies such as ICD, ICPC or DSM. This chapter covers this grey area.

CASE STUDY 1

Alan is 58 years old, and works as a linesman with a telecommunications provider. He works hard, although he exercises little outside work. His recreation is watching the football while drinking a beer. He smokes. He has a wife and one son. One evening, after going to bed, he develops chest pain that increases quickly in severity to the point where

---

he feels quite ill. He and his wife panic, fearing he is having a heart attack, and ring their doctor, who comes quickly and arranges an ambulance. By the time Alan arrives in hospital, the ECG shows ST changes confirming ischaemia and likely ensuing infarction.

What happened here? Alan felt some physical discomfort (symptom perception). The intensity of it forced itself into his consciousness and he made a judgment that this was probably something serious, perhaps even a heart attack, which had caused the death of some of his friends (causal attribution). His level of concern, and that of his wife (illness worry), were such that he decided to do what one does when one is sick in Australia— call the doctor and/or go to hospital (illness behaviour). There seems nothing unusual in this (see Figure 11.1).

FIGURE 11.1 The process of recognising illness

Perceptions...   (of symptoms)

Attribution...   (of cause)

Concern or worry...   (about illness)

Illness behaviour

But let us consider some variations on this story. Could a person have a lower or higher threshold for pain, and how would this alter the story? Different people might make different causal attributions—one person to a serious disease, another attributing pain to stress or the gods. One person might have a low level of concern about disease (perhaps to the extent of illness denial) and another a high level of illness worry (for example, cardiac neurosis and cancer phobia). Finally, people have a whole range of behavioural responses that include going to the doctor or taking herbal remedies.

This chapter is all about people who have low sensitivity to somatic sensations and high illness worry and/or who readily make disease attributions and seek medical help. (Although perhaps we should be just as concerned about those people who have a high symptom threshold, low illness worry and who tend not to seek medical help, but they do not go to the doctor and therefore do not present a clinical dilemma.) This chapter is also about the system in which these patients find themselves: it includes the doctor; the structure of general practice, health funding and administration; and the social preoccupation with physical cures. Medicine often focuses on a disease and the search for a cure. Michael Balint reminds us that whether the patient presents saying they are depressed or have a pain, the illness is just the ticket to get in the door and be cared for. 'Every illness is also the vehicle for a plea for love and attention.'[4] Consider 'Case study 2', a case that illustrates some of the problems of somatisation.

CASE STUDY 2

Boris is a 62-year-old bookkeeper/accountant, who has worked for an energy company for the past eight years. Before that he worked for twenty years for the State Electricity

---

Commission until it was privatised. He has been a regular and frequent attendee at the same clinic for the past twenty years and has a very thick file, the result of numerous visits, mostly for recurring abdominal and chest pains. Boris has been married for thirty-two years; his wife is 60 and they have no children (he had a low sperm count and she had suffered from endometriosis). He is an only child. His father died twenty-five years ago at the age of 58 as a result of a myocardial infarction, and his mother died twelve years ago, aged 72, from peritonitis and septicaemia, the result of a ruptured colonic diverticulum. He is a non-smoker and social drinker.

Boris presents with abdominal pain that is generally right sided, sharp and colicky. It lasts for several hours to several days and is associated with loss of appetite, tiredness, excessive wind and occasional diarrhoea. It is noticeably associated with travel and deadlines. His chest pains are generally sharp, right sided, lasting from seconds to minutes. They are not related to exertion, but are sometimes associated with difficulty breathing. The symptoms have been thoroughly and repeatedly investigated and no physical cause has been found.

Boris remains concerned that he has an undiagnosed abdominal condition, possibly diverticular disease like his mother or Crohn's disease (a cousin had this condition), or perhaps he is carrying a germ that he contracted on a trip to South-East Asia. He also feels that there may be an undetected heart condition, given the sudden and unexpected death of his father many years ago.

The questions raised by this case study include:

- If you were taking over the management of Boris, what approach would you take the next time he visits you with a recurrence of similar symptoms?
- What are your diagnostic hypotheses?
- Do they include one or more psychiatric disorders, physical disorders or both?
- Boris had previously been managed symptomatically with antispasmodics and analgesics when required as well as occasional courses of metronidazole. How might your management differ?
- How many patients like this do you have in your practice? Can their management be improved? If so, how?

DEFINITION AND CLASSIFICATION OF SOMATISING DISORDERS

The classification of somatisation is clumsy in a number of ways. Whereas most psychiatric disorders are categorised according to the phenomena experienced by the patient—for example, mood, anxiety or psychotic symptoms—somatising disorders are grouped by their somatic focus. In fact, they include states where the most prominent 'phenomenon' is anxiety (hypochondriasis), overvalued ideas (hypochondriasis and body dysmorphic disorder), dissociation (conversion disorder) or seemingly inappropriate help-seeking behaviour (somatisation disorder). Furthermore, when patients present to doctors with either mood disturbance or chest pain from cardiac ischaemia, there is usually co-operation in sorting out the problem and a readiness to agree on a diagnosis and management plan. Patients are usually relieved to be given a diagnosis. This is rarely the case with somatisation. In fact, what defines somatisation is the disagreement between doctor and patient, with the patient believing they have a physical disease and the doctor not. This is why somatisation has been referred to as abnormal illness behaviour—the illness behaviour seems not to be appropriate to the objective disease state as determined by the doctor[5] (see Figure 11.2 for definitions of terms).

Somatisation is a theoretical notion—more 'in the eye of the beholder'—rather than a readily verifiable diagnosis. It is inferred when there are physical symptoms for which no underlying physical disease can be found. There are two problems with this. It is possible that the disease has just not declared itself fully, and GPs worry a lot about this possibility and often feel a need to keep investigating. On the other hand, just because a physical disease is found does not mean there are not significant psychosocial factors contributing to it. We know, for example, that stress and depression affect the autonomic system and platelet stickiness and are risk factors for myocardial infarction and sudden cardiac death. In fact, it is likely that psychological factors, as well as lifestyle factors, contribute significantly to most diseases. Recent epidemiological studies indicate that combined physical and psychiatric morbidity is the norm rather than the exception.

Medically unexplained symptoms are therefore the first clue to somatisation. The second requirement for making such a diagnosis is a relevant psychological factor—either a contemporaneous stressor or evident anxiety or depression. It should be possible to at least hypothesise a formulation in which psychological factors have led to the physical illness and help-seeking behaviour.

FIGURE 11.2 Definitions of terms

SOMATISATION The tendency to experience, conceptualise and communicate mental states and distress as physical symptoms or altered bodily function.

ILLNESS BEHAVIOUR Illness behaviour refers simply to the behaviour of the sick person. One person may be stoical, another dramatic. Some may seem to minimise symptoms, others exaggerate them. Illness behaviour depends on a person's perception and evaluation of the symptoms, perceived gains or risks, personality, modelling from family and others, and social norms.

SOMATOFORM DISORDER This umbrella term was created for the DSM-IV classification for many of the disorders outlined in this chapter (see Table 11.1).

CONVERSION DISORDER The presentation is of neurological symptoms (anaesthesia, blindness, paralysis). A psychological precipitant is identified and the condition is usually short lived.

SOMATISATION DISORDER An extreme condition, where a patient seeks treatment over many years for many physical symptoms that have no physical pathology. DSM-IV requires eight or more symptoms, including different types of pain.

HYPOCHONDRIASIS A persistent fear of contracting (phobia), or a preoccupation that one has (obsession), a serious physical disease based on a misrepresentation of bodily symptoms. The preoccupation persists despite medical evaluation and reassurance. It can occur as the predominant feature, or as part of a depressive illness, generalised anxiety, somatisation or psychotic disorder.

Table 11.1 summarises how DSM-IV[6] and ICD-10[7] classify the different syndromes that we include under the concept of somatisation. The main criteria for all include a presentation with physical symptoms where there is no physical disease but a presumption of a psychological cause. The third factor, which requires clinical judgment, is the level of consciousness of the process. In most cases, there is a presumption of an unconscious mechanism; however, often the GP wonders whether this person is deliberately feigning, and this possibility puts a completely different complexion on the consultation.

TABLE 11.1 Current major classification of somatisation

DSM-IV	ICD-10	DEFINING CHARACTERISTICS
Somatoform disorders ■ Conversion disorder ■ Chronic pain ■ Somatisation disorder	Somatoform disorders ■ Dissociative disorder of movement and sensation ■ Chronic pain ■ Somatisation disorder ■ Neurasthenia ■ Somatoform autonomic dysfunction	Physical symptoms, but no or minimal evidence of physical disease
Hypochondriasis	Hypochondriacal disorder	Illness worry or conviction (belief of having or fear of getting a disease) is most prominent
Psychological factors affecting medical condition	Psychological factors affecting medical condition	Psychophysiological disorders (e.g. heart disease, inflammatory bowel disease)
Malingering		Feigned illness or injury for obvious gain
Factitious disorder		Feigned illness or injury for no apparent gain

SOMATOFORM DISORDERS

The somatoform disorders are the archetypal somatising disorders.

CONVERSION DISORDER Conversion disorder is the old 'hysterical conversion', characteristically presenting with a single symptom, such as blindness, paralysis or aphonia. In psychoanalytic theory, the symptom arises from unresolved inner conflict and anxiety. and symbolically provides partial expression of the conflict (conversion). ICD-10 classifies the disorder with the dissociative disorders, together with dissociative fugue or amnesia and multiple personality. This reflects the idea that in each case the person is splitting off (dissociating) some part of their mental function (sensation, memory, identity) from their conscious self. The reason the person with hysterical anaesthesia cannot feel the pinprick is not because of any abnormality in the peripheral nervous system, nor indeed with central sensory registration areas (thalamus and sensory cortex), but because of higher cortical awareness processes. The type of illness that a person expresses may be partly a result of intrapsychic mechanisms—for example, representing the conflict in some way—but is also modelled on their experience of illness, either their own or others. One difficulty with diagnosing conversion disorder is that it may in fact occur together with physical disease. A common example of this is the co-occurrence of epilepsy and 'pseudoseizures' (now often called non-epileptic seizures).

CHRONIC PAIN Pain with a significant psychosocial contribution is difficult to categorise. It has traditionally been placed with somatoform disorders, inferring a similar mechanism to conversion disorder—for example, in a work stress situation, pain could be understood as a result of guilt, exacting punishment at the same time as achieving relief from the difficult situation. Clearly, psychological factors have a lot to do with pain. The experience of pain can be lessened by circumstance and psychological factors (consider a war or football injury, or hypnosis) and can presumably be worsened (for example, chronic pain arising from a trivial work injury). There are two major difficulties in considering pain. The first is the impossibility of being 100% sure that there is no physical contribution. The second is that, over time, many factors contribute to the maintenance of the pain. These may include physical factors (bad posture due to protecting the injury, and more serious secondary effects); social factors (a realignment of home and work duties); psychological factors (the shame of admitting later that there was no injury); and legal factors (embarking on compensation). These issues become like successive rings of an onion shielding the core, making it almost impossible to understand the psychological origins. Management of chronic pain therefore focuses more on understanding the maintaining factors rather than trying to work out the precipitants.

SOMATISATION DISORDER Somatisation disorder is a severe and chronic form of somatisation, with multiple unexplained symptoms occurring over a long period of time. DSM-IV requires eight or more symptoms, some of which are pain (see Table 11.2 on page 176 for the common types of unexplained symptoms). Despite being an uncommon disorder, these patients are frequent attendees to GPs.

HYPOCHONDRIASIS

As mentioned above, hypochondriasis primarily involves illness worry (that is, anxiety) and disease conviction (overvalued ideas). Its classic form can be found in persons with what was once called cardiac neurosis or cancer phobia. These patients are very similar to patients with somatisation disorder, although they may place less emphasis on the physical symptoms—which may be quite ordinary—and much more on fear and obsessional worrying.

PSYCHOLOGICAL FACTORS AFFECTING A MEDICAL CONDITION

The field of psychosomatics blossomed in the 1930s when, under the influence of Freudian psychoanalysis, the search was on to define particular personality types prone to particular diseases. There was a general clinical wisdom then that certain diseases occurred under stress in people predisposed to it by a particular psychological make-up or personality. This idea was called the 'specificity theory', and the so-called 'psychosomatic diseases' included dermatitis, hypertension, inflammatory bowel disease, asthma, thyrotoxicosis, peptic ulcer and rheumatoid arthritis. Unfortunately, despite advancing knowledge about the interaction between mind and body, empirical evidence for such specific associations has not been forthcoming. 'Psychological factors affecting a medical condition' is the rather cumbersome alternative for the term 'psychosomatic disorder'. It acknowledges that any disease may have significant psychological factors contributing, if not to the onset of the disease, then at least to its continuation. Although psychological factors are not often considered in the understanding and management of physical disease (part of our mind–body dualist heritage), there is now an enormous literature describing the association; four examples will be used.

Cardiovascular disease has perhaps the longest tradition of being understood as closely linked to the emotions—consider the concept of the 'broken heart', for instance. There is now a large amount of empirical evidence to support this. In particular, we know that people who are depressed or anxious are more likely to develop ischaemic heart disease, and patients with ischaemic heart disease and who are also depressed are more likely to suffer re-infarction or death.[8] The mechanisms for this most likely involve autonomic activity and platelet function, both of which are affected by depression.

Depression is a risk factor for stroke, as of course is hypertension, which is itself related to stress and lifestyle. Furthermore, for patients with stroke, depression confers increased risk for poor rehabilitation outcome and death.[9]

Asthma attacks often seem to be triggered by emotional events, and clinically, when patients present, it is often hard to know whether there is objectively determined worsening of disease status or just increased illness behaviour. Certainly we know that for people who present to hospital with severe asthma, they and their family have higher levels of depression and stress than those who do not.[10] Worsening of the condition could be mediated through the autonomic nervous system or the immune system, or behaviourally through loss of motivation and non-adherence to treatment.

Cancer is an intriguing area in which to consider principles of psychosomatics. Although defining a cancer prone personality has been a focus of research, the evidence for this is not particularly strong. Furthermore, defining such a personality serves to increase guilt in cancer patients rather than offer hope of remediation. Similarly, research into the relationship between life events and cancer is hampered by the technical difficulty of defining when the cancer process actually started. Nevertheless, a link between stress and cancer could be explained by hypercortisolaemia affecting the immune function. There is interesting research on the contribution of psychosocial effects on cancer progression. Preliminary evidence suggests that people who exhibit 'fighting spirit' as opposed to hopelessness, helplessness or stoic acceptance survive longer.[11] Patients with a non-assertive disposition have hastened cancer progression. There have been trials reported that suggest that psychological interventions, particularly group therapy, increase survival in patients with metastatic cancer.[12] Enticing as this is, not all trials have found this effect, and 'the jury is still out' on this issue. Despite this, there is clear evidence that as a result of the illness, people with cancer suffer from a range of emotional issues, including existential distress, demoralisation and body image disturbance as well as the more usual anxiety and depression. Consequently, some level of psychological treatment and support is often indicated in cancer patients.

MALINGERING AND FACTITIOUS DISORDER

Malingering and factitious disorder bring us to the tough end of somatisation. Medical practice is built on an assumption of mutual trust between the doctor and the patient. These 'disorders' challenge that assumption. Also GPs are often caught in a difficult situation—with a patient's request for a certificate, for example—where they may feel complicit in facilitating a patient's misrepresentation of their symptoms. Malingering is a fairly straightforward problem; it involves lying and feigning illness for obvious gain, such as time off work, compensation or other benefit. Factitious disorder is much more puzzling. Here patients lie or feign illness, or deliberately injure themselves, to gain hospitalisation or other levels of medical care; there is no other apparent gain, such as compensation. The psychological explanation for this behaviour is to infer a need for care (to be cared for) and masochism (punishing the self). Whatever psychological explanations are given, psychological therapies have not proven helpful; generally, what is required is tactful confrontation.

EPIDEMIOLOGY

The disorders described above are not particularly common. Conversion disorder, for instance, occurs in only 1% of neurology clinic attendees.[13] Somatisation disorder, although uncommon in the community, has a prevalence of 2.8% in those who attend a GP,[14] and is especially high (up to 20%) in patients who are high service utilisers.[15] Hypochondriasis is a diagnosis that is not often made, with a prevalence of 0.8% in general practice.[14] These data suggest that somatisation is not common, or that it is not well captured by the DSM and ICD classifications or the structured interviews developed for them.

If we take a different tack, and consider 'somatoform symptoms' rather than the defined syndromes, it is estimated that 15–30% of common symptoms presenting to GPs are not explained by a physical disease or by overt psychiatric disturbance, such as depression, panic or generalised anxiety[16] (see Table 11.2). Furthermore, when the incidence of depression and anxiety is correlated with the presence of somatoform (unexplained) symptoms, it is seen that the likelihood of depression and anxiety being present increases in proportion to the number of unexplained symptoms present (see Table 11.3).

Two facts are made clear by these data. First, somatoform, or unexplained, symptoms are common in general practice. Second, multiple unexplained symptoms are often associated with depression and anxiety. This supports the notion that somatisation is indeed an idiom of distress—the mind talking through the body. It also highlights the importance of having a good look at the emotional life of patients who present with unexplained symptoms, particularly multiple unexplained symptoms occurring on more than one occasion.

THE ENIGMATIC DISORDERS

The area of somatisation is bound in conflict. In the first instance, there is disagreement between the doctor and patient, the latter believing they have a physical disease while

TABLE 11.2 Common somatoform symptoms seen in primary care patients

SYMPTOM	PREVALENCE OF SYMPTOM IN PRIMARY CARE PATIENTS (%)	% OF SYMPTOMS UNEXPLAINED (i.e. SOMATOFORM)
Fainting	3.4	33.3
Menstrual problems	32.5	33.3
Headache	36.4	30.2
Chest pain	20.8	27.3
Dizziness	23.9	27.2
Palpitations	27.2	25.6
Sexual problems	6.4	25.0
Nausea, vomiting, indigestion	43.3	22.7
Constipation/diarrhoea	28.6	22.1
Abdominal pain	19.2	20.7
Dyspnoea	31.5	18.9
Fatigue	58.0	18.7
Insomnia	33.5	17.4
Joint or limb pain	58.7	17.1
Back pain	40.8	15.7

Source: Kroenke et al, 1994.[16]

TABLE 11.3 The occurrence of depression and anxiety with somatoform symptoms

NO. OF UNEXPLAINED PHYSICAL SYMPTOMS	DEPRESSION (%)	ANXIETY (%)
0–1	3	1
2–3	12	7
4–5	23	13
6–8	44	30
9 or more	60	48

Source: Kroenke et al, 1994.[14]

the former believing they do not. Mind–body dualism, which is deeply entrenched in Western thinking, then leads us to conclude that the problem must be in the mind. For whatever reason, this idea is frequently strongly resisted; perhaps it is because of the general stigma and shame attached to having a mental health problem. In any case, conflict remains, and this tends to lead to a polarisation—those who believe that psychological factors can cause physical disease, and those who do not. An important part of the management of these patients is not colluding with this polarisation, but holding the middle ground, but more will be said about that later.

There are a number of disorders that seem to be the repository for this continuing dispute. In the current era these are chronic fatigue syndrome (CFS), irritable bowel syndrome (IBS) and fibromyalgia. The cause of each of these is truly unknown, yet practitioners seem to divide into those who believe they are physical diseases and those who believe they are psychosomatic. The interesting thing about all these syndromes is that there is a lot of overlap. Epidemiological evidence suggests that people who have the symptoms of one often in fact have multiple physical symptoms. However, through the process of attribution described above, supported in some instances by involvement in groups that reinforce a particular illness identity, the focus often becomes directed on one small group of symptoms. Strong illness conviction by patients is a further thing these conditions have in common with the other somatoform disorders.

AETIOLOGY

Multiple factors can contribute to a strong disease conviction and illness behaviour. Somatisation is a process, and chronic somatising is a state that develops over time, reinforced by many things, including, perhaps, experience in the health system, and the reaction of family and lawyers. In understanding the patient, it is therefore important to try and construct a formulation or story explaining why this patient is ill in this way at this time. There will of course be patient factors, social and family factors, environmental factors (stress events) and health system factors.

BIOLOGICAL FACTORS

Clearly, biological factors are involved, especially those involving the autonomic, immune, pain and neuroendocrine systems;[17] however, the role of biological factors as causal agents is a little hypothetical at this stage. There is some evidence that people who somatise have a neural abnormality of failure to habituate that would explain increased sensitivity to sensory stimuli. There may be other neural mechanisms of somatosensory amplification as well. Viruses have been implicated in fatigue states. With the current state of knowledge, biological theories do not particularly assist in the management of patients.

FAMILY AND SOCIOCULTURAL FACTORS

A person's childhood experience of illness—the rewards and penalties, whether they received care or reprimand—are important in their development of an understanding of the meaning of illness. In addition, the types of illness they experience or witness in the family may provide a template for their later illness. Somatising illness can therefore be modelled on prior experience. The meaning of illness and of particular illnesses may be quite different in different families, but also in different cultural or racial groups. For example, in some circumstances a work injury may bring honour, but in other communities shame.

PERSONAL PSYCHOLOGICAL FACTORS

Sometimes an illness appears as an attempt to control or punish another person, or at other times to punish oneself. The latter could be precipitated by a guilt-inducing event, although often the proneness to guilt is long-standing and expressed as chronic feelings of low self-esteem and unworthiness. Sometimes poor self-esteem is disguised by a focus on achievement or obsessionality. Childhood sexual abuse often induces feelings of guilt and low self-esteem, and is strongly associated with somatisation.[18]

PERPETUATING FACTORS

The above causal factors are particularly important in the predisposition to, and precipitation of, somatisation. This is helpful in understanding the acute or short-term somatisers; however, it is far more useful in the management of people with chronic somatisation to have an understanding of what perpetuates the condition, or prevents recovery. As an illness persists, adjustment is made by the patient and family. The patient may come to see themselves as a 'sick person'. They receive care from the family—perhaps, for example, special attention from the grandchildren. The health system may reinforce the sick role, with patients with persistent symptoms being exposed to interventions of increasing invasiveness. Secondary physical effects may ensue, such as adhesions from abdominal surgery, or muscle atrophy and tiredness from disuse. If the sickness is a work injury, there may be lawyers and compensation matters involved, and recovery may be seen as evidence that the injury was not so bad after all. Finally, whatever the situation for the patient, there is usually never any real joy, and usually demoralisation, depression and irritability follow. An important part of the management of these patients will be to prevent, minimise or remove those factors that perpetuate the illness.

MANAGEMENT

It is important to remember the core feature of somatisation—illness conviction. Somatising patients are attending the GP for help. The ticket to get in to see the GP is a physical illness, which, as it turns out, has little basis in physical pathology. The GP infers a psychological or social causality for the illness. In the end, it will be the strength of a person's illness conviction that will determine their prognosis. If a person keeps insisting that they have a physical disease, one for which no cause can be found and therefore no treatment offered, they are consigning themselves to persistent illness. If, on the other hand, a patient acknowledges that possibly there are psychological and/or social factors contributing to the illness, or at least that the cause of the illness is unknown, then a number of avenues for intervention open up. Trying to find the psychological key that will magically cure the disease is an unproductive path. Rather, the important aspects of management are a clarification of diagnosis and formulation, reassurance, re-attribution (moving a person from a somatic conviction to consider psychological and somatic contributions) and case management, including behavioural planning for difficult and intractable cases. Once a diagnosis of somatisation is made, there are two important principles the GP should bear in mind:

■ Avoid or minimise physical treatment, including surgery and polypharmacy.
■ Do not desert the patient. Remember that the illness is just the patient's ticket to receive needed care.

Unfortunately, it is very difficult to do these two things. Patients are likely to feel rejected or not taken seriously if their requests for further investigation, drugs or referral to a specialist are denied. Second, if a GP stays working with the patient, at some point the pressure to do something physical or get another opinion can become intense. The art of successful management involves maintaining the tension of these two positions. For the GP, the art of maintaining good personal mental health while looking after such patients is realising that you cannot be successful in every case. (See Chapter 2.)

CLARIFICATION OF DIAGNOSIS AND FORMULATION

As described above, the diagnosis of somatisation requires the presence of symptoms or illness behaviour not adequately explained by physical disease. Clearly, a proper clinical history, examination and investigation needs to be carried out. The second requirement is an inference of psychogenicity. The discussion of aetiology above, describing the association of somatisation with sexual abuse; personality features of dependency, guilt and punishment; and the effect of modelling prior to illness demand that to understand the case a reasonably comprehensive family and personal history needs to be taken. Such a case history can be particularly helpful for the GP, providing a sense of understanding and reassurance about the case and the diagnosis.

REASSURANCE

Reassurance and the gentle art of persuasion are stock in trade for GPs. The first sign of a somatising patient is, of course, that they are not as easily reassured as other patients. Nevertheless, reassurance is an important part of the management of a somatising patient and, together with re-attribution (discussed below), will be an effective measure for the short illness or moderate disease conviction patients. Reassurance needs to be:

- realistic, being based on your best clinical understanding;
- offered after adequate attention has been given to the patient's symptoms through history, examination and investigation if necessary (this may mean not offering reassurance too early);
- given in the knowledge of, and tailored to, what you believe the patient will receive; and
- given for the patient's benefit and not the doctor's. This means not offering reassurance to dismiss the patient or to rid yourself of a difficult patient.

RE-ATTRIBUTION

Many patients who present with somatoform symptoms[19]—that is, come to the GP with physical symptoms assuming a physical cause—can be persuaded that there is a psychological or stress related cause. Re-attribution builds on reassurance. The four main steps are outlined below.

1 MAKE THE PATIENT FEEL UNDERSTOOD This is achieved by taking a full and proper history and physical examination as well as a targeted investigation if necessary. Also at this early stage, it is important to enquire about work and family stresses, feelings of depression or sadness, or any particular life events. A question such as: 'And has anything else been going on at this time?' may elicit useful information. It also gives the message to the patient that you are interested in psychosocial things and that they may be relevant. So often physical causes are examined first and when these are not found, doctors turn to examine the psychological. Done this way, patients often experience it as a rejection—that the doctor thinks there is nothing wrong. It is therefore important to emphasise the psychosocial from the start. Also, at this stage (the first consultation), health beliefs should be explored. Find out what the patient believes might be wrong with them and why they think that, and whether that gives them any particular concerns.

2 BROADEN THE AGENDA You have now completed your evaluation. You have found no physical cause for the symptoms. Probably you have identified some stressor or some feelings of depression (remember epidemiologic studies suggest that somatoform symptoms are often accompanied depression or anxiety). At this stage, you should just float the idea that the symptoms may be due to stress or depression (using whatever language for these you feel appropriate). This could be done in the second consultation. The steps are:

- Summarise the symptoms with which the patient has presented as well as the physical findings of the examination.
- Acknowledge the reality of the patient's symptoms.
- Remind the patient that they also have symptoms of depression or anxiety (if they have).
- Remind the patient of the context of the presentation—the life stresses that they told you about.

3 MAKE THE LINK—REFRAMING Present the hypothesis that these things might all be related. This needs to be both convincing and as reasonable as possible. You may need to describe how stress causes muscle tension, which can cause headache, or that chest pain and palpitations are very common with stress and anxiety when the heart jumps and goes a bit fast, or that people feel pain more exquisitely when they are under emotional stress.

4 AFTER RE-ATTRIBUTION What happens after the link is made and accepted is very important, although it depends on what has been uncovered. It is important to reassure the patient that the physical symptoms will resolve once the emotional issues are dealt with, and also that you will follow things up with the patient. Other management should be specifically targeted at the identified emotional difficulties and could include:

- counselling for loss, grief, interpersonal or work stresses (see Chapters 17 and 19);
- relaxation and/or short-term benzodiazepines for aroused anxiety states (see Chapter 17);
- antidepressants and counselling for prominent depression or specifically defined anxiety states—for example, panic disorder (see Chapters 8 and 9).

Some patients will not seem to be helped immediately by re-attribution. In these cases the situation needs to be re-evaluated, particularly with attention to the possible presence of depression and hopelessness, or the persistence of unresolved stress. After re-evaluation, re-attribution and reassurance can be tried again. If the hypochondriasis and disease conviction persist, the patient is at risk of becoming a chronic somatiser.

CASE MANAGEMENT

The management of chronic somatisation is similar to that of any chronic illness. In this situation, there is an acceptance that complete recovery is not possible or likely and the emphasis turns to maximising physical and social functioning and minimising harmful medical interventions. Because these patients are often searching for a cure, somatising patients quickly accumulate a large number of medical practitioners. If patients feel one doctor has dismissed their problems, they may go to another and maintain secrecy. Consequently, a new batch of investigations and referrals are embarked upon. The important role in this situation is that of the case manager, who has the trust of the patient, and communicates with all involved. This person must be clearly designated, and will usually be the GP. They will advocate for the patient, organise referrals when necessary, advise against specialist referrals when it would be unnecessary, oversee prescribing practice and generally, with the patient, define people's roles. Sometimes case conferences are required to allow everyone to share their views.

As in acute somatisation, the ultimate aim is to take the focus away from the physical symptoms. The reason for this is simple: a focus on symptoms will only lead to harmful interventions and no improvement. In chronic somatisation, it is unlikely that re-attribution will work; the illness conviction is relatively immutable. The emphasis should therefore be on encouraging an acceptance of the illness, a re-evaluation of life's priorities in the context of the limitations of the illness, minimising harmful interventions and maximising social functioning. Monitoring a range of behaviours with the aim of increasing capacities might be helpful. These could include sleep, walking, standing and staying out of hospital. Just taking the focus away from the symptoms can be helpful. In addition, showing that small gains are possible is encouraging. Maintaining hope for both doctor and patient is critical, while at the same time refusing the promised cure is a difficult but important task. Referral to a specialist in psychosomatic medicine (of which there are very few) may provide encouragement and reassurance to the GP.

REVISITING CASE STUDY 2

We'll return to our patient Boris, who has recurrent bouts of chest pain and abdominal pain. As the new GP taking over his care, it is essential that you begin by building a trusting doctor–patient relationship and demonstrating a willingness to continue a therapeutic role, regardless of the clinical outcome. The diagnosis is most likely somatisation with associated anxiety, but depression would need to be excluded. It is likely that Boris already has a thick file of negative investigations, so avoiding further and unnecessary tests is essential, even though this may pose some difficulties in establishing a new relationship with a patient such as Boris.

It may be necessary to spend the initial consultation establishing the relationship. Over the next two consultations, set out a management plan that focuses on broadening the agenda to help the patient reframe the physical symptoms as having a psychological basis. You will need to explain the nature of mind–body connections. The process known as re-attribution is the key to assisting Boris to accept the notion that if there is a psychological basis to the symptoms, then psychological rather than symptomatic pharmacological interventions are the appropriate form of treatment. If Boris accepts this, then you may institute cognitive behavioural therapy or interpersonal therapy, if you have been trained in these, or refer him to a trained psychologist or psychiatrist for several sessions. Naturally, you will need to make decisions regarding the judicious use of anxiolytics or antidepressants. As the GP responsible for continuing care, you will need to maintain vigilance to ensure that concurrent and intercurrent physical conditions are investigated and managed. That includes investigation of subtle changes to the presenting symptoms. Boris should never feel abandoned.

CONCLUSION

Somatising disorders are among the most difficult for doctors to manage, and lead to substantial health costs, disability and iatrogenic complications. The central core of the phenomena is a difference in illness attribution between doctor and patient. The emphasis of the doctor must be a concentrated effort to maintain a therapeutic relationship.

REFERENCES

1. Murtagh J. General Practice. Sydney, Australia: McGraw-Hill, 1998.
2. Stephens GG. The Intellectual Basis of Family Practice. Tucson, Arizona: Winter Publishing Co., 1982.
3. Pauli HG, White KL, McWhinney IR. Medical education, research and scientific thinking in the 21st century (Part Two of three). Education in Health 2000;13:165–72.
4. Balint M. The Doctor, His Patient and the Illness. London: Pitman Medical, 1957.
5. Pilowsky I. Abnormal Illness Behaviour. Chichester: John Wiley & Sons, 1997.
6. American Psychiatric Association. Diagnostic and Statistical Manual of Mental Disorders. 4th edn. Washington DC: American Psychiatric Association, 1994.
7. World Health Organization. The ICD-10 Classification of Mental and Behavioural Disorders. Geneva: WHO, 1992.
8. Jiang W, Krishnan RRK, O'Connor CM. Depression and heart disease: evidence of a link and its therapeutic implications. CNS Drugs 2002;16:111–27.
9. Ramasubbu R, Patten SB. Effect of depression on stroke morbidity and mortality. Canadian Journal of Psychiatry 2003;48:250–7.
10. Zielinski TA, Brown ES. Depression in patients with asthma. Advances in Psychosomatic Medicine 2003;24:42–50.
11. Morris T, Pettingale KW, Haybittle J. Psychological response to cancer diagnosis and disease outcome in patients with breast cancer and lymphoma. Psycho-Oncology 1992;1:105–14.
12. Spiegel D, Kato PM. Psychosocial influences on cancer incidence and progression. Harvard Review of Psychiatry 1996;4:10–26.
13. Trimble MR. Functional diseases. British Medical Journal 1982;2:1768–70.
14. Gureje O, Simon GE, Ustun TB, Goldberg DP. Somatisation in a cross-cultural perspective: a World Health Organization study in primary care. American Journal of Psychiatry 1997;154:989–95.
15. Katon W, VonKorff M, Lin E, Lipscomb P, Wagner E, Polk E. Distressed high utilizers of medical care: DSM-III-R diagnoses and treatment needs. General Hospital Psychiatry 1990;12;355–62.
16. Kroenke K, Spitzer RL, Williams JBW, Linzer M, Hahn SR, deGruy FV, Brody D. Physical symptoms in primary care: predictors of psychiatric disorders and functional impairment. Archives of Family Medicine 1994;3:774–9.
17. Rief W, Barsky AJ. Psychobiological perspectives on somatoform disorders. Psychoneuro-endocrinology 2005;30:996–1002.
18. Hulme PA. Theoretical perspectives on the health problems of adults who experienced childhood sexual abuse. Issues in Mental Health Nursing 2004;25:339–61.
19. Goldberg D, Gask L, O'Dowd T. The treatment of somatization: teaching techniques of reattribution. Journal of Psychosomatic Research 1989; 33:689–95.

CHAPTER 12
PSYCHOSES

N Keks, R O'Bryan and A Stocky

Canst thou not minister to a mind diseas'd,
Pluck from the memory a rooted sorrow,
Raze out the written troubles of the brain,
And with some sweet oblivious antidote
Cleanse the stuff'd bosom of that perilous stuff,
Which weighs upon the heart?
...
Throw physic to the dogs; I'll none of it.

WILLIAM SHAKESPEARE, *Macbeth, Act V, Scene III, c. 1606*

CASE STUDY

Justin's parents are concerned about his changed behaviour and they bring him to your surgery. Justin, aged 19, is a university student living at home. He is a bright but shy young man. His mother reports that over the past few weeks Justin has become withdrawn, irritable and verbally aggressive, spending most of his time in bed listening to music through his earphones. At night he is disturbing the family's sleep by wandering aimlessly about the house. Justin is seeing none of his friends, refuses to come to the family meal table and eat, and is neglecting to wash himself. He has become pale, and he has lost a lot of weight. His parents have detected a sickly sweetish smell coming from his bedroom and they suspect that he is smoking 'pot'. They have finally come for help because Justin has declared he is dropping out of his university course.

You are struck by Justin's untidy appearance and by his withdrawn and sullen demeanour. With some difficulty you entice Justin to talk to you about how he feels. He denies that there is anything wrong. He has dropped out of his course because he has lost interest and cannot concentrate on his studies. As an aside he adds that one of his lecturers has been picking on him and talking about him behind his back. He is not suicidal and has no aggressive intentions.

From the limited clinical evidence presented to you by Justin and his parents, you suspect that Justin's condition is most likely to be the manifestation of an early onset psychosis. While the definitive diagnosis is unclear, there is plentiful evidence that Justin is presenting with a 'schizophrenia spectrum' disorder, in the broad sense for therapeutic purposes. Justin agrees to take medication to reduce stress and anxiety, and to improve sleep. You prescribe amisulpride 200 mg bd and temazepam at night. He agrees to let his parents help with the tablets. You contract with Justin to cease using cannabis, to eat and sleep properly, to look after his hygiene and to exercise.

You arrange an appointment for him to see a psychiatrist as soon as possible. With Justin's parents you discuss the diagnosis of early psychosis, and its possible underlying causes, using patient information brochures and a website to emphasise the nature and management of psychosis. It is important to stress that psychosis is due to a chemical imbalance in a part of the brain and needs to be corrected with medication.

KEY FACTS

■ Schizophrenia, bipolar mood disorder, schizoaffective disorder and psychotic depression may affect up to 5% of the population during their lifetimes. Most general practitioners (GPs) have 4–5 such patients in their practice.

■ Men and women from all social classes are equally affected, and age of onset is usually between 15 and 30 years of age. There is a significant genetic component.

■ The boundaries between psychotic disorders tend to be blurred, and it is useful to evaluate patients in terms of key symptoms—positive, negative, elevation, depression and psychosocial deterioration.

■ The prodrome of schizophrenia and related psychoses is often fairly non-specific initially, until frank psychotic symptoms develop. A high index of suspicion is needed, particularly in adolescents.

■ Early psychosis usually responds well to treatment, and the vast majority of patients recover.

■ The prognosis tends to worsen with repeated episodes, and eventually one-third of patients with psychoses manifest chronic symptomatology that does not fully respond to treatment.

■ Psychoses are disorders of the brain, usually involving dysfunction of the neurotransmitter dopamine. The cornerstone of treatment involves dopamine antagonist (antipsychotic) medication.

■ Antipsychotic medication has allowed the vast majority of patients with psychoses to live in the community. Many patients suffer severe disability and require case management and psychosocial support. Rates of non-adherence to treatment are high, as is alcohol and/or drug abuse comorbidity.

■ GPs have a crucial role in monitoring patients during long-term treatment, with particular emphasis on physical health in areas such as weight, smoking, blood glucose, lipids, Pap smears and other preventive measures.

INTRODUCTION

Psychoses are major mental disorders in which, at some stage during the course of the illness, the patient's capacity to appreciate reality becomes impaired. The appearance of symptoms such as delusions, hallucinations, disordered thinking and bizarre behaviour constitutes strong evidence for the presence of psychosis (see Figure 12.1). The diagnosis of psychoses is entirely clinical. Despite many indicators of neurobiological dysfunction in psychoses, there are no diagnostic tests except for those disorders where there is a physical cause (see Figure 12.2). Appropriate investigations are needed to exclude organic disorders.

FIGURE 12.1 Symptoms and manifestations of psychoses

1 POSITIVE SYMPTOMS

  (a) Delusions
  (b) Hallucinations
  (c) Formal thought disorder

2 NEGATIVE SYMPTOMS

  (a) Flat effect
  (b) Poverty of thought
  (c) Lack of motivation
  (d) Social withdrawal

3 COGNITIVE SYMPTOMS

  (a) Distractibility
  (b) Impaired working memory
  (c) Impaired executive function

4 MOOD SYMPTOMS

  (a) Depression
  (b) Elevation (mania)

5 ANXIETY/PANIC

6 AGGRESSION/HOSTILITY/SUICIDAL BEHAVIOUR

7 IMPAIRED FUNCTION IN OCCUPATIONAL/SOCIAL ROLES, LOSS OF SKILLS

8 ALCOHOL/DRUG ABUSE OR DEPENDENCE

CLASSIFICATION

A number of disorders are classified as psychoses (see Table 12.1). The DSM-IV[1] disorders and the first seven ICD-10[2] categories of psychoses are broadly equivalent, but the ICD then includes a number of disorders that do not appear in the DSM as discrete entities. Schizophreniform disorder is a schizophrenia-like illness that has been in evidence less than six months.

FIGURE 12.2 Physical (organic) causes of psychosis

- Amphetamines/stimulants
- Hallucinogens
- Cannabis
- Temporal lobe epilepsy
- CNS infections (for example, HIV)
- Huntington's disease
- Cerebral trauma
- Cerebrovascular disease
- Brain tumours
- Cushing's disease, steroids
- Thyrotoxicosis
- Hyperparathyroidism
- Systemic lupus erythematosus
- Wilson's disease

TABLE 12.1 Current major classification of psychoses

DSM-IV	ICD-10
Schizophrenia	Schizophrenia Schizotypal disorder
Schizophreniform disorder	Schizophreniform disorder not otherwise specified
Delusional disorder	Persistent delusional disorders
Brief psychotic disorder	Acute and transient psychotic disorders
Shared psychotic disorder	Induced delusional disorder
Psychotic disorder due to general medical condition	Organic hallucinosis Organic catatonic disorder Organic delusional disorder
Substance induced psychotic disorder	Psychotic disorder due to psychoactive substance abuse
Schizoaffective disorder	Schizoaffective disorder
Psychotic disorder not otherwise specified	Other non-organic psychotic disorders Unspecified non-organic psychosis
Major depression with psychotic features	Severe depressive episode with psychotic symptoms
Bipolar disorder with psychotic features	Mania with psychotic symptoms Bipolar affective disorder with psychotic symptoms

SCHIZOPHRENIA

Schizophrenia is a psychosis that is not due to a mood disorder and that tends to be characterised by the occurrence of positive symptoms initially, and subsequently negative symptoms and cognitive dysfunction. While positive symptoms tend to respond to antipsychotic medication, negative symptoms are associated with serious deterioration in functioning and disability.[3] About a third of patients develop severe treatment resistant illness, characterised by ongoing positive and negative symptoms. Many patients also become depressed. Diagnostic criteria and boundaries of schizophrenia differ between different diagnostic systems: a comparison of the DSM-IV criteria and the ICD-10 is presented in Table 12.2. There are a number of diagnostic systems in use and most patients with a psychosis will have disorders diagnosable within the 'schizophrenia spectrum'.

TABLE 12.2 Comparison of DSM-IV and ICD-10 definitions of schizophrenia

DIAGNOSTIC CRITERIA	DSM-IV	ICD-10
Characteristic symptoms	Delusions, hallucinations, disorganised speech, disorganised or catatonic behaviour, negative symptoms	Thought interference, passivity delusions, hallucinations, thought disorder, catatonic behaviour, negative symptoms, deterioration into self-absorbed behaviour
Duration	6 months	1 month (12 months for simple schizophrenia)
Mood change	Brief periods of mood change only	Schizophrenic symptoms must antedate any mood disorder
Other exclusions	No overt brain disease; not during intoxication or withdrawal	Not due to the direct physiological effects of a substance or a general medical condition

PSYCHOTIC DEPRESSION

A small proportion of patients with major depression develop psychotic symptoms, such as delusions of guilt, poverty and hypochondriasis ('mood congruent' delusions). Hallucinations can also occur, and frequently there is psychomotor agitation and suicidal thinking. About half of these patients eventually develop bipolar mood disorder over the following fifteen years.

BIPOLAR MOOD DISORDER

By definition, bipolar illness requires the occurrence of a manic episode. Characteristic symptoms are elevated and/or irritable mood, hyperactivity, overspending, disinhibited and dangerous behaviours, high energy, lack of need for sleep, grandiosity, pressured speech and flight of ideas. When delusions and/or hallucinations occur, these are typically grandiose or 'mood congruent' in nature. Patients usually recover fully but proceed to have further episodes of depression or mania.[4]

SCHIZOAFFECTIVE DISORDER

Some patients have symptoms of both schizophrenia and bipolar disorder, either simultaneously or in different episodes. On the whole, prognosis is better than schizophrenia but worse than bipolar illness.

DELUSIONAL DISORDERS

This is a group of disorders that are characterised by the occurrence of specific delusions while the personality remains intact and other psychotic symptoms, such as hallucinations and thought disorder, do not occur. Examples include delusional jealousy, erotomania and dysmorphophobia. The disorders can be highly resistant to treatment and also associated with behaviour harmful to others and self.

ORGANIC PSYCHOSES

These are illnesses with a clear physical cause, and can include the dementias, where some patients manifest psychotic symptoms. While uncommon, particularly in younger patients, the possibility of such disorders should be borne in mind, especially as some— for example, Wilson's disease—are highly treatable if detected early.

CLINICAL PERSPECTIVE

A recent Australian study found that 81% of patients with psychosis had seen a GP at least once in the preceding year.[5] Surveys of GPs indicate that most practices see three or four patients with known psychosis, while some GPs with a special interest in mental health see large numbers of patients with psychoses, and often extensively manage the illness without specialist support. Many rural practices provide the sole medical support for these patients.

In addition to bipolar mood disorder, psychotic depression, schizoaffective disorder and delusional disorders, schizophrenia is a major cause of psychoses. Together these illnesses may affect about 5% of the population during their lifetime. Since antipsychotic medications tend to be helpful for psychotic symptoms due to psychotic disorders in general, and the boundaries between the various illnesses are not distinct, many clinicians consider all psychoses to be schizophrenia related disorders.

AETIOLOGY

Schizophrenia remains an idiopathic psychosis. It is well recognised, however, that genetic factors and the occurrence of perinatal complications are risk factors for the development of the illness. First degree relatives of patients with schizophrenia have a ten-fold increase in risk for the disorder. A child with two parents who have schizophrenia has a 40% chance of illness. Twin studies reveal monozygotic concordance of about 53% versus 15% for dizygotic pairs. Therefore, despite the importance of genetic factors, a third of the liability for schizophrenia is attributable to environmental influences, and there may be considerable variability between patients due to illness heterogeneity.

The best established environmental factor in the vulnerability to schizophrenia is the occurrence of obstetric complications, usually involving hypoxia. This association clearly carries the possibility of primary prevention through improved obstetric services. Schizophrenia is also associated with winter birth, suggesting the possibility of a link with intrauterine viral infections such as influenza in the second trimester. The use of cannabis may also be a risk factor, but the most clinically relevant effect of this drug is in worsening the illness course and treatment response of users.

The onset of schizophrenia may be triggered in vulnerable individuals by psychosocial stress and negative life events. At a clinical level, substance and alcohol abuse often appear to play a role in the precipitation of illness. Other patients appear to be using substances for symptom relief. Amphetamines, cocaine, cannabis and hallucinogens have all been linked to psychosis.

Various neuroimaging techniques have made possible studies that have revealed the anatomy of schizophrenia. Temporal lobe abnormalities have been linked to auditory hallucinations. The hippocampus and the basal ganglia have also been implicated in abnormalities of thinking. It is apparent that negative manifestations of schizophrenia constitute a partial frontal lobe syndrome, with amotivation and apathy being characteristic of medial surface lesions. Hypofunctioning of the prefrontal cortex has been consistently demonstrated in schizophrenia.

At a neurochemical level, it has been long understood that dysfunction of dopaminergic mechanisms in the brain is linked to the pathophysiology of schizophrenia—the dopamine hypothesis. This theory emerged from knowledge of the effects of stimulants (which cause psychosis) on dopamine, the postulated mode of action of antipsychosis drugs, the finding of increased dopamine receptors in post-mortem schizophrenic brains as well as endocrine evidence of dopamine D2 receptor overactivity. All effective antipsychosis medications are dopamine D2 receptor antagonists. More recently, evidence concerning the involvement of brain serotonergic and glutaminergic dysfunction in the illness has emerged.

PHASES OF ILLNESS

Psychoses tend to begin with an initial episode that is variably preceded by a prodrome. The illness is usually controlled but, not uncommonly, relapses occur. Treatment may prevent further relapses in a minority of patients, but usually there are recurrent episodes, and symptoms may become increasingly resistant to treatment. About a third of patients develop chronic positive and negative symptoms, and remain severely disabled. Treatment is conveniently divided by illness phase: first episode, relapse prevention, acute relapse and long-term maintenance therapy.

MANAGING FIRST EPISODE PSYCHOSIS

Early detection and treatment of psychoses is likely to improve the long-term outcome for a patient, partly by minimising psychosocial handicaps, but possibly also by inhibiting illness progression. Early or prodromal symptoms of psychosis are given in Figure 12.3.

The principles for management of patients with early psychosis are outlined in Figure 12.4. Most GPs will elect to refer a patient presenting with a first episode of psychosis to specialist services.

FIGURE 12.3 Early or prodromal symptoms of psychosis

- Reduced concentration, attention
- Irritability
- Reduced drive and motivation, anergia
- Social withdrawal
- Depressed mood

- Deterioration in role functioning
- Suspiciousness
- Anxiety
- Sleep disturbance

FIGURE 12.4 Guidelines for management of patients presenting with first episode psychosis

- Assess patient's danger to self and others; determine need for hospitalisation.
- Consider involving specialist treatment options—for example, psychiatrist, crisis outreach community psychiatric service.
- Exclude physical illness and drug related causes.
- Use new generation antipsychotic (see also Chapter 20):
  — risperidone 1 mg nocte increasing to 1 mg bd
  — olanzapine 2.5–10 mg nocte
  — quetiapine 25 mg bd (day 1), 50 mg bd (day 2), 100 mg bd (day 3), 100/200 mg bd (day 4), 200 mg bd (day 5)
  — amisulpride 100 mg bd
  — aripiprazole 10 mg daily
- If no response after two weeks, may need to gradually increase dose over next two weeks:
  — risperidone 2–4 mg
  — olanzapine 10–20 mg
  — quetiapine 400–600 mg
  — amisulpride 800 mg
  — aripiprazole 30 mg
- Monitor for extrapyramidal side effects (EPS), reduce dose if necessary.
- Treat anxiety, agitation and insomnia with diazepam 5–10 mg, repeated as required.
- Provide supportive psychotherapy/crisis intervention (for patient and family), designed for early psychosis.
- After stabilisation, continue out-patient management using pharmacotherapy and individual supportive psychotherapy (including cognitive behavioural therapy) to promote reintegration; family therapy/psychoeducation; and vocational rehabilitation as needed.
- Case management and/or assertive community treatment may be helpful.
- Continue pharmacotherapy for at least one year, and if the patient has been symptom-free over that period, consider a slow discontinuation (over 3–6 months) observing for signs of relapse.

Although specialist services will usually take a leading role in treatment, the GP should continue to see the patient and particularly the family. Apart from providing physical care, the GP may offer family therapy, focusing on psychoeducation about the illness, treatment, problem solving and conflict minimisation. Ensuring that the side effects of medication are minimised and providing supportive psychotherapy with elements of cognitive behavioural therapy will also assist treatment adherence.[6]

MANAGING RELAPSE

REVISITING THE CASE STUDY It is two years since you last saw Justin. He arrives unannounced in your rooms with his distressed parents. They have brought him back from Queensland, where he has been living an isolated existence in a rooming house for the past three months.

Justin's mental health and physical wellbeing have deteriorated markedly. He exhibits florid global symptoms of schizophrenia, hypomania, bizarre somatic concerns and suicidal ideation; and he is in a state of extreme self-neglect. He has received no psychiatric treatment for over a year, and has resumed smoking cannabis.

You recognise that Justin is highly vulnerable to self-harm, and that he is therapeutically inaccessible. As a matter of urgency you decide to involve the emergency outreach team of the local community mental health service in his management. Despite this intervention, Justin is eventually hospitalised as an involuntary patient.

The incidence of relapse following successful treatment of a first episode psychosis is high, and is commonly associated with withdrawal of antipsychotic medication by the patient's treating GP or psychiatrist, or by the patient's non-compliance with prescribed medication. Cannabis use may precipitate a relapse in schizophrenic symptomatology, whether or not the patient continues to adhere to prescribed antipsychotic medication. Apart from alcohol or substance abuse, other causes of relapse include family difficulties and psychosocial stress.

The principles of managing relapse are given in Figure 12.5. It is often possible to manage acute relapse without hospitalisation, especially if community outreach services are available 24 hours a day. Patient outcomes are substantially improved if early warning signs of relapse (usually attenuated symptoms) are recognised by the patient or carers. Careful physical assessment is essential and alcohol/drug abuse may also need to be addressed separately.[7]

As with first episode patients, it is appropriate to use novel antipsychosis medications as treatments of choice due to their favourable side effect and efficacy characteristics. Many patients who relapse due to non-compliance with conventional antipsychotics will find novel medications less unpleasant. Minimising side effects is important for improving treatment adherence. In addition, a reduction in negative symptoms and an improvement in cognition will also enhance drug compliance.

Patients who have experienced more than one episode of illness generally require increased doses of antipsychosis medication in order to control their clinical state. It is also usual for the time it takes the patient to improve to lengthen with each episode until the patient has reached the stable illness phase. The dosage recommendations in Figure 12.5 are therefore approximate, and need to be established individually for each patient.

For many patients, it is essential to plan comprehensive long-term management that will address issues such as the establishment of a social network (which may need to be the community psychiatric service in the first instance), access to financial support, accommodation, assistance with basic living skills, and vocational rehabilitation if possible. The complex mix of services needed usually requires the patient to be supported by a case manager.

FIGURE 12.5 Guidelines for managing acute relapse of psychoses

- Assess danger to self/others and the need for hospitalisation.
- Assess physical state and consider the possibility of substance abuse.
- Consider specialist treatment options—for example, psychiatrist, or involvement of mobile community outreach psychiatric services.
- Antipsychotic medication—new generation medications risperidone, olanzapine, quetiapine:
  — risperidone 1 mg bd, increasing over a few days to 2 mg bd
  — olanzapine 10 mg nocte
  — quetiapine 25 mg bd (day 1), 50 mg bd (day 2), 100 mg bd (day 3), 100 mg mane and 200 mg nocte (day 4), 200 mg bd (day 5)
  — amisulpride 300–400 mg bd
  — aripiprazole 15 mg daily
- If response is inadequate in three weeks, the dose can be increased (unless significant extrapyramidal side effects occur):
  — risperidone to 3 mg bd or 6 mg nocte
  — olanzapine to 20 mg nocte
  — quetiapine 400–750 mg daily
  — amisulpride 400–600 mg bd
  — aripiprazole 20–30 mg daily
- Treat anxiety, agitation and insomnia with short-term diazepam; repeated as required.
- Consider the use of long-acting injectable risperidone if adherence is unlikely, despite psychosocial interventions, or if the patient fails to achieve the optimal response from oral therapy.
- If depression persists, adjunctive antidepressants may be necessary.
- Engage the patient in supportive psychotherapy and case management. Family therapy and cognitive behaviour therapy may also be indicated.
- Consider social interventions—housing options, resources, social supports.
- Evaluate functional status and consider vocational rehabilitation options.

LONG-TERM MANAGEMENT

REVISITING THE CASE STUDY Justin returns to your care three months after his admission to hospital. He was hospitalised for three weeks and then managed as an out-patient at the local community psychiatric centre. You are asked to manage him in collaboration with his psychiatrist, case manager and other allied carers.

He has returned to live with his parents. He no longer uses cannabis or alcohol, but he still smokes cigarettes. His physical health is good, he is eating satisfactorily, sleeping better, and he is no longer moody. However, he is not interested in social activities, and he takes very little exercise. He has no potential to work or study. He has been granted a disability support pension.

His maintenance medication is risperidone long-acting intramuscular injection 25 mg fortnightly, quetiapine 100 mg nocte, valproate 1500 mg nocte and temazepam as needed. Your tasks are to monitor Justin's mental state and particularly his physical condition, as well as to administer the injectable long-acting risperidone. The patient also sees his clinic case manager every three weeks and is reviewed by a psychiatrist every three months.

Perhaps about a third of patients who initially present with psychoses proceed over the next five years to develop chronic illness, where symptoms continue, despite treatment. The principles of long-term management of patients with chronic psychoses are presented in Figure 12.6.

FIGURE 12.6 Guidelines for maintenance therapy of schizophrenia

- Monitor mental state, physical state and substance abuse.
- Observe for medication side effects, depression/suicidality, anxiety/panic.
- Foster therapeutic alliance through supportive psychotherapy.
- Access case management services, behavioural therapies, vocational rehabilitation, housing support options and social interventions as necessary.
- Antipsychotic medication: use new generation medications (risperidone, olanzapine, quetiapine, amisulpride, aripiprazole) at minimal effective dose (which may be less than doses needed for acute treatment).
- For patients who have failed to respond adequately to other antipsychotic medications, use of clozapine may be instituted by a psychiatrist.
- Consider use of long-acting injectable risperidone if psychosocial interventions fail to achieve compliance.
- Treat depression, suicidality, anxiety/panic and substance abuse as necessary.
- Consider indefinite continuation of maintenance therapy for multiple episode patients.

One of the key roles for the GP will be the physical care of patients (see Figure 12.7). If possible, on first contact, a thorough clinical history should be taken, and an on-couch physical examination should be performed. Examination should include an estimation of the Body Mass Index, dental and oral examination, examination for any external evidence of self-harm, and office urinalysis. A plain X-ray of the chest is desirable.

Physical health problems commonly seen in patients with psychosis are obesity, hypertension, diabetes mellitus, electrolytic disturbances (in association with psychogenic polydypsia), disturbed bowel function, dermatoses, tinea pedis, dental caries and poor oral hygiene. Ongoing physical health management must be undertaken in conjunction with psychiatric management, and both require patient cooperation, which may be difficult to obtain to an optimal degree.[6]

Patients with schizophrenia and schizophrenia-like psychoses often seem to ignore, or have a high threshold of tolerance to, physical discomfort, and may not volunteer significant symptoms of physical ill health. On the other hand, they may present with delusional somatic symptomatology, sometimes necessitating multiple and repetitive investigations.

There are many tasks and issues for the GP managing a patient with psychoses. These can include the following.

- Address the patient's poor compliance with treatment. This can be due to grandiosity, deficient insight into presence of illness and need for treatment, intolerable side effects, poor motivation, cost, disorganisation and peer pressure. Strategies include

FIGURE 12.7 Physical monitoring of patients with psychoses

BASELINE EVALUATION

1 Physical examination: general examination, including cardiovascular (looking for evidence of arrhythmias and ischaemic heart disease), neurological (tardive dyskinesia), fundoscopic exam through undilated pupil (lens opacities) and weight
2 Calculate Body Mass Index (BMI): weight in kilograms divided by height in metres squared (x kg/x m^2)
3 Random blood glucose—baseline needed due to subsequent increased diabetes risk with some atypical antipsychotics
4 Lipids—increased risk of cardiovascular disorders
5 B12 and folate
6 Calcium, phosphate
7 Full blood examination, erythrocyte sedimentation rate (ESR)
8 Urinary drug screen—looking for illicit drugs, alcohol, benzodiazepines
9 Liver function tests—alcohol, medication effects
10 Prolactin
11 Chest X-ray

SIX MONTHLY INVESTIGATIONS (UNLESS SPECIAL RISK IN PATIENT OR DRUG TREATMENT)

1 Fasting blood glucose
2 Fasting lipids
3 Full blood examination, ESR
4 Liver function test
5 Thyroid function tests
6 Urea and electrolytes
7 ECG—cardiovascular risk and QTc effects of some therapies
8 Urinary drug screen—regularly if there is indicative history
9 Other investigations as appropriate (for example, Pap smear)

adjusting medication for optimal illness control, psychoeducation for patient and carers about the illness and its management, minimising the side effects of treatment, cognitive behavioural therapy and family therapy.

■ Assess the use of long-acting, injectable antipsychotic medication that can assist compliance. Conventional depots cause high rates of extrapyramidal side effects, and risperidone injection is now preferred. Close liaison between the GP and a psychiatrist to plan the treatment is necessary.

■ Re-evaluate the efficacy of existing psychopharmacological treatment and, when necessary (usually in collaboration with the patient's psychiatrist), adjust the current dose schedule or change the medication.

■ Recognise and respond to the side effects of the prescribed antipsychotic medication, particularly akathisia and tardive dyskinesia. Other problems include anticholinergic effects, sedation, postural hypotension, weight gain and hyperprolactinaemia.

■ Identify and therapeutically respond to symptomatology indicative of comorbid psychological disturbances, such as mood instability, irritability, agitation, anxiety, depression, phobic disorders, somatic delusions and insomnia.

- Recognise and address issues arising from substance abuse, such as nicotine, alcohol, cannabis, amphetamine and opiates. Referral to specialist services may help.
- Make the appropriate specialist psychiatrist referral when deterioration in the patient's psychosis occurs, evidenced by worsening psychotic symptomatology, or symptoms suggestive of self-harm or harm to others.
- Encourage and facilitate engagement with case managers and other community based carers. Good communication between you and the mental health services will enable a collaborative agreement between the service and yourself. This agreement should specify the roles of each party, timelines for intervention and a contingency plan in event of a crisis. The patient and carers should participate in any such agreement.
- Report to the psychiatrist: at times the collaborative care arrangements for the patient in the community are mandated by a legal order. The GP may then have reporting obligations to the legally authorised psychiatrist to ensure follow-up occurs appropriately.
- Detect any substance abuse and dependence that will greatly worsen outcomes for the patient.
- Recognise that although implementing treatment strategies is usually difficult, it is also vital. Optimal control of psychosis is the aim, and referral to specialist services may be necessary.
- Liaise with and, if possible, re-link the patient with their family, close friends or associates to help address a patient's social isolation.
- Assess and address the patient's welfare needs: housing, nutrition, clothing, personal hygiene, physical exercise, social and recreational interests and outlets, interpersonal relationships, and dental and foot care are especially relevant and important.
- Deal appropriately with language and cultural issues that may hinder diagnosis and management.
- Educate the patient about the nature of psychosis, and the patient's need for continuing and long-lasting care and self-care.
- Ensure continuity of care when the patient undertakes management with another GP.

CONCLUSION

The treatment of a patient with psychosis presents the GP with multiple challenges. There is the need for early detection as well as maximum effort to facilitate recovery. Subsequent to detection, relapse prevention assumes top priority. For patients who have developed chronic illness, optimal control of the illness rather than cure becomes the aim of management.

The GP needs to be committed to the long-term treatment of a patient; to be prepared to accept and respond caringly to patient irrationality, negativity, apathy, hostility and rejection; and to have a realistic expectation of the limitations in treatment outcomes.

Psychopharmacology, although often spectacularly beneficial in its clinical effects, does neither address nor resolve the totality of lifestyle and social problems that can beset the patient with psychosis.

Collaborative care, involving the GP and other health and welfare providers in the field of community psychiatry, is an essential and indispensable aspect of the management of a patient with psychosis.

REFERENCES

1. American Psychiatric Association. Diagnostic and Statistical Manual of Mental Disorders. 4th edn. Washington DC: American Psychiatric Association, 2000.
2. World Health Organization. The ICD-10 Classification of Mental and Behavioural Disorders. Geneva: WHO, 1992.
3. Blashki G, Keks N, Stocky A, Hocking B. Managing schizophrenia in general practice. Australian Family Physician 2004;33(4):221–7.
4. Joyce PR, Mitchell PB. Mood Disorders: Recognition and Treatment. Sydney: UNSW Press, 2004.
5. Jablensky A, McGrath J, Herman H, Castle D, Gureje O, Morgan V, Korten A. National Survey of Health and Wellbeing. Report 4. People Living with Psychotic Illness: An Australian Study 1997–1998. Canberra: Commonwealth Department of Health and Aged Care, 1999.
6. Keks N, Stocky A, Aufgang M, Blashki G. Managing Schizophrenia. A Guide For General Practice in Australia. Sydney: PharmaGuide, 2003.
7. RANZCP Clinical Practice Guidelines Team for the Treatment of Schizophrenia and Related Disorders. RANZCP clinical practice guidelines for the treatment of schizophrenia and related disorders. Australian and New Zealand Journal of Psychiatry 2005;39:1–30.

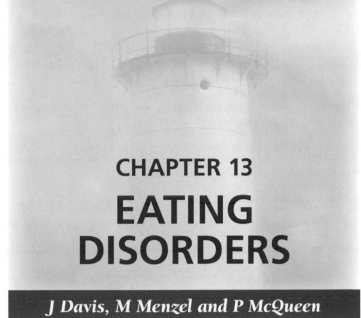

CHAPTER 13
EATING DISORDERS

J Davis, M Menzel and P McQueen

What is food to one, is to others bitter poison.

LUCRETIUS, 99–55 BC

CASE STUDY

Sally is a 17-year-old girl in year 12. Accompanied by her worried mother, she is reluctant to see you. Her mother is concerned because Sally has lost weight and 'is not eating enough and has become vegetarian'. Her mother says Sally has become withdrawn and irritable. When interviewed alone, Sally reports that she is stressed about her study and worries that her marks will not be high enough to allow her to study medicine. She started a low carbohydrate diet and exercise regimen several months ago to get 'fitter and healthier'. She stopped eating meat and 'junk food' because they were 'fattening'. She has lost 8 kg over six months and her Body Mass Index (BMI) is 17. She says she is fat and needs to lose more weight. She denies bingeing, vomiting or using laxatives or diuretics. She runs 5 km every day to help her lose weight. Her periods have become lighter and irregular.

KEY FACTS

- Eating disorders must be differentiated from the common dieting and weight reduction behaviours in the community.

- Alongside diabetes and obesity, anorexia nervosa is one of the most serious chronic diseases of adolescent girls and young women in developed countries.

- Eating disorders have medical complications that require the attention of the general practitioner (GP).

---

continued overleaf

KEY FACTS *continued*

■ Comorbid depression, anxiety and substance abuse are common.

■ Biological (especially genetic), psychological, social and cultural factors are important in the development of eating disorders.

■ These disorders often follow a relapsing and remitting or chronic course.

■ Treatment requires a multidisciplinary approach.

■ A GP should always be involved in management.

■ The mortality rate from anorexia nervosa in the long term is about 20%.

■ Early intervention is essential before behaviours become entrenched and physical problems severe.

INTRODUCTION

Eating disorders are often thought to be a twentieth century Western phenomenon. This is not so: patients with features consistent with anorexia nervosa have been described for over a thousand years. Early descriptions are found in religious literature, and case examples of anorexia nervosa were described but not named by physicians in the seventeenth century. In the nineteenth century, two physicians, William Gull[1] and Charles Lasegue,[2] independently described cases of the disorder and coined the term 'anorexia nervosa'.

Bulimia nervosa was identified and described as a distinct disorder by Gerald Russell in 1979.[3] However, historical texts clearly document cases of rapid ingestion of food, secret eating, bingeing and vomiting occurring prior to the nineteenth century.

It is stated that 5% of women registered with a GP have an eating disorder, with most patients presenting with potential or partial syndromes.

CLASSIFICATION

Anorexia nervosa (AN) and bulimia nervosa (BN) are generally grouped together as eating disorders. In addition, a variety of other disorders, characterised by disturbances in eating behaviour and associated with psychological or behavioural syndromes, may be included in the category of eating disorders (see Table 13.1). It should be noted that obesity is generally regarded as a medical condition rather than a psychiatric disorder.

EPIDEMIOLOGY

Eating disorders are most common among females in late adolescence and early adulthood. The female to male ratio is approximately 10:1.[4] The diagnosis of AN may be missed more often in males, where there is no obvious marker such as cessation of menstruation. BN is more common than AN. Among adolescent and young adult females, BN affects 1–4% and AN 0.5–1%.[5] Notably, there appears to be an increase in the prevalence of eating disorders in the last 50–60 years.[6]

TABLE 13.1 Current major classifications of eating disorders

DSM-IV	ICD-10
Anorexia nervosa	■ Anorexia nervosa
Bulimia nervosa	■ Bulimia nervosa
Eating disorder not otherwise specified (EDNOS)	■ Atypical anorexia nervosa ■ Atypical bulimia nervosa
	■ Overeating associated with other psychological disturbances ■ Vomiting associated with other psychological disturbances ■ Other eating disorders — Pica of non-organic origin — Psychogenic loss of appetite ■ Eating disorder, unspecified

AETIOLOGY

In common with most psychiatric disorders, eating disorders are currently regarded as involving sociocultural, biological and psychological factors in their causation

SOCIOCULTURAL FACTORS

In the 1980s, eating disorders were widely regarded as an extreme manifestation of society's obsession with thinness. Eating disorders are well described in affluent Western cultures, and there are several studies showing that individuals from poor countries who are transposed to Western societies are at increased risk of an eating disorder compared with their cohorts who remained in their countries of origin.[7] There are groups of people—such as gymnasts, ballet dancers, elite athletes and models—known to be at high risk of eating disorders.[4]

In the 1990s, causality has focused more on gender dynamics, and subsequently there has been an interest in worldwide cultural dynamics, including cultures in transition and confused gender identities. However, the contribution of these sociocultural factors must be re-evaluated in the light of our increasing knowledge of the genetic contribution to the development of these disorders.

BIOLOGICAL FACTORS

The starvation studies conducted in America on service personnel in the 1950s[8] demonstrated that excessive dieting leads to distortion of body image, preoccupation with food and further dieting behaviours—a vicious cycle.

Exciting developments in the area of epidemiological and genetic studies have occurred in the last decade. Previous theories of the development of eating disorders, in particular AN, gave little credence to the possibility of a biological contribution, despite animal models showing eating disorder behaviours to be present in animals with various types of hypothalamic lesions.

Family studies have shown that AN runs in families, with a first degree relative of an affected individual at an increased risk of developing AN by a factor of up to 12.[9] This is comparable to the risk for first degree relatives shown in family studies of schizophrenia and bipolar affective disorder.

Twin studies have led to a dramatic re-evaluation of the long-standing emphasis on the social and cultural explanations of eating disorders. Bulik and colleagues[10, 11] have demonstrated that many traits related to eating disorders—including binge eating, self-induced vomiting, the drive for thinness and dietary restraint—have a heritable component. It is postulated that additive multiple gene effects may be operative in about half of all cases of AN and BN.

Contrary to previously held views, twin studies have shown common or shared environmental factors, reflecting that cultural and social drivers appear less significant in causation. However, individual lifestyle factors contribute about one-quarter of the heritability of these disorders.[12]

These are important new findings, as they point to these disorders being complex in their causation and not just the result of social conditioning. Further gene linkage studies are trying to determine what gene loci and chromosomes may be operative.

PSYCHOLOGICAL FACTORS

Almost without exception, persons with AN are obsessional in character, with perfectionist personality traits often associated with a compulsion to succeed at all things in life. Childhood striving and perfectionism, antedating the development of AN by several years, is often seen.[13] Compulsivity and obsessionality have been linked to restricting AN sub-types, whereas novelty-seeking personality characteristics have been linked to bingeing. Individuals with both AN and BN show features of high harm avoidance in their personality construct.[14]

It is possible that the genetic predisposition, as already described, may be manifested in part or whole through the development of the various personality constructs, which then leads to eating disorder behaviours. The biological and psychological risk factors may prime a person to develop an eating disorder in response to stress or sociocultural changes or challenges.

In the past families, and in particular mothers, were blamed for these disorders, leading to much apprehension about seeking help and much anger within the family towards the individual or to those who felt responsible. Like most other psychiatric disorders, these disorders are complex, with many operative factors. This highlights the fact that there will not be one particular treatment strategy available for eating disorder sufferers, and that a treatment plan addressing all the possible factors in the causation, overseen and monitored by the GP, is essential.

CLINICAL FEATURES AND COURSE

There is still some dispute over what exactly constitutes the syndromes of AN and BN. In addition, the syndromes can overlap at any one time or over the longitudinal course, and progression from one to the other is common.

ANOREXIA NERVOSA

The key features of AN are behaviours that wilfully lead to excessive weight loss associated with a refusal to maintain body weight at a healthy level (that is, body weight is 15% or more below standard weight for height tables). An intense fear of putting on weight, despite objective evidence of emaciation, is combined with a disturbance in the way body weight or shape is subjectively experienced. In those patients who have commenced menstruation, amenorrhoea for at least three consecutive menstrual cycles, reflecting hypothalamic pituitary dysfunction, is also required to make the diagnosis of classical AN. In clinical practice, the BMI (weight (kg)/[height (m)]^2) is used for assessment and monitoring. BMIs of less than 17 indicate a risk situation of emaciation.

The DSM-IV describes two sub-types, depending on which behaviours are engaged in to maintain the weight loss: the restricting type, where the person restricts food as the predominant means of weight loss; and the binge eating/purging type, where the person regularly engages in self-induced vomiting or the misuse of laxatives, diuretics or enemas, while also having features of AN.[5]

The average duration of AN is somewhere between 7 and 10 years. A full spectrum of outcomes is seen. Approximately one-quarter to one-third fully recover, usually after a period of several years. Approximately one-quarter develop a chronic refractory illness with associated significant medical comorbidity. The other 50% show a relapsing and remitting course or improvement, but not full recovery. It is important to note that development of solid lung tumours from excessive smoking is seen at an alarming rate in chronic AN cases in patients over the age of 40. Despite the presence of an illness that is potentially so incapacitating, the vast majority of patients manage to function reasonably well in social and work settings, with the exception of those who are severely chronic and refractory.

In Western countries, alongside diabetes mellitus and asthma, AN is the most serious chronic illness affecting adolescent females. Long-term studies have shown a mortality rate of 20%.[15] While studies show that many patients with AN will die from the complications of the disorder itself, it is important to note that the risk of suicide in this group is high.

BULIMIA NERVOSA

The key features of BN are: episodes of binge eating (that is, eating in a discrete period of time an amount of food that is definitely larger than most individuals would eat under similar circumstances); and inappropriate compensatory behaviour, such as self-induced vomiting, excessive exercise, and misuse of laxatives, diuretics and enemas. An essential aspect, which can lead to a diagnosis of BN, is the feeling of loss of control during the binge-eating episode and that self-esteem and self-worth are linked to body shape and weight. It is important to realise that the vast majority of bulimic patients do not have significant weight loss or if there is weight loss, it is of mild degree.

The DSM-IV describes two sub-types—purging and non-purging—depending on the presence or absence of the regular use of purging methods as a means to compensate for the binge eating.[5]

Like AN, BN usually begins in late adolescence or early adult life. Prolonged dieting behaviours often precede the development of binge vomiting (bulimia). Treatment generally requires several years, with about 50% of diagnosed cases recovering after 5–10 years. Approximately a quarter of patients may show earlier improvement, but of concern is the 25% who proceed to a more chronic course. Relapse is common, with a third to a half of those who have recovered from BN relapsing at some stage in the future. The mortality rate for BN is much lower than that of AN, with rates between 0 and 3% being reported in the literature.[16]

EATING DISORDERS NOT OTHERWISE SPECIFIED

This category, ENDOS, describes a range of variants that are frequently seen in clinical practice. These may include women who have:

- all the features of AN but still have regular menses;
- typical but infrequent episodes of binge eating and inappropriate compensatory behaviours;
- all of the features of AN but current weight in the normal range; or
- recurrent episodes of binge eating without regular use of inappropriate compensatory behaviours.

COMPLICATIONS OF EATING DISORDERS

Eating disorders may result in a variety of secondary problems. These include medical comorbidity and secondary psychological and social problems. The severity of complications will depend on the duration and severity of the eating disorder.

Figure 13.1 lists the main physiological, psychological and social effects of AN. Some of these complications, particularly electrolyte and gastrointestinal problems, will also be seen in BN.

It is perplexing for GPs that patients with AN see themselves as overweight when everyone else sees them as being emaciated. This perceptual distortion (one of the cognitive complications) is not demonstrated in the anorexic patient's assessment of other persons' weight and shape. It is important to note that the cognitive deficits improve once refeeding is established.

As shown, depression, anxiety and substance abuse are recognised complications of eating disorders. Depression and anxiety are reported in approximately 50% of eating disorder sufferers.[17] It is also important to note that in these patients substance abuse may include abuse of prescription medication.

As indicated above, a variety of eating related behaviours are associated with AN; these are listed in Figure 13.2.

Family relationships are usually significantly disturbed, with parents feeling alienated, frustrated and helpless. The family coping and attributional style that has been described in the literature in the past as contributing to AN is probably more the result of families coming to grips with this problem than being an antecedent cause. Frustration and intolerance frequently develop, and it is not uncommon for all family problems to be displaced onto the patient. It is also not unusual for frustration to boil over onto those who are trying to assist the patient.

FIGURE 13.1 Physiological, psychological and social complications of eating disorders

PHYSIOLOGICAL EFFECTS

These may result from a combination of emaciation, electrolyte imbalance (from vomiting and laxative abuse) and dehydration.

Cardiovascular
- Hypotension, arrythmias (brady/tachycardias, ectopics), ECG changes (prolonged QT interval, T and U wave changes)
- Cardiac arrest
- Heart failure and oedema

Renal
- Renal failure
- Electrolyte anomalies

Endocrine
- Amennorhoea
- 'Sick euthyroid syndrome' (low TSH, T3 and T4)
- Low testosterone levels (males)
- Loss of libido
- Hypercortisolaemia

Gastrointestinal
- Tooth enamel destruction
- Nausea, abdominal pains, bloating, constipation
- Enlarged parotid glands
- Sore throat/dysphagia
- Dyspepsia/oesophageal and peptic ulcers
- Oesophageal perforation (vomiting)

Haematological
- Anaemia, neutropenia, pancytopenia
- Low transferrin, iron, B12, folate

Neurological
- Cramps and paraesthesiae (low calcium)
- Peripheral neuropathy
- Cerebral atrophic changes

Skeletal
- Osteopenia, osteoporosis, pathological fractures

Metabolic
- Hypokalaemia, hyponatraemia
- Metabolic hypokalaemic alkalosis (vomiting)
- Low zinc, magnesium

continued overleaf

FIGURE 13.1 *continued*

Dermatological
- Dry skin, alopecia, carotenedermia, lanugo hair

PSYCHOLOGICAL EFFECTS

Cognitive effects
- Impaired concentration, poor memory
- Obsessional thinking
- Impaired judgment and problem-solving ability
- Perceptual distortions

Personal and behavioural effects
- Heightened personality characteristics (for example, increased perfectionism)
- Feelings of inadequacy
- Increased low self-esteem
- Eating related behaviours (see Figure 13.2)
- Psychiatric complications—depression, anxiety, substance abuse
- Self-harming behaviours (particularly BN), suicide attempts

SOCIAL EFFECTS

- Withdrawal and isolation
- Interpersonal difficulties, especially with family
- Reduced sexual interests/relationships
- Development of interests relating to food

FIGURE 13.2 Eating related behaviours associated with anorexia nervosa

- Refusal to eat
- Measurement of food quantities
- Minimal conversation at meals
- Eating slowly/quickly
- Difficulty choosing foods
- Excessive use of condiments
- Using inappropriate utensils
- Fussiness about food
- Desire to talk about food frequently
- Excessive interest in recipes/cooking
- Pushing food around plate or 'playing' with food
- Claiming to dislike or react to feared foods
- Feeling full after eating small amount
- Obsessional calorie counting
- Reluctance to eat with others
- Eating different food from family
- Cutting food into tiny pieces
- Excessive water consumption
- Unusual food combinations
- Eating food in a specific sequence
- Excessive use of diet food
- Excessive handling of food
- Leaving table frequently during meals
- Secretly disposing of food during meal
- Excessive interest in what others are eating

Source: Treatment Protocol Project, 2000.[18]

PRESENTATION IN GENERAL PRACTICE

Patients with eating disorders rarely present to a general practice complaining of this problem. Parents, partners and friends are often not aware of the behaviours characteristic of AN and BN patients. For example, it is not uncommon for bulimic patients to engage in binge vomiting episodes for years before others become aware of them. AN may be more obvious to families because of the preoccupation and rituals associated with food preparation and eating and also the excessive exercising; ultimately, the loss of weight becomes manifest.

Common modes of presentation to the GP include:

- symptoms of depression and/or anxiety;
- concern at the loss of control associated with binge vomiting episodes;
- seeking benzodiazepines to deal with anxiety or to minimise the effects of withdrawal from comorbid illicit substance dependence;
- requests for laxatives or appetite suppressants;
- feelings of nausea, bloating, flatulence, vomiting and constipation (such gastrointestinal complaints voiced to a concerned parent may elicit consultation with a GP);
- nicotine dependence (in chronic cases the pulmonary complications of chronic obstructive airways disease, recurring bronchitis and pneumonia may occur; in older AN patients who smoke the possibility of solid lung tumours must always be considered, as this is a significant cause of mortality in this group);
- physical damage from excessive exercise in more severe cases of AN; and
- stress fractures and bone pain in the significantly malnourished.

In both AN and BN, the most dramatic presentations will be when an emergency supervenes from the medical complications of these disorders—for example:

- Dehydration may cause postural hypotension, with giddiness and feelings of collapse.
- Electrolyte anomalies may predispose to cardiac arrhythmias, which may produce palpitations, weakness or syncopal episodes.
- Chronic tiredness and weakness from anaemia, dehydration, hypokalaemia or endocrine disturbance may occur.
- Oesophageal and gastric erosions producing haematemesis or acute perforation of the oesophageus may occur.
- In AN, occult infection, including septicaemia, can occur without significant fever and may underlie profound tiredness, exhaustion, physical weakness or collapse.
- In AN, the patient may experience shortness of breath from pleural or pericardial effusions or complain of development of oedema.
- Finally, family discord associated with dealing with a child with AN may be the reason why the GP becomes involved. Often families live with these problems for a considerable period of time before they seek help. By this time, family dynamics have been significantly altered, with much frustration and blaming occurring. The GP may be consulted to try and deal with the disturbed family harmony and interpersonal functioning.

ASSESSMENT BY THE GP

The assessment of a person suspected of AN will usually depend upon the presenting complaint. For example, if the initial presentation is for weight loss, then most GPs will have their own checklist for excluding organic causes of weight loss. The following need to be assessed for exclusion:

- bowel disease (for example, Crohn's disease, coeliac disease, ulcerative colitis)
- infectious diseases (for example, HIV)
- endocrine disturbances (for example, diabetes, thyroid disease)
- Addison's disease
- malignant tumours (for example, lymphomas, kidney tumours, brain tumours)
- autoimmune diseases (for example, rheumatoid arthritis)
- liver and kidney disease—hepatitis B and C
- recurring urinary tract infection

Psychological causes of weight loss include depression, anxiety and substance abuse.

The diagnosis of an eating disorder is made when physical and other psychiatric possibilities are excluded and the person fulfils the criteria for an eating disorder already outlined. It is important that adequate consultation with the patient and possibly other corroborative sources, including family, occurs.

The following questions may assist in assessing a patient for an eating disorder:

- Are you happy with the way you look?
- Do you obsess over certain foods or your body weight?
- Are you always on a diet?
- Do you agree that the whole Western world seems obsessed with diets and weight loss?
- Do you compare yourself to others a lot?
- Are you happy to eat with other people—family, friends—at restaurants?
- Do you prepare all your own food?
- Do you read lots of diet books, recipe books or beauty magazines?
- Do you check all food labels?
- How long does it take to do your food shopping?
- Do you exercise every day?
- Do you sometimes feel so anxious or bloated that you vomit or take laxatives?

INVESTIGATIONS FOR EATING DISORDERS

Based upon the clinical assessment, the GP will order specific tests to assist in diagnosis (for example, to exclude organic causes of weight loss) and detect physical complications. Even in clinically mild cases of AN, abnormalities in blood chemistry may occur, and conversely, in moderate or severe cases blood chemistry may be normal. The possible investigations for an eating disorder are listed in Table 13.2.

It goes without saying that an estimation of BMI is an essential part of the initial assessment and monitoring of patients with AN. A BMI under 17 indicates significant undernutrition, and lower levels may indicate the need for hospitalisation. Remember to

TABLE 13.2 Investigations for eating disorders

INVESTIGATION	LIKELY ABNORMALITY	ACTION
Full blood count	Low haemoglobin	Refeed, consider iron supplements
	Low white cell count	Refeed, monitor if below 2000/mm^3. Consider admission for haematological investigation and refeeding
	Low platelet count	Refeed, monitor
Biochemistry	Uraemia	Refeed, monitor. Check fluid intake, creatinine and creatinine clearance
	Hypokalaemia	Refeed, monitor. Consider potassium supplements. If below 3.0 mmol/l, consider admission for bed rest and refeeding
	Hypophosphataemia	Unlikely to be a problem with gradual refeeding, but monitor if admitted for high-calorie diet, and consider oral supplementation if levels are severely depressed
	Hypomagnesaemia	Refeed. Supplement if refractory hypocalcaemia or hypokalaemia present
	Low D12 and folate	Exclude pernicious anaemia or malabsorption; folate and B12 supplementation
	Low zinc	Zinc supplementation
	Abnormal iron studies	Check for gastrointestinal blood loss, exclude iron storage diseases or bone marrow problems; iron supplementation
	Low creatinine clearance	Refeed, monitor
	Hypoproteinaemia	Refeed, monitor. If present with marked oedema, admit for refeeding or intravenous protein replacement in an emergency
	Raised creatinine kinase	May be an indication of severe starvation and autodigestion of cardiac and skeletal muscle (measure cardiac and skeletal muscle fractions)
Urinalysis	Proteinuria	Monitor. If severe or chronic, consider referral to renal physician

continued overleaf

TABLE 13.2 *continued*		
INVESTIGATION	**LIKELY ABNORMALITY**	**ACTION**
Electrocardiograph	Bradycardia	Refeed, monitor. If hypotension present, consider bed rest and elevation
	Prolonged QT interval	Consider admission for refeeding and cardiac monitoring
	Other arrhythmias	Refeed, monitor. If symptomatic, admit for refeeding and cardiac monitoring
T3, T4, TSH	Low T3	Refeed, monitor. Thyroid supplements not indicated
Bone density scan	Low	Exclude metabolic bone disease. Refeed, monitor. If below 0.8g/cm^3, caution against strenuous exercise. Consider calcium supplements and/or oestrogen replacement

Source: Modified from Freeman, 1995.[16]

weigh the person (after voiding), if possible stripped to their underwear. AN patients are very good at water loading to put on some weight before the weighing occurs. Or they may wear baggy and loose clothing, not only to conceal their change in body habitus but also to conceal the carrying of weights of various sorts.

REVISITING THE CASE STUDY

Sally denies there is a problem and resents her mother for 'making her' attend the appointment. The GP is empathic in approach and is careful not to be authoritarian or judgmental.

The GP does the following:

- weighs Sally and shows her a BMI chart to demonstrate that she falls on the edge of 'very underweight' and AN categories;
- explains to Sally and her mother that there are physical problems that can occur at this weight and therefore tests will need to be done;
- explains that even if Sally does not want help, she needs to come back in a week to get the test results;
- informs them of the need for a hospital admission if her weight gets too low;
- explains the effects of starvation—for example, poor concentration and mood lability and how this will affect her study;
- stresses the importance of a balanced diet while acknowledging that eating is difficult for Sally;
- stresses the importance of no more weight loss, but stabilisation, before insisting on weight gain;
- gives them written information on eating disorders and healthy eating; and
- makes an appointment for a week's time.

MANAGEMENT

If a diagnosis of an eating disorder of significant severity is established, a multidisciplinary team will be required for managing the medical, nutritional/dietary and psychological issues.

Medical stabilisation and monitoring are an important part of patient management. All patients require thorough medical assessment to identify any medical complications. Patients with significant medical complications may require hospitalisation, including refeeding. The assistance of a gastroenterologist should be sought when refeeding because of the risk of hypophosphataemia developing. This can result in death (refeeding syndrome). Significant metabolic and electrolyte abnormalities, dehydration, syncopal episodes and cardiac arrythmias will usually require hospitalisation for management. Once the patient is stabilised, ongoing monitoring by the GP is essential.

Admission to a psychiatric inpatient service is required for severe depression and/or anxiety, significant self-harm or suicide attempts, or when out-patient treatment of AN has failed and the BMI is falling (<16). Liaison between the GP, inpatient medical staff and mental health professionals is essential for the development of a comprehensive treatment plan.

Most patients with eating disorders are managed in the community. The GP is vital in co-ordinating various professionals (for example, psychiatrist, dietician, physician) and in delivering psychological therapy and psychoeducation. The GP's role also includes monitoring the eating disorder, conducting surveillance for complications and treating or detecting psychiatric comorbidities. Specific areas of management for the GP include:

- psychoeducation about the disorder and the effects of starvation;
- nutritional education, development of a balanced meal plan and dietary monitoring provided by a dietician with expertise in eating disorders (a target weight and expected weekly weight gain should be agreed by both the dietician and the GP, who will usually monitor the expected weight gain);
- psychological treatment, usually necessary for recovery except in mild, uncomplicated cases. Common modalities are cognitive behavioural therapy (see Chapter 17), interpersonal therapy (see Chapter 17) and psychodynamic therapy. The efficacy of cognitive behavioural therapy and interpersonal therapy for BN is well established, and evidence is mounting for their application to AN.[19] Group therapy is particularly effective for BN[20] (and is likely to be effective for adults with AN). Psychological therapies for more severe cases are probably best undertaken by psychologists, psychiatrists or GPs who have undertaken specific training;
- family therapy, which should be the first priority for adolescents. The gold standard model of family therapy for AN that has been shown to be efficacious is that produced by specialists at the Maudsley hospital in London;[21] and
- medication, which may be indicated for comorbid depression or anxiety. It's worth noting that no drug has been found to be efficacious for AN. However, fluoxetine has been shown to produce a short-term reduction in bulimic symptoms.[22]

Other management strategies the GP may employ include motivational interviewing (see Chapter 10) and focused psychological strategies (for example, relaxation, self-monitoring, stress management, problem solving—see Chapter 17), guided self-help and general supportive psychotherapy. Liaison with a psychologist will be helpful in delivering this area of management.

The GP should act as case manager, and in undertaking this role, they must clearly identify for the patient and the family who is the point of contact for information and liaison with other health professionals involved in the case.

The patient may need to be referred to a specialist mental health service or private practitioner if:

- there is diagnostic uncertainty;
- he or she fails to respond to treatment;
- medical treatment is complicated by side effects or the development of significant complications;
- assessment and advice on management of comorbid problems (for example, depression, anxiety, substance abuse) is required;
- nutritional assessment and recommendations from a dietician (for example, meal planning for weight restoration) is required; and
- if individual and/or family psychotherapy is required.

LONG-TERM MANAGEMENT

Eating disorders are commonly chronic conditions. Patients are likely to experience exacerbations at times of stress, including significant life events (for example, pregnancy) or if they develop comorbid psychiatric problems. Eating disorder sufferers frequently exhibit features of other eating disorder problems over the longitudinal course. Thus, management needs to be flexible and reviewed frequently, and to continue for the long term. Chronic illness is associated with increased medical and psychiatric morbidity and higher risk of mortality.

REVISITING THE CASE STUDY

During Sally's second visit, the GP asks her what she thinks about the information she was given, and checks how her eating has been in the past week. She says she has had a look at the information but does not think she has an eating disorder. She has continued to restrict her food intake. The GP weighs her. She has lost 300 g. The GP reiterates the consequences of continued weight loss and suggests referral for out-patient treatment. He explains the importance of regular consultations with the GP for monitoring potential medical problems, even if she does not want dietary or psychological help. They negotiate how Sally will get to appointments (with Mum, Mum to drop off or alone); the GP encourages independence but stresses the importance of her getting to appointments. Sally is reluctant to see a therapist and does not think she needs to see a dietician, but agrees it would be better than going to hospital.

After the assessment is completed, the GP informs Sally and her family that co-ordination of treatment will be conducted by the GP and that a clinical psychologist, dietician and family therapist will be involved in ongoing management. A written management plan is developed and agreed to by Sally and her parents, and it is signed by all parties. The members of the treating team will keep each other informed of Sally's progress or of any problems on a regular basis.

Sally sees a dietician once a month for help with developing a balanced meal plan to maintain her at a healthy weight, and for education about nutrition and weight recovery.

Sally sees a clinical psychologist for cognitive behavioural therapy an hour a week. Each week she is given tasks to complete at home, such as monitoring her thoughts (in a diary), introducing new foods, modifying her eating behaviours, engaging in social activities and modifying how she relates to others. She learns to challenge her negative thoughts about food, body and self through cognitive restructuring. She is guided through a graduated behavioural change regimen to normalise her eating and exercise patterns. She learns relaxation strategies to help her cope with the anxiety associated with eating and weight gain and her studies. She also learns to express her feelings and assert her needs to others. Once she has normalised her eating and exercise patterns and established and maintained a healthy weight, the frequency of sessions is reduced to monthly. She learns how to identify early warning signs of relapse, and agrees to consult her GP and request a booster session with her psychologist.

Sally and her family see a family therapist once a month. They learn to appreciate each other's perspective on the illness, and work towards fostering recovery and improving communication within the family.

Sally sees her GP monthly to monitor her weight, blood pressure and pulse rate, state of hydration and medical complications. Regular blood tests for assessing known complications are conducted.

CONCLUSION

Eating disorders are common, and most GPs are likely to be required to assess and/or manage these patients. Early detection and effective treatment, preferably involving a multidisciplinary team, are required to treat the multiple short- and long-term problems that occur in individuals with an eating disorder.

RESOURCES

INFORMATION FOR HEALTH PRACTITIONERS

ANZAED Clinical Practice Guidelines for Anorexia Nervosa, downloadable from
www.cedd.org.au/cpg/cpg_guid.html

New South Wales Centre for Eating & Dieting Disorders (CEDD)
www.cedd.org.au
email: info@cedd.org.au

Victorian Centre of Excellence in Eating Disorders (CEED)
www.ceed.org.au
email: ceed@mh.org.au

TEXTBOOKS AND TREATMENT MANUALS

Brownell KD, Fairburn CG. Eating Disorders and Obesity: A Comprehensive Handbook. New York: Guilford, 1995.

Freeman C. Eating Disorders: A Guide for Primary Care. Edinburgh: Cullen Centre, Royal Edinburgh Hospital, 1995.

Garner DM, Garfinkel PE. Handbook of Treatment for Eating Disorders. 2nd edn. New York: Guilford, 1997.

Jacob F. Solution Focussed Recovery from Eating Distress. London: BT Press, 2001.

Lock J, Le Grange D, Agras WS, Dare C. Treatment Manual for Anorexia Nervosa: A Family-Based Approach. New York: Guilford, 2001.

RESOURCES FOR PATIENTS AND CARERS

Centre for Eating and Dieting Disorders (NSW)
www.cedd.org.au/index.html
email: info@cedd.org.au

Eating Disorders Association of Queensland
www.uq.net.au/eda
email: eda.inc@uq.net.au

Eating Disorders Association of South Australia
www.communitywebs.org/edasa
email: edasa@internode.on.net

Eating Disorders Foundation of New South Wales
www.edf.org.au
email: edf@edf.org.au

Eating Disorders Foundation of Victoria
www.eatingdisorders.org .au
email: edfv@eatingdisorders.org.au

SELF-HELP BOOKS

Crisp AH, Joughin N, Halek C, Bowyer C. Anorexia Nervosa: A Wish to Change. New York: Psychology Press, 1996.

Cooper PJ. Bulimia Nervosa and Binge-Eating: A Guide to Recovery. New York: New York University Press, 1995.

Fairburn C. Overcoming Binge Eating. New York: Guilford, 1995.

Schmidt U, Treasure J. Getting Better Bit(e) by Bit(e). New York: Psychology Press, 1993.

GUIDES FOR PARENTS AND FRIENDS

Treasure J. Anorexia Nervosa: A Survival Guide for Families, Friends, and Sufferers. New York: Psychology Press, 1997.

REFERENCES

1. Gull WW. Anorexia Nervosa. In: Kaufman RM, Heiman M, eds. Evolution of Psychomatic Concepts: Anorexia Nervosa: A Paradigm. New York: International Universities Press, 1964.

2. Lasegue C. De L'anorexie hystérique. In: Kaufman RM. Heiman M, eds. Evolution of Psychosomatic Concepts: Anorexia Nervosa: A Paradigm. New York: International Universities Press, 1964.

3. Russell GFM. Bulimia nervosa: an ominous variant of anorexia nervosa. Psychological Medicine 1979;9:429–448.

4. Farmer A, Treasure J, Szmukler G. Eating disorders: a review of recent research. Digestive Diseases 1986;4:13–25.

5. American Psychiatric Association. Diagnostic and statistical manual of mental disorders. 4th edn. Washington DC: American Psychiatric Association, 1994.

6. Hoek IIW. Review of the epidemiological studies of eating disorders. International Review of Psychiatry 1993;8:61–75.

7. McCarthy M. The thin ideal, depression and eating disorders in women. Behaviour Research Therapy 1990;28:205–12.

8. Keys A, Brozek J, Henschel A, Mickelson O, Taylor HL. The biology of human starvation. Minneapolis: University of Minnesota Press, 1950.

9. Lilenfeld LR, Kaye WH, Greeno CG, Merikangas KR, Plotnicov K, Pollice C, Rao R, Strober M, Bulik CM, Nagy L. A controlled family study of anorexia nervosa and bulimia nervosa: psychiatric disorders in first degree relatives and effects of proband comorbidity. Archives of General Psychiatry 1998;55:603–10.

10. Bulik CM, Sullivan PF, Wade TD, Kendler KS. Twin studies of eating disorders: a review. International Journal of Eating Disorders 2000;27:1–20.

11. Bulik CM, Devlin B, Bacanu SA, Thornton L, Klump K, Ficter M, Halmi K, Kaplan A, Strober M, Woodside DB, Bergen AW, Ganjei JK, Crow S, Mitchell J, Rotondo A, Mauri M, Cassano G, Keel P, Berrettini WH, Kaye WH. Significant linkage on chromosome 10p in families with bulimia nervosa. American Journal of Human Genetics 2003;72:200–7.

12. Bulik CM. Proceedings of Annual Conference of the Australasian Society for Psychiatric Research, Christchurch, NZ, December 3–5, 2003.

13. Connan F, Campbell IC, Katzman M, Lightman SL, Treasure J. A neurodevelopmental model for anorexia nervosa. Physiology and Behaviour 2003;79:13–24.

14. Karwatz A, Troop NA, Rabe-Hesketh S, Collier DA, Treasure JL. Personality disorders and personality dimensions in anorexia nervosa. Journal of Personality Disorders 2003;17:73–85.

15. Theander S. Long-term prognosis of anorexia nervosa: a preliminary report. In: Darby PL, Garfinkel PE, Garner DM, Coscina DV, eds. Anorexia Nervosa: Recent Developments in Research. New York: Alan R. Liss Inc. 1983;441–2.

16. Freeman C. Eating Disorders: A Guide for Primary Care. Edinburgh: Cullen Centre, Royal Edinburgh Hospital, 1995.

17. O'Brien KM, Vincent NK. Psychiatric comorbidity in anorexia and bulimia nervosa: nature, prevalence and causal relationships. Clinical Psychology Review 2003;23:57–74.

18. Treatment Protocol Project. Management of Mental Disorders. 3rd edn. Sydney: World Heath Organization Collaborating Centres for Mental Health and Substance Abuse, 2000:423–58.

19. Fairburn CG, Jones R, Peveler RC, Carr SJ, Solomon RA, O'Conner ME, Burton J, Hope RA. The psychological treatments for bulimia nervosa. Archives of General Psychiatry 1991;48:163–469.

20. Fettes PA, Peters JM. A meta-analysis of group treatments for bulimia nervosa. International Journal of Eating Disorders 1992;11:97–110.

21. Lock J. Treating adolescents with eating disorders in the family context. Empirical and theoretical considerations. Child and Adolescent Psychiatric Clinics of North America 2002;11:331–42.

22. Hay P, Bacaltchuk J. Bulim000000ia nervosa. Clinical Evidence 2003;10:1070–84.

CHAPTER 14

COMMON MENTAL HEALTH PROBLEMS IN CHILDHOOD

L Ciechomski, G Blashki and B Tonge

Children are remarkable for their intelligence and ardor, for their curiosity, their intolerance of shams, the clarity…of their vision.

ALDOUS HUXLEY, *1894–1963*

CASE STUDY

Michelle, a 9-year-old girl, is brought in by her mother Louise, who describes a two-month history of escalating resistance to attending school. Michelle is a shy girl who has some trouble making friends, but was previously well and settled at school. Problems emerged two months ago, after a bout of gastroenteritis kept her at home for three days. Michelle experiences marked anxiety and lower abdominal pains associated with being taken to school in the morning; on several occasions, arrangements were made for Michelle to go home at lunchtime. Louise has tried to return her daughter to school in the afternoon but with no success. Michelle's symptoms appear to subside during the day, and she is happy and well at home. Michelle's teacher had requested a medical assessment.

KEY FACTS

- Childhood emotional and behavioural disorders are prevalent in the community and are associated with increased risk of depression and other mental health and adjustment problems in adolescence and adulthood.

- Common disorders in children include separation anxiety disorder and school refusal, depression, attention deficit hyperactivity disorder and conduct disorder.

- Although each disorder has distinct core symptoms, research has consistently found high comorbidity with an overlap of symptoms between these disorders.

- A multidimensional approach, whereby information is gathered from a number of sources—for example, parents and teachers—is regarded as best practice in the recognition and management of childhood mental health problems.

- General practitioners (GPs) have a key role to play in the early recognition of problems, since children with psychiatric disorders are frequently brought to primary care.

- Common initial complaints involve somatic symptoms, such as headaches and abdominal pain, rather than seeking help for a psychological problem.

- GPs are in an ideal position to administer a brief screening tool such as the Strengths and Difficulties Questionnaire (SDQ) for the preliminary detection of specific mental health problems in children.

- In the majority of cases, GPs need to liaise with specialist mental health services who have the expertise for dealing with complex childhood mental illnesses.

- There is evidence for the effective use of psychological treatments for many childhood mental health problems—for example, cognitive behavioural therapy.

- Psychotropic drugs may also be effective in the treatment of some childhood psychopathologies, but they are usually used in combination with psychological and educational interventions.

INTRODUCTION

Mental disorders in childhood are common in the community. Community samples have found prevalence rates of around 5% for emotional disorders and 5–6% for behavioural disorders in school aged children.[1, 2] The prevalence of autism (pervasive developmental disorders) has increased from 0.1% to 0.6% or even higher over the past twenty years, but this may be due to improved case finding and changes in diagnostic criteria. The prevalence of attention deficit hyperactivity disorder (ADHD) has been estimated to be 2.4% in children aged 5 to 11.[3] This chapter will examine the presentation, detection and management of childhood mental illness in general practice settings.

Prevalence figures for psychiatric disorders in general practice are hard to find; however, an early study reported that almost a quarter of children aged between 7 and 12 years seen in general practice have psychiatric disorders.[4] Many children with mental illness suffer a mixture of emotional and behavioural problems, such as anxiety, phobias, depression and ADHD. It has been suggested that rates of behavioural problems such as conduct disorder are even higher among children who are frequent attendees—that is, four or more consultations a year—to primary care.[5]

Recent studies suggest that children with ADHD in particular often present to GPs. A United Kingdom study reports that a GP may have regular contact with 2–4 children receiving treatment for ADHD.[6] One survey involving 150 GPs found that 85% were currently managing at least one child with ADHD, although a further 13% suspected ADHD in children seen in their practice.[7] In a cross-sectional survey of 399 Australian GPs, over 90% saw more than five children a week and most diagnosed 1–5 cases of

ADHD per year.[8] Another study suggests that GPs identify an average of five childhood mental health problems within a six-month period.[9]

DIAGNOSIS OF CHILDHOOD DISORDERS

The current classification of common childhood mental illnesses is specified either by the widely used Diagnostic and Statistical Manual of Mental Disorders (DSM-IV)[10] or the similar International Classification of Diseases (ICD-10)[11] (see Table 14.1). Figure 14.1 outlines the defining features of common childhood disorders according to the DSM-IV. Some of these disorders—such as separation anxiety disorder and ADHD—are first diagnosed in childhood, but most, such as obsessive-compulsive disorder and post-traumatic stress disorder, are not specific to childhood. These are more common in adolescence or adulthood.[10]

TABLE 14.1 Current major classifications of childhood disorders

DSM-IV	ICD-10
DISORDERS FIRST DIAGNOSED IN CHILDHOOD	**DISORDERS FIRST DIAGNOSED IN CHILDHOOD**
Attention deficit hyperactivity disorder	**Hyperkinetic disorders**
■ Primarily inattentive type	■ Disturbance of activity and attention
■ Primarily hyperactive type	■ Hyperkinetic conduct disorder
■ Combined type	■ Other hyperkinetic disorders
	■ Hyperkinetic disorder, unspecified
Conduct disorder	
■ Childhood onset type	**Conduct disorders**
■ Adolescent onset type	■ Conduct disorder confined to the family context
Oppositional defiant disorder	■ Unsocialised conduct disorder
	■ Socialised conduct disorder
Adjustment disorders with depressed mood	■ Oppositional defiant disorder
	■ Other conduct disorders
■ Anxiety	■ Conduct disorder, unspecified
■ Conduct disturbance	■ Mixed disorders of conduct and emotions
■ Mixed emotions and conduct	
Elimination disorders	**Other behavioural and emotional disorders**
■ Encopresis	■ Non-organic enuresis
■ Enuresis	■ Non-organic encopresis
Pervasive developmental disorders	**Pervasive developmental disorders**
■ Autistic disorder	■ Childhood autism
■ Asperger's disorder	■ Overactive disorder associated with mental retardation and stereotyped movements
■ Pervasive developmental disorder not otherwise specified	■ Asperger's disorder

TABLE 14.1 *continued*

DSM-IV	ICD-10
OTHER DISORDERS OF CHILDHOOD OR ADOLESCENCE ■ Separation anxiety disorder ■ Selective mutism ■ Reactive attachment disorder of childhood	**DISORDERS OF SOCIAL FUNCTIONING WITH ONSET SPECIFIC TO CHILDHOOD AND ADOLESCENCE** ■ Elective mutism ■ Reactive attachment disorder of childhood ■ Disinhibited attachment disorder of childhood
DISORDERS NOT SPECIFIC TO CHILDHOOD **Depressive disorders** ■ Major depressive disorders ■ Dysthymic disorder	**DISORDERS NOT SPECIFIC TO CHILDHOOD** **Depressive episode with or without psychotic features** **Dysthymic disorder**
Eating disorders ■ Anorexia nervosa ■ Bulimia nervosa ■ Eating disorder not otherwise specified (EDNOS)	**Eating disorders** ■ Anorexia nervosa ■ Bulimia nervosa ■ Eating disorder not otherwise specified (EDNOS)
Sleep disorders (parasomnias) ■ Nightmare disorder ■ Sleep terror disorder ■ Sleepwalking disorder ■ Related to another mental disorder	**Non-organic sleep disorders** ■ Non-organic insomnia ■ Non-organic hypersomnia ■ Sleepwalking ■ Sleep terrors ■ Nightmares
Anxiety disorders ■ Panic disorder ■ Specific phobia ■ Social phobia ■ Obsessive compulsive disorder ■ Post-traumatic stress disorder ■ Generalised anxiety disorder	

	EMOTIONAL DISORDERS WITH ONSET SPECIFIC TO CHILDHOOD
	■ Separation anxiety disorder of childhood
	■ Phobic anxiety disorder of childhood
	■ Social anxiety disorder of childhood
	■ Sibling rivalry disorder
	■ Other childhood emotional disorders
	  — Identity disorder
	  — Overanxious disorder
	■ Childhood emotional disorder, unspecified

FIGURE 14.1 Defining features of common childhood mental illnesses based on DSM-IV

ANXIETY DISORDERS

SEPARATION ANXIETY Developmentally inappropriate and excessive worry concerning separation from parent and home; school refusal; reluctance to be home alone; nightmares and physical complaints

GENERAL ANXIETY Excessive anxiety and worry; difficulty controlling the worry; restlessness; fatigue; difficulty concentrating; irritability; muscle tenseness; and sleep disturbance

SPECIFIC PHOBIA Excessive and unreasonable fear of objects or situations (for example, heights, animals, injections, loud noises); exposure to object/situation provokes anxiety response (for example, crying, clinging), and the object/situation is avoided or endured with intense anxiety

ATTENTION DEFICIT HYPERACTIVITY DISORDER

ADD Difficulty sustaining attention; often does not listen, avoids difficult tasks, easily distracted, disorganised and forgetful

AHD Often fidgets, often leaves seat in classroom, often runs about or climbs in inappropriate situations, has difficulty playing quietly, has problems waiting turn and often interrupts others

ADHD Combination of symptoms of ADD and AHD

DISRUPTIVE BEHAVIOUR DISORDERS

OPPOSITIONAL DEFIANT DISORDER Often loses temper, argues with adults, refuses to comply with adult rules, touchy and easily annoyed by others, often angry, spiteful or vindictive

CONDUCT DISORDER Often bullies, initiates physical fights; has been physically cruel to people or animals; has stolen; forced sexual activity with others; deliberately set fires or destroyed property; often lies, runs away and is truant

DEPRESSIVE DISORDERS

MAJOR DEPRESSION At least two weeks of persistent depressed and/or irritable mood with loss of usual interests; significant increase or decrease in appetite and weight gain or loss or failure to maintain weight gain of childhood; insomnia or hypersomnia; agitation or lethargy; feelings of worthlessness; inability to think or concentrate; and thoughts of death or suicide

DYSTHYMIC DISORDER Persistent depression and/or irritability for at least twelve months, associated with disturbed appetite and/or sleep, lethargy and loss of interest, feelings of hopelessness, low self-esteem and poor concentration and school performance

Source: Based on the DSM-IV, 4th edn, 2000.[10]

SEPARATION ANXIETY DISORDER AND SCHOOL REFUSAL

REVISITING THE CASE STUDY A thorough GP assessment of Michelle, including physical examination and stool micro and culture, has been unremarkable. The GP informs Louise that school refusal is a common occurrence after illness. The GP encourages Louise in her efforts to return her daughter to school, and provides some advice on management, suggesting that Louise try not to make home too comfortable a place for Michelle on the days she is at home from school—for example, she should try not to let Michelle engage in activities that reinforce her desire to stay home, such as watching television or movies. Louise is encouraged to liaise with Michelle's teacher so she can help with Michelle's school attendance, and a referral is made to the school psychologist for further assessment and behaviour management strategies.

For clinical diagnoses of anxiety disorders, several symptoms outlined in Figure 14.1 need to be present for a minimum of six months, and cause significant disturbance in the child's routine, in at least two areas of functioning—for example, social and academic. Children with separation anxiety disorder need only to have had symptoms for a four-week period. Like other common childhood disorders, anxiety is best treated early, as there is a high risk of disorder in adulthood. For example, childhood anxiety in the form of social inhibition or avoidance may be a risk factor for depression.[12] Long-term school refusal can affect academic achievement and the development of peer relationships.[13]

School refusal differs from truancy. Parents of school refusers are usually aware of the child's absence from school and the child is compliant—for example, willing to do school work at home—whereas truants frequently conceal school absence from parents and do not stay at home.[14] Symptoms of school refusal may emerge after a holiday or illness, as in the case of Michelle. For some children, attendance might be sporadic, whereas others have been absent from school for weeks or months.[15] School refusers experience a range of anxiety symptoms—for example, excessive worries regarding school attendance and physiological symptoms, such as abdominal pain, nausea, diarrhoea and sore throat. The presence of physiological symptoms means that an evaluation by a GP is important to rule out any underlying medical illness.[14]

Presentation of anxiety disorders in general practice is most likely to be in the form of somatic complaints, and gastrointestinal symptoms are particularly common in older children with separation anxiety disorder.[13] Parents may report changes in their child's mood—for example, withdrawal from normal activities, and increasing school absence.[14] In addition, teachers may convey their concerns to parents—for example, a decline in academic performance.

Some research has also found that complaints of headaches and musculoskeletal pains appear to be associated with anxiety disorders in females—for example, separation anxiety disorder—and disruptive behavioural disorders in males—for example, conduct disorders.[16] Although mood and anxiety disorders are more common among females than males,[4] gender differences are less pronounced in young children. For example, the rate of school refusal is similar between boys and girls,[15] and it is likely that this equal gender distribution of anxious children is reflected in general practice settings.

DEPRESSIVE DISORDERS

Children are vulnerable to depression if they have a depressed parent, or experience a range of social and physical stressors, such as the threat of school failure, or loss, abuse, rejection or abandonment by primary caregivers.[17] Children with depression can vary greatly in presentation; however, all have depressed mood and/or irritability as well as at least one of the other symptoms listed in Figure 14.1. The rate of depression in a child with a depressed parent is as high as 30% by the end of adolescence.[18] Children who experience depression are at increased risk for depression in adulthood.[19] There is a frequent association between anxiety and depressive disorders in childhood, as well as depression and behavioural disorders such as ADHD and conduct disorder.[17] Parents may not recognise that their child is depressed, but may be aware that something is troubling their child or they may observe a decline in school performance.[20] The child's irritable behaviour is usually a stress on family relationships.

PRESENTATION OF CHILDHOOD DEPRESSION Preschool children experience the same symptoms of depression—for example, sadness, anhedonia and lack of energy—that characterise depression in older children, adolescents and adults,[21] but common symptoms are also headaches and stomach aches.[22] Young children with depression frequently experience disorganised and unsupportive environments and physical neglect and/or sexual or physical abuse.[23] Changes in behaviour indicative of depression in very young children include: a loss of interest in play, or sad pretend play; irritability and excessive whining and crying; social withdrawal; low energy; and failure to gain weight.[24]

Children may not be able to fully conceptualise or communicate their depressed feelings to others but their depression is obvious in their behaviour. The behavioural consequences of depression include a loss of confidence, a drop in academic performance, loss of interest in usual activities and isolation from family and friends.

DUMPS is a useful acronym that covers most of the DSM-IV criteria for the manifestations of childhood depression. It is summarised in Table 14.2.[22]

TABLE 14.2 DUMPS: manifestations of childhood depression	
D—duration of symptoms	There is a change in the child's mood over a number of weeks or months.
U—undeniable	There is often an undeniable drop in the child's educational achievement/grades or interest in school.
M—morbid	The child has suicidal ideas and morbid play, thoughts, writings and drawings.
P—pessimism	Prominent symptoms are low self-esteem, negative self-statements and lack of confidence.
S—somatic symptoms	Abdominal pain and headaches, appetite change and sleep disturbance are common presenting symptoms to general practice.

ATTENTION DEFICIT HYPERACTIVITY DISORDER

Most often, the diagnosis of ADHD is made by paediatricians and child psychiatrists.[25] Few GPs diagnose ADHD,[8] preferring to refer children with suspected ADHD to specialists (for example, paediatricians, psychiatrists) for assessment and pharmacological treatment. However, GPs play a significant role in educating parents about ADHD, collaborating and liaising with the child's school and making referrals for behaviour and family therapy.[8]

Any professional who does diagnose ADHD needs to gather information about problems in at least two areas of daily functioning, not only from the child's parents or caregiver, but also from others, such as teachers.[10]

The GP should be alert to the possibility of ADHD in disruptive male children because ADHD is more common in males.[3] Children with ADHD, particularly those who also have conduct disorder, are at risk of substance use disorders, and drug related antisocial and illegal activity in adolescence.[26] Although many young people recover from ADHD as they mature, symptoms—of inattention in particular—may persist into adulthood.[27]

CONDUCT DISORDER

Children with disruptive disorders are particularly challenging for professionals, due to frequent aggressive and destructive behaviour, especially among males. Presentation of conduct problems in female children is less well understood, as research has tended to focus on males.[28] A pattern of disruptive behaviour such as tempers and non-compliance from early childhood is usually found in children with conduct disorder.[29] These children tend to experience rejection by most of their peers and seek out friendships with other antisocial aggressive children. Truancy is common and is often associated with academic problems.

Children diagnosed with conduct disorder have at least three persistent symptoms (see Figure 14.1) for a period of twelve months. Family factors may contribute to the onset of conduct disorder, including parental conflict and violence, inconsistent care and control, and neglect.[29] Conduct disorder in male children is a predictor of employment and relationship problems, as well as antisocial personality disorder, in adulthood.[30] If they consult a GP, parents are likely to present concerns regarding disruptive, out of control behaviour or truancy.

COMORBIDITY

In clinic samples of children with anxiety disorders, the majority are diagnosed with at least one other disorder, frequently depression or another anxiety disorder, including specific phobia, social phobia, generalised anxiety disorder and separation anxiety disorder, providing some support for a general anxiety syndrome.[31] Comorbidity among the behavioural and disruptive disorders is also common—for example, many children with ADHD have anxiety or conduct problems in adolescence.[26]

FIRST CONTACT WITH GPs
INITIAL PRESENTATION IN GENERAL PRACTICE

Initial presentations of mental disorders in primary care are likely to be in the form of changes in behaviour, such as loss of interest in usual activities, refusal to go to school, irritability, aggression or defiance; and somatic complaints, such as dizziness, back pain, abdominal pain, headaches,[2, 13, 32] sleep problems or eating problems.[33] There is a particular set of problems that parents present to GPs that may be indicative of an underlying mental disorder in their child: a description of the child as being in poor health, with low energy levels and physical illness when under stress.[5]

SCREENING TOOLS

Time constraints on practice visits and competing health concerns are two major obstacles in the screening of child mental health problems in general practice.[34] However, recent research suggests that children with mood and anxiety disorders may be missed unless screening instruments are used in general practice settings.[33] Many checklists have been developed in the last few decades for psychiatric assessment of depression anxiety[35] and for behavioural and disruptive disorders.[36, 37]

TOOLS SUITABLE FOR GENERAL PRACTICE

INSTRUMENTS FOR ASSISTING INTERVIEWS WITH CHILDREN Gathering information from children themselves is important, especially as they tend to provide different information from their parents.[38] Children with school refusal may be reluctant to identify factors that have led to or are maintaining their school refusal; therefore building up some rapport with them is crucial.[15] The Barkley scales[39] are brief and closely follow the DSM-IV criteria for ADHD. Other instruments have been designed to tap into specific problems such as school refusal—for example, the School Refusal Assessment Scale.[40] One quick and effective method of assessing anxiety intensity is to administer a feelings thermometer. This is a pictorial rating scale, which simply consists of a straight line (that is, one end represents 0 and the other 100), on which a child can indicate their current level of anxiety or fear.[35] Alternatively, the Child Functioning Scale is a brief 6-item, 3-point scale with pictures that taps into feelings about relationships at home and at school.[38]

The Children's Depression Inventory (CDI)[41] can be very useful as an aid to identifying depression, although it should always be used in conjunction with a clinical interview.[42]

QUESTIONNAIRES TO USE WITH PARENTS There are a number of checklists that may be suitable for use in general practice. The Strengths and Difficulties Questionnaire (SDQ)[43] is a 25-item instrument that can detect common emotional and behavioural problems, such as conduct disorder, ADHD, depression and some anxiety disorders in children aged 4–16 years. The SDQ is completed by parents, teachers and by older children themselves within approximately five minutes. Although specificity and sensitivity is good (94.6% and 63.3%, respectively), the SDQ is only the first stage of screening for general symptomatology. A second stage clinical assessment must be conducted to confirm the diagnosis of a disorder.[44] The SDQ, including scoring sheets, can be downloaded from the internet (www.sdqinfo.com).

ASSESSMENT AND MANAGEMENT OF CHILDHOOD MENTAL ILLNESSES

A multidimensional approach, whereby information is gathered from a number of sources— for example, parents and teachers—is regarded as best practice, given the complexity of these disorders[14] (see Figure 14.2). Assessment and management usually requires collaboration between the family physician, school staff, parents and a mental health professional.[25, 35] Useful questions to ask parents are listed in Figures 14.3, 14.4 and 14.5.

Psychological management includes: parent education in behaviour management; teacher education; counselling for the child; and strategies to assist with learning difficulties.[25] Referral to paediatricians or child psychiatrists is generally required to initiate pharmacological treatment, if this is necessary—for example, for ADHD. Childhood mental illness is rarely diagnosed from a fifteen-minute consultation,[27] questionnaire responses or the report of a single observer;[45] however, obtaining a history of the problem, whether in relation to anxiety depression, ADHD or disruptive behaviour, in addition to having a parent complete a brief questionnaire, is achievable in a GP setting, and can guide decisions about the best course of action.

FIGURE 14.2 Preliminary assessment of mental health problems in children

WITH PARENTS

- Define the problem(s) and obtain specifics—that is, when did they become concerned? Did any specific events occur in the family around this time? Has this problem occurred before? For how long? Are others (for example, teachers) aware of the problem?
- Obtain a brief developmental history—for example, early health/separation problems.
- What types of changes (for example, in diet, sleeping) have they observed in their child?
- Ask parents to be as specific as possible—for example, change in mood, reluctance to go to school, learning difficulties.
- Ask parents to complete a brief screening instrument, and explain that the purpose is to gather more information and to clarify what type of problem their child may be experiencing.
- Enquire about supports and any services they are currently using and ask about their effectiveness.

WITH CHILDREN

- Use play and drawing with a younger child.
- Ask the child about how they are feeling and any worries that they might have.
- Consider asking the child to write a list of worries or wishes (some children may prefer to do this activity with a parent).
- Ask about how things are going at home and school—for example, do they cope okay with schoolwork? Do they have friends?
- Consider a brief interview with the child alone if parent–child conflict is obvious.
- Ask the child if they would complete a brief questionnaire, and explain the purpose.
- Observe the child and be mindful of any co-ordination problems or clumsiness when they are writing that may contribute to learning difficulties.

FIGURE 14.3 Useful questions to ask parents for identification of anxiety related to school refusal

- Would your child rather be with you than go to school?
- Would your child like to be home with you or your partner more than other kids their age?
- How often does your child feel they would rather be with you?
- Does your child report feeling sick or nervous at school?
- How often does your child have bad feelings about school?
- Does your child have many friends?
- Does your child stay away from school because it is hard for him/her to speak with other kids at school?
- Would it be easier for your child to go to school if you went with him/her?

> **FIGURE 14.4** Useful questions to ask parents for preliminary identification of ADHD
>
> - Does your child appear to have trouble listening to you?
> - Does your child appear to have difficulty following through on tasks?
> - Does your child interrupt you and have problems waiting his/her turn?
> - Does he/she appear easily distracted or forgetful?
> - Does he/she appear to be hyperactive or constantly on the go?
> - Is he/she often fidgety or does he/she run or climb excessively?
> - For all of the above, do you believe that your child shows these symptoms more than other kids his/her age?

> **FIGURE 14.5** Useful questions to ask parents for preliminary identification of conduct disorder
>
> - Does your child often lose his/her temper?
> - Does your child often argue with adults/actively defy rules?
> - Does your child often blame others for his/her mistakes (beyond norms such as sibling rivalry)?
> - Is he/she touchy or easily annoyed by others?
> - Does he/she often bully or threaten/get into fights with others?
> - Is he/she often truant from school?
> - Is he/she physically cruel to people/animals?
> - Has he/she run away from home? How often?

ROLE OF THE GP

Very little research has been conducted on the management of childhood mental health disorders in primary care settings, although some attention has been given to the management of ADHD.[46] A recent survey involving 150 GPs revealed that the majority were comfortable with ongoing prescribing and physical monitoring of children with ADHD, but felt that specialists should initiate pharmacological treatment and provide clinical monitoring of the child.[7] The presence of additional disorders can complicate assessment and treatment.[47] Recent media attention given to the suspected problems with overdiagnosis and overtreatment of ADHD may affect attitudes in primary care regarding use of stimulant medication, and possibly increase anxiety regarding management.[6] We advocate that GPs do not try and manage these cases alone, but liaise with and refer to specialists as needed.

Given the number of professionals who may be involved in managing children with ADHD—including teachers, psychologists and speech pathologists—GPs have a key co-ordination role to play in the care of children with mental health disorders.[48] Having a keen interest in child mental health and access to a good multidisciplinary team appear to be crucial factors in a GP's willingness to be the primary care provider for children with ADHD.[49]

INVOLVEMENT OF SPECIALISTS AND SHARED CARE

There is a continuum of GP involvement in the care and management of children with mental health disorders, ranging from GPs referring a patient for management with little ongoing involvement, to those more actively involved in the shared care of patients. In the majority of cases, GPs need to liaise with specialist mental health services who have the expertise and time to deal with complex childhood mental illnesses.[8] Barriers to effective referrals by GPs include lack of awareness of services[50] or of specific therapies available, long waiting periods[51] and costs to the patient.[52] As with other areas of mental health care, the systems of care are a critical determinant of referral patterns, and influence the type of service GPs can access for patients and their families (see Chapter 22).

A number of models of care currently exist, including shared care,[48] employment of an onsite counsellor[51] and specialist clinics.[50] The shared care model has been trialled in Western Australia and has led to better management of children with ADHD.[48] This model involves the establishment through co-ordinated care meetings of a strong network of health and educational professionals—for example, GPs, psychologists and teachers, who work together to detect and manage children with ADHD. An assessment involves gathering information from several sources—for example, school reports and rating scales—and then referring the patient to a specialist for confirmation of the diagnosis. If the diagnosis is confirmed, a shared care, multimodal treatment program may commence, with a review a few weeks later and subsequent monthly reviews. Implementation of shared care arrangements, whereby GPs integrate with other health service providers, may help increase GP confidence in the detection of mental health problems and facilitate more appropriate referrals to specialists.

Another model that may also improve collaboration between GPs and mental health specialists involves employing a counsellor in a GP surgery who has links with a child mental health team, including child psychiatrists and psychologists.[51] The aim of this model is to encourage good communication between all three parties, to provide training to staff at the GP surgery and to provide good continuity of care to families.

PSYCHOLOGICAL INTERVENTIONS

There is growing evidence of the efficacy of and empirical support for the psychological treatment of childhood mental health problems. For example, cognitive behavioural treatment (CBT) of anxiety in children with and without comorbid disorders leads to a clinically significant reduction in pre-treatment diagnoses and symptoms.[31] CBT for anxiety is effective in a group or individual format, and parental involvement enhances treatment effectiveness.[35] Child therapy and caregiver training is also effective in the treatment of school refusal,[53] and is recommended for parents of children with ADHD.[25] The treatment of school refusal may involve relaxation training to reduce physiological symptoms, and cognitive work to identify and modify anxiety-producing self-talk, so that the child is mobilised towards coping with school attendance.[15]

CBT is the first choice in the treatment of depression in children and adolescents[54] (see Chapter 17). The treatment of anxiety and depression in children needs to consider the developmental level of the child, comorbidity and severity of the disorder, and involve the family and other support systems, such as school staff.[55] The treatment of a child with recent onset anxiety or depression might involve education on improving sleep and increasing exercise, practical coping skills and family interventions with frequent and supportive contact.[56] If they have been truant, getting children back to school and promoting participation in activities and social situations is important.[57] CBT for childhood depression and anxiety targets depressive and anxiety symptomatology through recognition and labelling of emotions, enhancement of social skills, and training in relaxation and stress management techniques.

GPs may refer children with anxiety and depression to a clinician trained in family therapy. Family therapy may be particularly beneficial for young children, for those whose mothers are depressed and for adolescents in families with poor communication and problem solving skills.[58] Play therapy can also be effective, especially for very young children.[17] There is some overlap between the treatment modalities. For example, family therapy may contain elements of CBT, as it focuses on problem solving and improving communication and interaction among family members.[58]

PHARMACOLOGICAL INTERVENTIONS

Psychotropic drugs may be effective in the treatment of childhood psychopathology, but only when used in combination with other psychological and educational interventions. The role of the GP should be to support specialist paediatricians and child psychiatrists in the prescription and regular monitoring of response, compliance and side effects.

There is good empirical evidence for the efficacy of stimulant medication such as dexamphetamine in reducing the distractibility and hyperactivity of ADHD.[59] Side effects such as anorexia, insomnia, irritability and emotional disturbance can be troublesome and prohibit the use of this treatment. Sometimes the addition of clonidine in the evening may counteract the insomnia and also have a positive, but not always persistent effect, on ADHD symptoms. It is necessary to monitor the patient for any hypotensive effects.

Recent randomised placebo controlled trials demonstrate that atomoxetine, an inhibitor of the pre-synaptic norepinephrine transporter, is as effective as methylphenidate in the treatment of inattention and hyperactivity.[60, 61] Side effects that may cause discontinuation include vomiting, anorexia, somnolence, irritability and dermatitis.

Some anxiety disorders, such as separation anxiety and school refusal, may respond to the anxiolytic effect of imipramine (10–25 mg nocte), but the child should have a normal electrocardiogram (ECG) and no history of heart disease because of the tendency for imipramine to prolong the P-R interval.[62] There is relatively weak evidence that selective serotonin reuptake inhibitors (SSRIs) reduce anxiety in adolescents, but they may be an effective treatment of obsessive-compulsive disorder.

There is equivocal evidence that SSRIs are effective in the treatment of depressive illness in young people[63] (see the guidelines in Chapter 15). In the UK there is concern that SSRIs, apart from fluoxetine, may increase suicide risk. Therefore, only fluoxetine is authorised for use in young people attending primary care.[64] However, given the disabling effects of adolescent depression and the associated risk of suicide, a trial of fluoxetine should be considered by Australian GPs if CBT has failed.[65]

Low dose neuroleptic drugs (haloperidol and risperidone) may be effective in the management of disruptive and aggressive behaviour in children with intellectual disability or autism.[66]

CONCLUSION

Children experiencing mental illness often present to GPs in the first instance, frequently with somatic symptoms, or disruptive behaviour at home or at school. Perhaps, more than in any other field of psychiatry, GPs need to work closely with other health professionals, often collaborating with psychiatrists, psychologists and/or school counsellors. Psychological approaches such as CBT are effective for many childhood mental illnesses. Pharmacological treatments also have a place but need to be used with care to minimise side effects.

REFERENCES

1. Costello JE, Mustillo S, Erkanli A, Keeler G, Angold A. Prevalence and development of psychiatric disorders in childhood and adolescence. Archives of General Psychiatry 2003;60:837–44.
2. Burke AE, Silverman WK. The prescriptive treatment of school refusal. Clinical Psychology Review 1987;7:353–62.
3. Gomez R, Harvey J, Quick C, Scharer I, Harris G. DSM-IV AD/HD: confirmatory factor models, prevalence, and gender and age differences based on parent and teacher ratings of Australian primary school children. Journal of Child Psychology and Psychiatry 1999;40:265–74.
4. Garralda ME, Bailey D. Children with psychiatric disorders in primary care. Journal of Child Psychology and Psychiatry 1986;27:611–24.
5. Garralda ME, Bowman FM, Mandalia S. Children with psychiatric disorders who are frequent attenders to primary care. European Child and Adolescent Psychiatry 1999;8:34–44.
6. Thapar A, Thapar A. Is primary care ready to take on attention deficit hyperactivity disorder? BMC Family Practice 2002;3:7.
7. Ball C. Attention-deficit hyperactivity disorder and the use of methylphenidate. A survey of general practitioners. Psychiatric Bulletin 2001;25:301–4.
8. Shaw KA, Mitchell GK, Wagner IJ, Eastwood HL. Attitudes and practices of general practitioners in the diagnosis and management of attention-deficit/hyperactivity disorder. Journal of Paediatric Child Health 2002;38:481–6.
9. Luk ES, Brann P, Sutherland S, Mildred H, Birleson P. Training general practitioners in the assessment of childhood mental health professionals. Clinical Child Psychology and Psychiatry 2002;7:571–9.
10. American Psychiatric Association. Diagnostic and Statistical Manual of Mental Disorders. 4th edn. Washington DC: American Psychiatric Association Press, 2000.
11. World Health Organization. The ICD-10 Classification of Mental and Behavioural Disorders. Geneva: WHO, 1992.
12. Parker G, Wilhelm K, Mitchell P, Austin MP, Roussos J, Gladstone G. The influence of anxiety as a risk to early onset depression. Journal of Affective Disorders 1999;52:11–17.
13. Bernstein GA, Massie ED, Thuras PD, Perwien AR, Borchardt CM, Crosby RD. Somatic symptoms in anxious-depressed school refusers. Journal of the American Academy of Child and Adolescent Psychiatry 1997;36:661–8.
14. Fremont WP. School refusal in children and adolescents. American Family Physician 2003; 68:1555–60.
15. Heyne D, King NJ, Tonge BJ, Cooper H. School refusal. Epidemiology and management. Paediatric Drugs 2001;3:719–32.
16. Egger HL, Costello EJ, Erkanli A, Angold A. Somatic complaints and psychopathology in children and adolescents: stomach aches, musculoskeletal pains and headaches. Journal of the American Academy of Child and Adolescent Psychiatry 1999;38:852–60.

17. Sabatino DA, Webster BG, Vance HB. Childhood mood disorders: history, characteristics, diagnosis and treatment. In: Vance HB, Pumariega AJ, eds. Clinical Assessment of Child and Adolsecent Behavior. New York: John Wiley & Sons, 2001.

18. Downey G, Coyne JC. Children of depressed parents: an integrative review. Psychological Bulletin 1990;180:50–76.

19. Roza SJ, Hofstra MB, Ende J, Verhulst FC. Stable prediction of mood and anxiety disorders based on behavioral and emotional problems in childhood, adolescence and young adulthood. American Journal of Psychiatry 2003;160:2116–21.

20. Wagner KD. Major depression in children and adolescents. Psychiatric Annals 2003;33:266–70.

21. Luby JL, Heffelfinger AK, Mrakotsky C, Brown KM, Hessler M, Wallis JM, Spitznagel EL. The clinical picture of depression in preschool children. Journal of the American Academy of Child and Adolescent Psychiatry 2003;42:340–8.

22. Carlson GA. The challenge of diagnosing depression in childhood and adolescence. Journal of Affective Disorders 2000;61:S3–8.

23. Voelker R. Researchers probe depression in children. Journal of the American Medical Association 3003;289:3078–9.

24. Luby JL, Heffelfinger A, Koenig-McNaught AL, Brown K, Spitznagel E. The preschool feelings checklist: a brief and sensitive screening measure for depression in young children. Journal of the American Academy of Child and Adolescent Psychiatry 2004;43:708–17.

25. Australian Psychological Society Working Group. Attention Deficit Hyperactivity Disorder in Children. A Guide to Best Practice for Psychologists. Victoria: The Australian Psychological Society Ltd, 1997.

26. Barkley RA, Fischer M, Smallish L, Fletcher K. Young adult follow-up of hyperactive children: antisocial activities and drug use. Journal of Child Psychology and Psychiatry 2004;45:195–211.

27. Goldman LS, Genel M, Bezman RJ, Slanetz PJ. Diagnosis and treatment of attention-deficit/hyperactivity disorder in children and adolescents. Journal of the American Medical Association 1998;279:1100–7.

28. Kann RT, Hanna FJ. Disruptive behavior disorders in children and adolescents: how do girls differ from boys? Journal of Counseling and Development 2000;78:267–74.

29. Holmes SE, Slaughter JR, Kashani J. Risk factors in childhood that lead to the development of conduct disorder and antisocial personality disorder. Child Psychiatry and Human Development 2001;31:183–93.

30. Barry L, Fleming MF, Manwell LB, Copeland LA. Conduct disorder and antisocial personality in adult primary care patients. Journal of Family Practice 1997;45:151–8.

31. Kendall PC, Brady EU, Verduin TL. Comorbidity in childhood anxiety disorders and treatment outcome. Journal of the American Academy of Child and Adolescent Psychiatry 2001;40:787–94.

32. Garralda E. Child and adolescent psychiatry in general practice. Australian and New Zealand Journal of Psychiatry 2001;35:308–14.

33. Wren FJ, Scholle SH, Heo J, Comer DM. Pediatric mood and anxiety syndromes in primary care: who gets identified? International Journal of Psychiatry in Medicine 2003;33:1–16.

34. Gardner W, Kelleher KJ, Pajer KA. Multidimensional adaptive testing for mental health problems in primary care. Medical Care 2002;40:812–23.

35. Velting ON, Setzer NJ, Albano AM. Update on and advances in assessment and cognitive-behavioural treatment of anxiety disorders in children and adolescents. Professional Psychology: Research and Practice 2004;35:42–54.

36. Collett BR, Ohan JL, Myers KM. Ten-year review of rating scales: V: Scales assessing attention-deficit/hyperactivity disorder. Journal of the American Academy of Child and Adolescent Psychiatry 2003;42:1015–37.

37. Collett BR, Ohan JL, Myers KM. Ten-year review of rating scales: V: Scales assessing externalizing behaviours. Journal of the American Academy of Child and Adolescent Psychiatry 2003; 42:1143–70.

38. Wildman BG, Kinsman AM, Smucker WD. Use of child reports of daily functioning to facilitate identification of psychosocial problems in children. Archives of Family Medicine 2000;9:612–16.

39. Barkley RA. Attention-Deficit Hyperactivity Disorder. A Handbook for Diagnosis and Treatment. New York: Guilford Press, 1990.

40. Kearney CA. Identifying the function of school refusal behavior: A revision of the School Refusal Assessment Scale. Journal of Psychopathology and Behavioral Assessment 2002;24:235–45.

41. Kovacs M. The Children's Depression Inventory. North Tonawanda, NY: Mental Health Systems, 1992.

42. Jones-Hiscock C. Using depression inventories: not a replacement for clinical judgment. Canadian Journal of Psychiatry 2004;49:646–7.

43. Goodman R. The Strengths and Difficulties Questionnaire: a research note. Journal of Child Psychology and Psychiatry 1997;38:581–6.

44. Goodman R, Ford T, Simmons H, Gatward R, Meltzer H. Using the Strengths and Difficulties Questionnaire (SDQ) to screen for child psychiatric disorders in a community sample. British Journal of Psychiatry 2000;177:534–9.

45. Luk ESL. Four pertinent issues in treatment. Australian and New Zealand Journal of Psychiatry 2002;36:479–81.

46. Duggan CM, Mitchell G, Nikles CJ, Glasziou PP, Del Mar CB, Clavarino A. Managing ADHD in general practice. N of 1 trials can help! Australian Family Physician 2000;29:1205–9.

47. Waxmonsky J. Assessment and treatment of attention deficit hyperactivity disorder in children with comorbid psychiatric illness. Current Opinion in Pediatrics 2003;15:476–82.

48. Pedlow K. Incorporating the management of ADHD into your practice. Can it be done? Australian Family Physician 2000;29:1210–14.

49. Shaw K, Wagner I, Eastwood H, Mitchell G. A qualitative study of Australian GPs' attitudes and practices in the diagnosis and management of attention-deficit/hyperactivity disorder (ADHD). Family Practice 2003;20:129–34

50. Emmerson B, Frost A, Powell J, Ward W, Barnes M, Frank R. Evaluating a GP consultative psychiatric service in an Australian metropolitan hospital district. Australasian Psychiatry 2003;11:195–8.

51. McNicholas F. Attitudes of general practitioners to child psychiatry services. Irish Journal of Psychiatric Medicine 1997;14:43–6.

52. Pryor AMR, Knowles A. The relationship between general practitioners' characteristics and the extent to which they refer clients to psychologists. Australian Psychologist 2001;36:227–31.

53. Heyne D, King NJ, Tonge BJ, Rollings S, Young D, Pritchard M, Ollendick TH. Evaluation of child therapy and caregiver training in the treatment of school refusal. Journal of the American Academy of Child and Adolescent Psychiatry 2002;41:687–95.

54. Carr VAJ, Boyd CP. Efficacy of treatments for depression in children and adolescents. Behaviour Change 2003;20:103–8.

55. Saxe L, Cross T, Silverman N. Children's mental health: The gap between what we know and what we do. American Psychologist 1988;43:800–7.

56. Garland EJ. Facing the evidence: antidepressant treatment in children and adolescents. Canadian Medical Association Journal 2004;170:489–91.

57. Shoaf TL, Emslie GJ, Mayes TL. Childhood depression: diagnosis and treatment strategies in general pediatrics. Pediatric Annals 2001;30:130–7.

58. Cottrell D. Outcomes studies of family therapy in child and adolescent depression. Journal of Family Therapy 2003;25:406–16.

59. Tonge B. Common child and adolescent psychiatric problems and their management in the community. In: Keks NA, Burrows GD, eds. Medical Journal of Australia Practice Essentials: Mental Health. Sydney: Australasian Medical Publishing Company Limited, 1998:63–70.

60. Kratochvil CJ, Heilingenstein MD, Dittman R, Spencer TJ, Biederman J, Wernicke J, Newcorn JH, Casat C, Milton D, Michelson D. Atomoxetine and Methylphenidate treatment in children with ADHD: a prospective, randomized, open-label trial. Journal of the American Academy of Child and Adolescent Psychiatry 2002;41(7):776–84.

61. Kelsey DK, Sumner CR, Casat CD, Coury DL, Quintana H, Saylor KE, Suttin VK, Gonzales J, Malcolm SK, Schuh KJ, Allen AJ. Once-daily Atomoxetine treatment for children with Attention-Deficit/

Hyperactivity Disorder, including an assessment of evening and morning behaviour: a double-blind placebo-controlled trial. Paediatrics 2004;114(1):1–8.

62. King NJ, Ollendick TH, Tonge BJ. School Refusal: Assessment and Treatment. Boston: Allyn & Bacon, 1995.

63. Whittington CJ, Kendall T, Fonagy P, Cottrell D, Cotgrove A, Boddington E. Selective serotonin reuptake inhibitors in childhood depression: systematic review of published versus unpublished data. Lancet 2004;363:1341–5.

64. Wessely S, Kerwin R. Suicide risk and the SSRIs. Journal of the American Medical Association 2004;292:379–81. http://www.mca.gov.uk/ourwork/monitorsafequalmed/safetymessages/ssriewginterimreportfinal.pdf

65. Rowe L, Tonge B, Melvin G. When should GPs prescribe SSRIs for adolescent depression? Australian Family Physician 2004;33(12):1005–8.

66. Findling RL, Aman MG, Eerdekens M, Derivan A, Lyons B. Long-term, open-label study of risperidone in children with severe disruptive behaviors and below-average IQ. American Journal of Psychiatry 2004;161:677–84.

CHAPTER 15
COMMON MENTAL HEALTH PROBLEMS IN ADOLESCENCE

L Sanci, A Vance, D Haller, G Patton and A Chanen

...Good medical care of the adolescent does not depend on the speciality of the provider, but on the sensitivity of the physician to the enormous physical and psychological changes that are taking place during the teenage years.

CE RAPP Jr, 1983[1]

CASE STUDY

It's a busy Monday morning and 15-year-old Kelly Smith, accompanied by her mother, is your next patient. While you have looked after the Smith family for many years, you have not seen Kelly in the clinic since her immunisation booster two years ago. However, you do recognise her as the girl arguing loudly with a teacher when you picked up your own daughter from school last week.

Kelly looks reluctant to be in the clinic this morning. She is in school uniform but is wearing a jumper even though it is a warm day, her hair is messy and she is gazing down at her shoes. Her mother looks very concerned as she opens the discussion with her reason for bringing in Kelly. Kelly makes little eye contact with you as her mother tells the story.

Kelly has been experiencing headaches frequently over the past few weeks and has missed more than five days of school. She has been very moody and irritable at home, and prefers to spend time in her room listening to music rather than join her family at mealtimes or in the evening. She does not eat properly and stays up late. While she refuses to go places with her family, she seems happy enough to attend parties with her friends.

Mrs Smith is wondering if Kelly is putting on these headaches to get her own way.

KEY FACTS

■ Most adolescents go through the teenage years without major mental health problems, yet a significant 1 in 4 will have a problem.

■ Among those presenting to primary care, over a third have symptoms of depression and anxiety.

■ Confidentiality, along with understanding psychosocial developmental issues in adolescents, is an important aspect of effective adolescent health care.

■ Presentation of emotional problems in adolescents may take the form of behavioural (for example, irritability, binge drinking) or somatic problems (for example, tension headaches).

■ The HEADSS screen is useful for quickly capturing a global psychosocial picture of an adolescent.[2]

■ When prescribing medication, monitoring for side effects within the first 24 hours, and then within the next 7–10 days, is essential. Monitoring should be continued regularly throughout treatment.

■ Management of mental disorders in adolescence should include a suicide risk assessment at each visit.

■ Where possible, involve parents in management.

■ Attending to the effects of mental disorder on family, school and peer relationships is an important aspect of management.

■ After recovery, follow-up visits provide an opportunity to identify any recurrence.

INTRODUCTION

Mental health problems are not uncommon during adolescence yet symptoms are frequently under-recognised by the adolescents themselves, their families and health professionals. Delays in seeking and obtaining professional help may contribute to poorer outcomes. This chapter aims to heighten awareness of the common and important mental health problems that occur in adolescence, how they may present in general practice and how they can be managed. With most adolescents visiting a general practitioner (GP) once a year, there is an important contribution general practice can make in the detection and management of mental health problems.

PREVALENCE OF ADOLESCENT MENTAL HEALTH PROBLEMS
POPULATION STUDIES

Recent community surveys of Australia's young people confirm that psychosocial problems form the greatest burden of disease for young people.[3] In the Australian National Survey of Mental Health and Wellbeing, 12% of youth aged 12–17 years had either depressive, conduct or attention deficit hyperactivity disorder (ADHD) symptoms in the past year.[4] ADHD was the most prevalent (8%), followed by depressive disorder (4%) and conduct disorder (3%). Because these diagnoses were based on *parent* report, they probably underestimate the prevalence of internalising mood disorders, which are generally higher using *adolescent* self-report.[5]

International studies suggest that between 1 in 3 and 1 in 4 teenagers have had a mental disorder by the age of 16, with mood and anxiety disorders, substance use disorders and behavioural disorders being the most common in this age group.[5-7]

Some groups of adolescents are more at risk of mental health problems than others, namely: young offenders and the homeless; Australian Aboriginal people and Torres Strait Islanders; those with a family history of a psychiatric disorder or family conflict (for example, hostile, critical, rigid, scape-goating) and those with a history of childhood abuse or learning problems.[8] A good relationship (for example, warm, sensitive, attuned, empathetic, nurturing and confiding) with at least one parent, good peer relationships (confiding and nurturing) and being employed are known protective factors.[8]

Youth suicide remains a major health problem in Australia. In 2001, 14%, or 349 of the 2452 deaths from suicide in all age groups were among young people aged 12–24 years.[9] This represents a suicide rate of 15.2 per 100 000 young people compared to an overall population suicide rate of 11.8 per 100 000 persons. In 1982, 8.7 per 100 000 young people died by suicide and in 1997 it peaked at 24.2 per 100 000 young people. Males comprised 81% of the deaths of young people due to suicide in 2001. In the Australian National Survey of Mental Health and Wellbeing, about 12% of adolescents aged 13–17 had experienced suicidal thoughts and 4% had made an attempt, with 1% requiring medical care.[4] Suicidal thoughts were much more common in those with severe mental health problems (42%) compared to those with few problems (2%).[4]

Substance use problems are also common in adolescence. Bonomo has summarised the epidemiology of adolescent substance use.[10] Alcohol use is occurring earlier in adolescence, with 90% having consumed alcohol by 15 years of age and over 70% by 13 years of age.[10] Binge drinking is common, with about 40% of young people drinking at levels that put them at risk of short-term harm. Regular smoking (at least weekly) usually begins between 12 and 19 years of age, while about 15% of teenagers smoke daily. Cannabis is the most commonly used illicit drug among teenagers, with 40–50% of 16–24-year-olds in Australia having tried cannabis at least once. Of young Australians, 10%, 7% and 1% use amphetamines, ecstasy and opiates, respectively. Reasons for abuse of substances by teenagers are complex but include peer group or family influences, coping with stress or mental health symptoms, personality traits, age of onset of use under 15 years, availability of substances and perceived social norms.[10]

Psychotic disorders are also becoming an increasingly important condition requiring diagnosis and intervention early in adolescence. Eighty per cent of first episodes of psychoses occur between the ages of 16 and 30 years, and the burden of disease from psychosis is the third highest of all diseases worldwide.[11] Nearly 40% of men and 20% of women experience onset of psychotic symptoms before 19 years of age.[12] Psychotic disorders affect around 1% of Australians.

PRIMARY CARE STUDIES

Despite the great prominence of mental and behavioural disorders in young people, the majority of consultations to GPs by young people are for physical complaints (respiratory, musculoskeletal and dermatological).[3] Only 25% of adolescents with a psychiatric disorder in Australia actually seek professional help, most often from the GP.[4] However, Australian work suggests that around 40% of young people attending the GP have significant levels of emotional distress, with 22% having had suicidal thoughts.[13] One United Kingdom study revealed that only 2% of youth aged 14–16 years and attending GPs presented with a psychiatric complaint, yet when interviewed, 38% had had a psychiatric disorder in the previous year.[14] Most of these (84%) had depressive or anxiety disorders.

Hence, while the population prevalence of mental health disorder in youth is around the 20% mark, the prevalence of disorder in youth actually attending general practice is likely to be at least double this figure. While behavioural disorders and substance abuse are significant problems at a population level, depression and anxiety predominate in young people attending primary care.

Given that most young people access GPs for health care at least once a year, the GP visit presents an ideal opportunity to detect hidden psychosocial health burdens, yet sometimes there are barriers to recognition and diagnosis of mental illness (see Chapter 1). In addition, inaccurate historical perceptions that 'storm and stress' is normal in adolescence may act against early recognition of mental health problems in troubled youth. Moreover, youth value free and easy to access services, especially where no appointment is needed and services are confidential and anonymous. Fears about lack of confidentiality are a major barrier to seeking help.[15]

UNDERSTANDING ADOLESCENCE

Temporary deviations in mood that may last several days and involve risk taking or even delinquent behaviour are common in adolescence.[16] The duration and severity of the symptoms or associated risk-taking behaviour and the impact of the symptoms or behaviour on the adolescents' life (for example, school, home, relationships, activities) determine whether they become a problem.[16]

In assessing an adolescent for the presence or severity of a mental health problem, it is helpful to have a working definition of adolescence and an understanding of the normal key developmental tasks adolescents undertake in making the transition from childhood to adulthood. In the presence of a mental health problem, achievement of these tasks is likely to be impaired.

A useful definition of adolescence is as follows: the distinct developmental period between childhood and adulthood—beginning with the biological changes associated with puberty and ending with the social markers of acquisition of adult roles and responsibilities.[17]

CHRONOLOGICAL AGE

To allow international epidemiological comparisons, the World Health Organization (WHO) defines adolescence as being between 10 and 19 years; youth as those between

15 and 24 years; and young people as the entire age range (10 to 24 years of age).[18] However, there is variability in the rates of physiological, psychological and social maturation of young people, hence chronological age is not always a sound marker of maturation. Even within the one person, each facet of development may occur at differing rates—for example, someone physically quite mature may be emotionally immature. Therefore it is helpful to assess the stage of maturation in a biopsychosocial framework, taking into account the psychosocial as well as the biological markers.

PSYCHOSOCIAL DEVELOPMENT IN ADOLESCENCE

Understanding a young person's psychosocial development provides a guide for judging their capacity for informed consent and for choosing strategies of communication most likely to be effective in management. Clinicians should also take the time to understand the cultural expectations of the adolescent patient with whom they are consulting, as these may present a source of conflict for a young person living in a dominant culture that differs from that of their family of origin. (See Chapter 5.)

Some critical psychosocial developmental tasks of adolescence have been proposed:

- adjusting to changing body image;
- achieving ability to reason and think abstractly;
- joining peer groups;
- achieving greater emotional autonomy from parents;
- adopting a sex role congruent with self-concept and body image;
- internalising a sense of morality or ethical system; and
- taking a career choice congruent with self-concept, attitudes, values and ability.[19]

Adolescence can arbitrarily be separated into three stages, with some of the above tasks being more characteristic of particular stages:

1 EARLY STAGE (ABOUT 10–14 YEARS) Key question: 'Am I normal?'
- At this stage, the young person is coming to terms with puberty and body shape and change.
- The individual is beginning the struggle for independence, and is often moody.
- Cognitively, they can still be concrete in their thinking and have less appreciation for future time. Communication may require more focused questions, and health promotion needs to be relevant to the present.
- The major transition from primary to high school can make this a vulnerable period.

2 MIDDLE STAGE (ABOUT 15–17 YEARS) Key question: 'Who am I?'
- Cognitively, their capacity for abstract thought is more developed, and they can communicate more easily on abstract concepts such as health.
- There is a strong need for peer group acceptance.
- They experiment more and take more risks.
- They have new sexual drives, and they can find their emerging sexual identity confusing.
- There is a strong need for privacy; they may be struggling to balance the demands of peers and family.

3 LATE STAGE (ABOUT 18+ YEARS) Key question: 'Where am I going?'

■ At this stage, they are tending to form more intimate one on one relationships.

■ Their capacity for abstract thought and their sense of future time is more developed, hence they are inclined to communicate abstract concepts, respond to open-ended questions and have an appreciation of present actions affecting them in the future.

■ They are becoming more independent from parents.

■ Around this time, they are considering their future career or study goals.

■ They may be finding transition from high school to work or further study challenging.

NEUROBIOLOGY OF ADOLESCENT DEVELOPMENT

Adolescence is characterised by continuing brain development, with maturation of the frontal lobe (involved in organisation, prioritising, planning and inhibition of behaviour, thoughts and feelings) and much greater activity in the limbic system, which underpins emotional reactions.

Three aspects of adolescent brain development are particularly relevant for the management of mental health problems. First, the serotonin neurotransmitter system develops by middle childhood, while the noradrenaline and dopamine neurotransmitter systems reach maturity by early adulthood.[20–23] The most commonly prescribed antidepressant medications, selective serotonin reuptake inhibitors (SSRIs), act to increase serotonin functional activity to 're-balance' the serotonin, noradrenaline and dopamine systems. These SSRI medications may work well in some adolescents, but not in others, because of individual differences in the rate of maturation of these three neurotransmitter systems. Furthermore, adverse reactions to these medications differ between individuals, particularly in adolescence, for the same reason. Therefore, the use of these medications in adolescents must be initiated carefully, and there should be regular ongoing monitoring for side effects such as increased agitation or suicidality.

Second, the presentation and consequences of mental disorder may differ at different stages of brain development. The hippocampus, for example, is an important integrating centre that depends on mature frontal lobe connections and amygdala control of 'limbic' activity functions which develop later. Hippocampus size and function in adults decreases in direct proportion to how long a major depressive disorder continues untreated. Effectively treating major depressive disorder in children and adolescents may be even more important in preventing structural brain changes with longer term adverse effects. [24, 25]

Third, there are aspects of the 'architecture' of sleep that are specific to adolescence: slow wave activity begins to decline during adolescence and generally declines throughout the remainder of the life cycle.[26] The establishment of healthy sleep patterns appears important in facilitating the optimal development of the emerging frontal lobe and amygdala connections. Therefore, ensuring that the sleep–wake cycle is normalised in young people is an important clinical intervention that may reduce the later morbidity associated with all psychiatric disorders arising in adolescence.

CLINICAL APPROACH TO THE PSYCHOSOCIAL ASSESSMENT OF AN ADOLESCENT

As we have discussed, adolescents rarely present to GPs primarily for their mental health problems, therefore doctors may need to conduct an opportunistic screen when an adolescent presents for other reasons.

The HEADSS mnemonic (see Figure 15.1) provides a framework for taking a psychosocial history from an adolescent, covering all the major areas of risk. It is not designed to be used as a checklist of questions; many of the sensitive areas—such as home, depression, sexuality or drug use—require building a rapport with the adolescent before the doctor can delve into them. Readers are encouraged to access the original paper or the update to learn sensitive ways of asking these questions;[2, 27] some examples are given in Figure 15.1.

Communication skills with adolescents are therefore crucial for developing the necessary rapport with the adolescent and for being able to conduct a psychosocial

---

FIGURE 15.1 HEADSS assessment

HOME: Where do you live? Who lives with you? How do you get along? Is there anyone you would go to with a problem?

EDUCATION/EMPLOYMENT: What do you like/not like about school? Have your grades changed recently? How do you get on with teachers/students? Does it worry you? Many young people experience bullying at school; have you ever experienced this? What was it that you experienced? How much does it worry or bother you (for example, on a scale of 1 to 10)?

EATING/EXERCISE: Sometimes when people get stressed they can over/under eat. Have you ever experienced such changes?

ACTIVITIES AND PEERS: What sort of things do you like to do in your spare time? Do you have hobbies or belong to clubs? Tell me what happens at parties these days?

DRUGS/CIGARETTES/ALCOHOL: Some young people are starting to experiment with [substance], I'm wondering if any of your friends are doing this, what about yourself? Have you ever had any regrets after your [substance] use?

SEXUALITY: Some young people are starting to get involved in sexual relationships. Have you had a sexual relationship with a guy or girl or both? Has anyone touched you in a way that has made you feel uncomfortable or has anyone used force on you? How do you feel about relationships in general? How do you feel about your own sexuality? [Explore protection against sexually transmitted infections (STIs) or unplanned pregnancy.]

SUICIDE/DEPRESSION/OTHER PSYCHOLOGICAL SYMPTOMS: How do you feel in yourself at the moment—on a scale of 1 to 10, where 10 is really happy and 1 the worst you have been? What sort of things do you do when you feel sad/angry/hurt? Some people who feel sad can feel like hurting themselves or even killing themselves. Have you ever felt this way? Have you tried before? Have you a current plan? [Assess suicidal thoughts, past attempts, current plans or actions.]

---

health risk assessment effectively. Explanations about confidentiality are also crucial. We have outlined below an example of how Kelly could be approached using sound communication skills. In addition, the resource for GPs by Chown et al[28] has useful step-by-step approaches to the adolescent.

REVISITING THE CASE STUDY: KEY STEPS IN ENGAGING AND SCREENING ADOLESCENTS FOR MENTAL HEALTH RISK

Kelly Smith has come to the surgery with her mother and both are in the consulting room with the doctor. The following steps may help the doctor engage Kelly and her parent.

1 Validate the accompanying parent's concerns, and check your understanding of these concerns with them: 'Thank you, Mrs Smith, I can see that you are very concerned about Kelly at the moment because she seems to be withdrawing from the family, not eating well, missing school a lot with these headaches and becoming more irritable. You are also perplexed that she can still go out with her friends despite feeling unwell at other times.'

2 Negotiate some time for interviewing the adolescent alone during the consultation and check with the young person that this is okay with them. Some young people, especially early adolescents, may not want to be alone with the doctor. It is important to build trust and confidence. You may need to set this up for the next consultation if the young person is reluctant. Alternatively, you could start the consult with the plan of speaking to both parent and adolescent together, then with the young person alone, then with the parent and adolescent again again: 'Kelly and Mrs Smith, it is my usual practice with young people to spend some time during the consultation speaking with the young person on their own. This will help me get to know Kelly a bit better so I can work out how best to help her. Is this okay with you, Kelly? Mrs Smith, after Kelly and I have had a chat, I'll ask you to come back in and we can talk about where to go to from here together. Kelly, is there anything you would like to say before your mother steps out of the room?'

3 Ascertain the adolescent's reactions about being brought along for this health issue, and empathise if you think they are uncomfortable about being brought in: 'Kelly, your Mum seems fairly concerned about you. I'm wondering how you're feeling about these headaches and also about being brought here by your Mum to talk about them. Sometimes that's a difficult position to be put in.'

4 Explain the terms of confidentiality and its common exceptions, and check their understanding. It is important for this to sound natural and not just a rehearsed or token explanation: 'Before we go much further, Kelly, I'd like to say something about confidentiality. I'm aware that many young people are concerned about confidentiality when they see a doctor, and I like to reassure all my patients that what we talk about will be kept private, between us. I'm not going to tell your parents or teachers or anyone else what we have talked about unless I have your permission. There are, however, a few situations where I might need to talk to other people if I believe you are in danger in any way—for example, if I were concerned that you may seriously harm yourself or

somebody else (for example, suicide/homicide) or if somebody was seriously harming you (for example, physical or sexual abuse). In any of those situations, I would need to talk to other people who could help keep you safe, and as far as possible I would work with you to contact those people together. Does that seem okay to you?'

If the young person could end up in court, it would also be important to outline issues around the subpoenaing of notes. If there is a risk of a notifiable infectious disease, it may be necessary to outline the need to notify the health department with the young person's initials and age. It may also be helpful to outline the terms of confidentiality when the parent is in the room: 'It's important, Mrs Smith and Kelly, that Kelly understands that what she and I talk about will be kept confidential unless her life or somebody else's life is in danger of being harmed or she is being abused in any way. This will help Kelly feel comfortable to discuss what may be going on for her. If she is in any danger of harm, we will take steps to protect her.'

5   Take a psychosocial history from the young person, eliciting their risk and protective factors from the key domains of: family, school, peer, community, culture and inner world. Use the HEADSS assessment as a guide for this process (see Figure 15.1): 'Kelly, I'd now like to ask you some questions about other aspects of your life that may be affecting your health. Some of these may be personal, so if you don't wish to answer, that's fine. Remember we talked about confidentiality…'

6   Perform a mental state examination (see Chapter 7).

7   If a physical examination is needed, be sensitive to the adolescent's possible sense of discomfort. Offer to have a chaperone present; examine the patient bit by bit rather than asking them to totally undress; keep a running commentary on any findings and reassure about normality.

8   Feed back to the young person your impression of their presentation: summarise the things they have told you that seem to be going well in their life and highlight the areas you feel require more attention. Compliment them on being able to share their problems with you.

9   Negotiate a management plan with the young person. In particular, discuss with them the content of the consultation you think needs to be discussed with the parent once they return to the room. Rehearse together what you or the patient may say. Sometimes they will be happy for the parent to know everything. At other times, however, they will be protective of some information, but over several consultations they may have built up enough trust in you to allow the parent to be involved, if appropriate.

10   You will probably need to gather information from other sources, particularly for adolescents with behavioural, learning or conduct disorders. Explain to the adolescent that it will be helpful for you to speak with other people who have spent time with them in other settings—for example, the school teacher or counsellor. Rehearse with the young person what you are going to ask these other people, and reassure them that you will not divulge any confidential information.

11   Discuss with the adolescent some resources they may use for help if necessary—for example, websites, 24-hour telephone help lines, hospital accident and emergency departments, and how to contact you at the clinic if necessary. Help the adolescent make a 'things to do when distressed list'. This may include contacting family

members or friends, calling a help line, visiting the doctor or walking the dog. It also helps to discuss with them how they can recognise themselves becoming more distressed so they can learn to take action early.

12 Some adolescents may need to be referred for specialist care. It is important to explain to the adolescent that you are referring because you feel the specialist service will have more skills to help them in a certain area. It often helps to schedule an appointment with them after they have been to the specialist service so you can see how it went. Ideally, explain to them how this service is likely to work and what to expect.

13 Before the adolescent leaves, ask them the best way to contact them if you need to—for example, mobile phone, house phone, by mail in a plain envelope or email.

14 Ensure they understand the appointment system and whether they need to pay or not before they leave. Keep in mind that young people attending GPs without the support of parents may be unable to pay for a consultation and will need to be bulk billed.

COMMON MENTAL HEALTH PROBLEMS IN ADOLESCENCE

Young people's mental health problems often do not fall neatly into the 'boxes' that we might use to diagnose adults. Blends of psychopathology do not make them any less serious. Severity should always be based upon an assessment of risk and of current psychosocial functioning. Whenever one risk factor or mental health problem is identified, the doctor should also exclude other coexisting mental health problems or risk factors. Coexisting conditions need to be treated in parallel. Some of the more common mental health problems of adolescence are discussed below.

DEPRESSION AND ANXIETY

See also Chapters 8 and 9.

CASE STUDY Kelly is irritable and argumentative, experiencing frequent headaches and spending more time on her own, yet she still goes to parties. This behaviour could be a sign of depression or anxiety.

DEFINITION The DSM-IV[29] criteria for diagnosing depression and anxiety in adults also apply to adolescents. Unlike adults, however, adolescents may not complain of sadness or low mood, rather they may feel irritable and bored and often want to be left alone. An adolescent's mood often varies during the day, and it is not unusual for depressed teenagers to retain one area of high involvement and interest, such as sports or outings with friends. This contrasts with the usual picture of total loss of interest seen in adults. Frequent somatic complaints—along with behavioural problems, school failure or school refusal—are also common manifestations of adolescent depression. A teenager's essays or other school work may carry depressed themes.

The symptoms of an anxiety disorder are the same in teenagers as in adults, but it may be more difficult to specify the anxiety disorder, since at this stage symptoms often still fluctuate. For example, teenagers may attribute symptoms of generalised anxiety to an exterior element such as school, leading to an inappropriate diagnosis of school phobia at the expense of managing the broader ranging syndrome.

School phobia is a rare but severe disorder, characterised by a persistent and irrational fear of going to school accompanied by marked anxiety symptoms—quite different from a mere dislike of school that is related to certain issues such as new teachers, exams or bullying[16] (see Chapter 14). Depression commonly coexists with anxiety related symptoms.

COURSE Most adults who suffer from anxiety or depression report that their symptoms began in adolescence.[30] For major depression, the mean age of onset is around 14 years of age, and episodes usually last 6–8 months.[5] Adolescents who have suffered from a first episode of depression are vulnerable to experiencing other episodes, which become increasingly severe.[31]

SCREENING In view of the high prevalence of mental health problems in young people attending primary care, it makes more sense for GPs to screen for depression than for them to measure their young patients' blood pressure. Currently, however, there is no evidence available to indicate whether screening adolescent patients for mental health disorders in primary care leads to improved outcomes.[32] The HEADSS framework includes questions the GP can ask during the consultation that will help diagnose depression, based on the symptoms outlined above.[2, 27] It is also important to screen whether the adolescent has been exposed to a recent life stress, such as bereavement, parental divorce or separation, or a severely disappointing experience.[33] The risks of depression associated with the event ,as well as family risk and protective factors, must be assessed. Simple psychometric scales such as the K-10[34] may also be helpful in screening teenagers who appear at risk, although this scale has not yet been specifically validated for use in teenagers (see Chapter 21).

MANAGEMENT OPTIONS Significant repercussions of the symptoms on school, family and social life are a good guide in deciding whether treatment is needed. For example, whereas the emotional turmoil of a first broken relationship may explain some fluctuation in school results, it is not commonly related to school failure. The latter should raise concerns about an emerging mood disorder. For mild depressive symptoms where there are no comorbid symptoms (for example, school or social breakdown) and no suicidal ideation, and where the adolescent does not want to be referred for specific counselling, a period of 'watchful waiting' after initial assessment and support may be appropriate, with a review within two weeks.[33] Persistence of depressive symptoms in mild depression to four weeks requires a specific psychological treatment.[33]

UK guidelines recommend specialist referral for all adolescents (under 18 years) who have moderate to severe depression or those with multiple risk histories for depression in one or more family members.[33] These guidelines are based on experts' clinical experience; no study has provided evidence on the effect of the use of these referral criteria on clinical outcomes. In addition, these guidelines do not reflect the current reality that specialist services are frequently scarce or overburdened. With common mental disorders so frequent in the community, it is a struggle to see how any health system could meet the demands emerging from referral of all individuals with moderate or severe mental disorders.

PSYCHOLOGICAL TREATMENTS Cognitive behavioural therapy (CBT) or interpersonal therapy (IPT) are treatments of first choice for both depression and anxiety disorders in adolescence[8] (see Chapter 17). In expert hands they should be of at least three months' duration.[33] CBT has been shown to be effective both in the treatment of depression and the prevention of relapses.[8] Specially trained psychologists may deliver this treatment, but there are an increasing number of training courses for GPs who wish to undertake this type of counselling. Computer based interactive treatment programs (such as 'Mood Gym'[35] or 'Beating the Blues'[36]) offer promising prospects.

IPT is another short-term psychological intervention that focuses on the social and interpersonal difficulties associated with the onset of depressive symptoms—for example, it may concentrate on problem areas such as grief or role transition.[37] In adolescents it involves parents and the school in therapy, and has been shown to be effective in two randomised trials.[37] There are comparatively few training courses in IPT for GPs; most treatments would be administered by psychologists.

MEDICATION Medication is considered in those teenagers with moderate to severe depression where psychological therapies have not improved mood within 4–6 sessions.[33] Unfortunately, research into the use of any medication during adolescence has suffered from the lack of recognition of adolescence as a biological and psychosocial stage that is significantly different from childhood and adulthood. However, despite the recent controversy around the use of SSRIs in childhood and adolescence,[38, 39] current evidence suggests a positive benefit to risk ratio, at least for fluoxetine, in the treatment of major depressive disorders.[40] Results of more appropriate research are anxiously awaited. In the mean time, we advise GPs to follow the guideline of Australia's Adverse Drug Reactions Advisory Committee (ADRAC) (see Figure 15.2) when prescribing fluoxetine to adolescents.

Regular monitoring is mandatory within 24 hours of starting medication or increasing the dose, in case serious adverse side effects develop (for example, suicidal behaviour, self-harm or hostility or other biological reactions); this monitoring may sometimes be made by telephone contact. Monitoring for adverse effects, mental state and general progress should be continued throughout treatment. The frequency of monitoring visits needs to be decided on an individual basis—for example, weekly for a month and, when stable, perhaps less often. Consider possible interactions with other drugs, alcohol and complementary medicines.[33]

Guidelines of the National Institute for Health and Clinical Excellence (in England) also recommend that antidepressant therapy be offered in conjunction with psychological therapy.[33] If the patient has refused psychological therapy, monitoring by the doctor will be even more critical. We do not recommend the use of anxiolytics for the treatment of adolescent anxiety and depressive disorders. Antidepressant medication should not be used for the initial treatment of adolescents with mild depression.[33] St John's wort is also not recommended for adolescent depression because of the lack of studies supporting its use, the extent of side effects and because of its significant interactions with other medications, such as the oral contraceptive pill.[33] For adolescents who do not tolerate fluoxetine, citalopram or sertraline are recommended second line treatments in the UK guidelines. Prescribing should only occur after discussion with the patient and carers about the associated risks.[33] If medication is started, it should be continued for at least six months after remission (defined as no symptoms and full functioning for at least eight weeks).[33] When discontinuing medication, it is recommended that it be gradually phased out over 6–12 weeks, with declining doses being titrated against level of withdrawal symptoms.[33]

FIGURE 15.2 Australia's Adverse Drug Reactions Advisory Committee (ADRAC) guidelines[41]

1   Any use of SSRIs in children and adolescents with major depressive disorder (MDD) and other psychiatric conditions should be undertaken only in the context of comprehensive patient management. Careful monitoring for the emergence of suicidal ideation and behaviour is important, especially early in therapy, if therapy is interrupted or if it is irregular because of poor compliance. CBT may enhance outcomes in MDD.

2   The choice of an SSRI for MDD in a child or adolescent should only be made after taking into account recent clinical trial data. Makers of fluvoxamine or sertraline (indicated for obsessive compulsive disorder) advise against use of these in treatment of adolescent MDD. Manufacturers of citalopram, escitalopram, paroxetine, venlafaxine and fluoxetine warn against their use in patients aged less than 18 years for any indication.

3   Children and adolescents being treated for MDD with an SSRI should not have their medication ceased abruptly.

Note: ADRAC is a national prescribing service, providing rational assessment of drugs and research: http://www.tga.gov.au/adr/adrac_ssri.htm[41] (accessed April 2005).

FAMILY INVOLVEMENT No evidence currently supports family therapy per se in the treatment of depression and anxiety in adolescence; however, one randomised trial comparing family therapy with CBT and supportive therapy did show a greater impact on reducing family conflict and parent–adolescent relationship problems in the family therapy group over the CBT group.[37]

GPs should at least always assess the strength and difficulties in the family, and involve parents and siblings in the management plan. In addition, psychoeducation of the family about their adolescent's problem, its treatment and advice on supporting the adolescent is important.[8] Adolescents are usually happy to have the doctor explain their problem to the family as long as specific details they may want kept confidential are not divulged—this should be discussed with the adolescent first. Management of school phobia, on the other hand, customarily involves the adolescent's whole family and the school along with CBT and sometimes SSRIs.[16]

MULTIDISCIPLINARY APPROACH School retention is a major goal in the treatment of any young person with a chronic illness. In the case of mental disorders, a co-ordinated approach involving the school counsellor, a mental health team and often a social worker is recommended, particularly in severe cases.

EATING DISORDERS

See also Chapter 13.

CASE STUDY Kelly is not eating well and is dressed in a jumper despite the warm day. It is possible she could either be cold from weight loss or covering up her weight loss.

DIAGNOSIS AND MANAGEMENT The diagnosis and management of eating disorders have been covered in Chapter 13. The DSM-IV diagnostic criteria are the same for adolescents as for adults. Severe dieting, which occurs in 7% of 15-year-old girls,[42] has been associated with an increased risk of developing an eating disorder, but there are other risk factors, such as low self-esteem, perfectionism, obsessionality, family history, exposure to intense competition in pursuits such as dancing and sport, and traumatic experiences, especially in childhood, including sexual or other abuse.[43, 44]

It is often difficult to detect eating disorders because the patient denies or plays down the symptoms. 'The single most important factor in the identification of eating disorders is for a health professional to consider the possibility of an eating disorder and be prepared to inquire in an empathetic and non-judgmental manner.'[44] One study has suggested some useful questions in the screening of eating disorders after rapport has been established:

- Do you ever eat in secret?
- Are you satisfied with your eating patterns?[45]

It is important to note that eating disorders frequently co-occur with other psychosocial conditions, such as depression. A full medical, psychological and dietary assessment is necessary. While there is a limited evidence base regarding the optimal management of eating disorders, there is general consensus that a multidimensional and multidisciplinary (or multiskilled) approach is essential for the care of individuals with eating disorders.[44]

CONDUCT DISORDER

See also Chapter 14.

CASE STUDY Kelly is arguing with the teachers and looking dishevelled, but there is not much else to suggest she could have a conduct disorder.

DEFINITION Conduct disorder is almost always preceded and accompanied by an oppositional defiant disorder. Conduct disorder is defined by the breaking of social, legal and moral/ethical mores, while oppositional defiant disorder is defined by oppositional patterns of behaviour that involve 'arguing back', 'wanting his/her own way' and generally structuring the environment to be predictable with attached 'low stress'.

ADOLESCENT SPECIFIC ISSUES In adolescence, conduct disorder is often associated with: alcohol and substance abuse and dependence disorders; depressive disorders (dysthymic disorder and major depressive disorder); language based learning difficulties associated with academic failure at school; deviant peer relationships that worsen the conduct disturbance; and a 'chaotic' family system with poor family role definition, problem solving and emotional communication. Very rarely, psychotic symptoms (usually auditory/visual hallucinations, persecutory/referential delusions and formal thought disorder, thought blocking and/or circumstantial thought forms) may herald the onset of a psychotic disorder.

TREATMENT Psychological treatment, usually undertaken in specialist settings, involves:

- parent–child dyadic therapy to develop consistent positive reinforcement strategies for desired behaviour;
- response cost procedures for undesired behaviour;
- social skills training to aid making and keeping friends;
- arousal and mood regulation skills; and
- problem solving, choice selection and victim empathy skills to maximise positive consequences for actions taken.

Medication to aid mood and arousal regulation can be tried if the above strategies are not helping. These medications include: (1) antidepressant medication and (2) clonidine. If impairing psychotic symptoms are present, then antipsychotic medication can be trialled (see Chapter 12). Careful monitoring—especially for the first 24 hours for side effects, the first 5–7 days for initial improvement and the first 4–6 weeks for a maintenance effect—is recommended. A formal psychiatric review is recommended if these medications are prescribed.

PERSONALITY DISORDER

See also Chapter 18.

CASE STUDY Kelly tells you of angry outbursts, 'mood swings' and attending lots of parties where she indulges in impulsive, unplanned and uncontrolled drinking and marijuana use. She also reveals that she has had many instances of unplanned, unsafe sex, both when she has been intoxicated and at other times. There are multiple cuts at various stages of healing on her left forearm. In this scenario, Kelly could have borderline personality disorder.

NEW EVIDENCE Despite the growing body of evidence suggesting that personality disorders (PD) can be reliably diagnosed prior to age 18 years[46, 47] and that they are valid,[46, 48–50] the diagnosis in young people remains controversial among some clinicians. Of all the PDs, borderline personality disorder (BPD) is clinically the most important[51] and is used here for illustrative purposes. However, as with all young people's mental health problems, blends of psychopathology are the norm and the most common co-occurring problems with any PDs are features of other PDs.[52]

BPD IN ADOLESCENCE Borderline personality disorder (BPD) has been defined in Chapter 18. There is evidence that DSM-IV BPD can be reliably diagnosed in adolescence,[46] along with evidence of its validity,[46–49, 53] similar stability to BPD in adults[54, 55] and serious morbidity, including self-harm and suicide, depression and substance abuse.[48–50, 56, 57] The prevalence of severe BPD in teenagers is somewhere between 1%[58] and 4%,[49] declining by age 19 to its adult prevalence of around 1%.[59, 60]

DIAGNOSIS The main task in diagnosing BPD (or any PD) in adolescence is taking a detailed enough history that allows the separation of 'state' (new features that might be out of character for Kelly) from 'trait' (Kelly's usual self). Young people experiencing major depression frequently display one or more features that resemble BPD, as described above, especially anger, mood instability and recurrent self-harm. However, when these are due to major depression (or other mental state disorders, such as bipolar disorder and psychosis), they are confined to the periods of abnormal mental state, such as pervasive depressed mood or anhedonia characteristic of major depression. This task of differentiation can be time consuming. However, it has important implications for management.

MANAGEMENT Because of the nature of the disorder, this group of patients is often stigmatised. 'Therapeutic nihilism' pervades many services, and referral options for GPs can often be limited. Moreover, the potential for iatrogenic harm in these patients is high, such that poor or misguided treatment can often be worse than no treatment.

SPECIALISED PSYCHOSOCIAL TREATMENT Specialised psychosocial treatment is currently the standard treatment for BPD,[51] based upon promising controlled psychotherapy trials in adults.[61, 62] However, there are no published controlled trials of treatments specifically for young people with BPD. Despite this, where specialised services are available, patients should be referred for treatment. Given the very limited availability of these services, there are important principles of management that can be implemented in general practice. Patients with BPD experience high rates of mental state disorders and these should not be seen as merely 'part of being borderline'. Correctly differentiating 'trait' from 'state' disorders, such as depression, will ensure that patients are not mislabelled and denied appropriate effective treatments for disorders such as depression. There is evidence in adults that conventional treatments for mental state disorders are effective in people with BPD[63] and there are also data suggesting the same in youth.[63] Finally, and most importantly, the building of a collaborative relationship that is structured and consistent and that focuses upon problem solving (using a conventional problem-solving model) is of considerable therapeutic value.[64]

EARLY PSYCHOSIS

See also Chapter 12.

CASE STUDY Kelly's behaviour, featuring increased irritability and a more dishevelled appearance, is regarded as out of character. Her symptoms may well be consistent with depression, but a prodromal phase of a psychotic episode is a possibility, especially if there is a family history.[65]

Possible causes, differential diagnosis management and prognosis of psychosis have been covered in Chapter 12. We will focus here more on the prodromal phase of psychosis.

DEFINITION Psychosis is regarded as losing touch with reality, characterised by hallucinations, delusions, disorganised thinking and bizarre behaviour.[12] Psychotic disorders that appear in adolescence or young adulthood include schizophrenia, bipolar disorder, schizoaffective disorder, major depression with psychotic features, drug induced psychosis, brief reactive psychosis and organic psychosis (for example, as a result of diseases affecting the brain).[66] The psychotic and mood features of schizophrenia have been described in Chapter 12. Schizoaffective disorder shares some of the disturbances of thought and perception found in schizophrenia (delusions and hallucinations) but the mood symptoms are more similar to those of bipolar disorder.[12] Psychotic symptoms that may occur in major depression are usually mood congruent (for example, voices morbidly derogatory) and the mood symptoms are typically sadness and helplessness, poor sleep and loss of appetite and suicidal thoughts.[12] Drug induced psychoses usually improve quickly as the substance is metabolised, but adolescents may continue to have symptoms of psychosis and even develop one of the psychotic illnesses. Brief reactive psychoses, lasting only a few days to weeks, may occur after accumulation of crises or major life change and result in full recovery.[66, 67]

The prodrome of psychotic illness, on the other hand, describes the non-specific symptoms that appear often one year or more before specific psychotic symptoms emerge.[12] These symptoms include decreased school or work performance, diminished attention abilities, social avoidance, peculiar behaviour, impaired personal hygiene, blunted or inappropriate emotional response, speech that is either over-elaborate or vague and impoverished, odd beliefs, lack of initiative and unusual perceptual experiences.[67] Parents' concerns need to be heeded and the young person's condition monitored, with ongoing enquiry into positive and negative symptoms of psychosis and suicidal ideation. These young people may be more likely to fail to attend appointments and it is helpful to have follow-up processes in place.

DIAGNOSIS What is of major importance to primary care clinicians is the need to be watchful for the above early prodromal signs of psychosis as well as the symptoms of the actual disorder. Early intervention improves prognosis: longitudinal studies show that outcomes at 2 years predict outcomes 15 years later.[11] Unfortunately, studies estimate there is usually 1–2 years between the onset of psychotic symptoms and treatment. Evidence is showing that the prognosis of first episode psychosis is related to the duration of untreated symptoms.[11, 68]

MANAGEMENT It has been estimated that most full-time GPs would see one or two new people with first episode psychosis per year.[11] The challenge is to have a high index of suspicion as possible symptoms evolve. Prompt referral of suspected prodromal or actual psychosis to specialist mental health services can allow for timely and appropriate assessment, investigation, monitoring and management. Where specialist services are not easy to obtain, management guided by a specialist in secondary consultation may be appropriate. Acute psychosis is a psychiatric emergency, where the safety of the person and those around him or her is paramount; admission to hospital may be necessary. In suspected psychosis it is critical to institute medical treatment with neuroleptic medication early; this is covered in Chapter 12. Once the psychotic symptoms are controlled, it is also critical to attend to psychotherapy and psychoeducation for the young patient and to support for the family.

BIPOLAR DISORDER

See also Chapter 8.

CASE STUDY Kelly's parents were initially relieved that her depressed mood had given way to quite a happy and effusive disposition that was quite out of character. They started becoming concerned again when Kelly was unable to concentrate on her schoolwork, was constantly on the go, barely sleeping, becoming irritable, and talking quickly and non-stop. She also began running up large expenses on the credit card and was saying she would rather leave school, as her talents were needed elsewhere. It is possible Kelly could have bipolar disorder.

DEFINITION Mid to late adolescent onset bipolar disorder (BD) has similar features to adult BD. More recently, there has been a wider acceptance that BD may begin in early adolescence or even in childhood.[69] Early adolescent BD may not present with the typical features. Chronicity with long episodes is common. Mixed mood states within episodes and/or rapid cycling between depressive and manic periods may occur. Irritability is common, and there is often a high rate of comorbid ADHD and anxiety disorders.[69]More usually, bipolar disorder presents in late adolescence, typically lasts many months and usually recurs. It occurs in less than 1% of adolescents.[8, 69]

SYMPTOMS The depressive symptoms are similar to those in unipolar depression, described above. BD often presents initially as a depressive episode, with about 20% of first depressive episodes in young people being a prodrome to BD.[8] Manic symptoms can begin quite mildly, but then progress such that the person acts in a more driven and disorganised way.[69] Elevated and/or irritable mood, high levels of energy, reduced need for sleep, grandiose thoughts, poor judgment, markedly increased sex drive and excess spending are all features, along with thought disorder or delusional ideas if the condition progresses.[70]

MANAGEMENT Young people diagnosed with BD are best referred, if possible, to a psychiatrist or specialist mental health service. Medications used to stabilise mood include lithium carbonate, and if that fails or is contraindicated, carbamazepine or sodium valproate.[8] Antidepressants may be needed during a depressive episode and an antipsychotic medication during manic episodes.[8, 70] ECT may be necessary for those unresponsive to other treatments. Psychosocial interventions, such as individual counselling for the young person and family, are important, along with the teaching of relapse recognition and prevention strategies.

SUBSTANCE USE

See also Chapter 10.

CASE STUDY With the changes in Kelly's behaviour, her moodiness and irritability, rarely spending time with her family, eating poorly and staying out late at parties, there is a possibility she could be abusing substances. She needs to be screened for alcohol, cigarette and other drug use when she is on her own with the clinician (part of the HEADSS assessment) and after the terms of confidentiality have been explained.

DIAGNOSIS If adolescents admit to using a substance, the history should cover the type of substance used, amount and frequency, social situation when consuming the substance, the way in which the substance is taken and the effects the substance produces on the young person, along with any regrets they have about using it. This will help establish how risky the use is. GPs should also enquire about consumption of over the counter drugs or prescribed drugs.

MANAGEMENT Dependence is rare in this age group and interventions should be aimed at preventing harms related to excessive drug and alcohol use. Brief interventions by primary health care providers have been shown to be effective in relation to alcohol and tobacco use.[71] A motivational interviewing approach or cognitive behavioural strategies in a brief intervention are adequate approaches.[72] The consultation would aim to cover: giving young people information about their drug problem, setting goals for change and setting a mutually convenient date for reviewing these goals. More complex issues require access to specialist services.

MENTAL DISORDER RELATING TO CHRONIC ILLNESS OR POST-VIRAL SYNDROME

CASE STUDY If Kelly had a chronic illness or a recent bout of glandular fever preceding her other symptoms, it is possible these could relate in some way to some of her mood changes.

DEFINITION There are a number of ways to understand how chronic illness or post-viral syndromes interface with a young person's mental health. These include:

- lowering the threshold for the onset of psychiatric disorders;
- prolonging their duration; and
- increasing the rates of non-response to psychological and/or medication treatments.

Further, changes to the young person's mental state can alter the response to the medical treatment provided for chronic illness or post-viral syndromes. Currently, the exact mechanisms for the above are the subject of research enquiry only.

MANAGEMENT Clinically, the assessment and treatment of each psychiatric disorder should occur on its own merits. The context for the management of these psychiatric disorders is always the existing medical disorder, which must be treated and monitored as a primary priority. Nevertheless, individual, parent–child and family psychological interventions, as well as educational and therapeutic groups for young people with their peer group, can aid the implementation of medical interventions for the existing medical disorder and each young person's compliance with them. However, psychotropic medications used to aid the management of psychiatric disorders in young people need to be administered carefully, given the potential for them to interact with the existing medical disorder treatment. In the case of chronic illness, consultation with a psychiatrist and the managing medical specialist would be preferable. A test for Epstein Barr and cytomegalovirus may be useful, along with more routine investigations, such as full blood examination and liver, renal and thyroid function.

MANAGEMENT PRINCIPLES FOR ADOLESCENT MENTAL HEALTH PROBLEMS

The key principles in managing adolescent mental health problems have been outlined in 'Key facts' and in the section on engaging adolescents and screening them for mental risk (see 'Revisiting the case study'); these can be used in conjunction with the general management principles that follow.

FEEDBACK AND NEGOTIATING A MANAGEMENT PLAN

Explaining to adolescents what you make of their presentation in terms they will understand will help maintain their engagement. It is also helpful to feed back positive information before explaining any issues about which you are concerned. It is best to be open and honest about your concerns. This also helps when discussing a management plan.

GPs often need to supplement a patient history with information from others (for example, family and teachers) to fully evaluate the adolescent's presentation. GPs must explain the rationale for this and obtain the adolescent's permission to contact others. It is important to rehearse with the adolescent what you will say to these other parties so the adolescent can give you their approval.

COMMUNICATING ABNORMAL FINDINGS

Even very significant symptoms can be discussed in such a way that adolescents do not feel hopeless. For example, if Kelly were hearing voices, you might say something like: 'Kelly, some people who become extremely stressed, worried or have used drugs experience voices in their head. This is a symptom that's very important and needs further assessment, because it could be a sign of a mental health problem that could make you more unwell if it continues; however, if it's detected, it can be treated and that will relieve your worries and distress.'

You may want to go on and name the symptom as a psychotic symptom, then carefully explain what this is and again reassure the patient that something can be done about it. Separating the symptom from the person is important so that their identity is not lost—for example: 'We can use medication to help you manage these psychotic symptoms' rather than 'You need medication because you are psychotic'.

INVOLVING PARENTS

Often adolescents do not want their parents to know they are unwell. It is important to explore their reasons for this. Many fear their parents will not understand or will be unduly burdened. You must ask enough history to understand whether or not the parents are an actual risk to the adolescent. If they are not, it is helpful to advise the adolescent that in your experience, most parents do understand once their son or daughter's condition is explained to them. You may offer to see the parents and explain the condition with the adolescent present. If the adolescent is still reluctant to involve their parents and there is a risk they will not return for care, it is better to respect their wishes and keep parental involvement as a goal for future consultations. As the young person starts to trust you, they may allow you to involve their family. This is particularly important where family support would help their mental health outcomes.

Parents or other carers must be involved, even against the adolescent's wishes, when the adolescent is not mature enough to understand the treatments or other management required, or if they are very unwell and a danger to themselves or others—for example, when they are severely depressed, suicidal or floridly psychotic. It is best to remind adolescents with one of these conditions that this is one of those situations where confidentiality cannot be kept and parents will need to be informed. To maintain their sense of empowerment, however, you can rehearse with the young person what you will tell the parents and offer them the choice of either you informing parents with the adolescent present or allowing the adolescent to talk to their parents with you present.

REFERRAL TO SPECIALIST MENTAL HEALTH SERVICES

In general, the more severe disorders such as psychotic disorders (including BD), severe depression, suicidality, self-harming behaviour, anorexia nervosa or complex comorbid conditions—such as mental illness with chronic illness or severe substance abuse—would need to be referred as soon as possible. In addition, mentally ill young people with little or no social supports and many social problems may also require management by a multidisciplinary team. In ADHD or conduct disorders, specialist care is also desirable for full access to treatment options.

The degree to which the adolescent engages with the GP's care may also influence whether a GP refers or not. Some young people may be reluctant or unlikely to visit another service, especially if it is not easily accessible. They often dislike having to repeat their story, and wonder about gaining trust in the new service. Sometimes it is appropriate to manage these young people by secondary consultation. However, young people may be more inclined to visit the service if the GP explains fully why this is necessary (for example, they will have access to the best skills to help them) and what to expect when they visit the service. If possible, ringing up the service to make the appointment while you have the young person in the consulting room, and preferably allowing the young person to speak to a service worker, can help engagement. GPs should offer to see the young person after the intended appointment to discuss their experience or to look for alternatives if it was negative or if they did not attend.

TREATMENT IN PRIMARY CARE

GPs intending to manage young people with mental health issues, particularly if starting them on medication, need to ensure appropriate follow-up and monitoring. For example, depressed young people probably need to be reviewed weekly or twice a week, depending on the severity of the illness, until they are stable. If medication is started, this is particularly important until an improvement in mood is established. With any start to medication or changes in dose, the GP should call the young person in 24 hours to ensure they are not experiencing severe adverse side effects; preferably, they should ensure that someone in the young person's world is aware that they are taking a new medication.

CRISIS PREVENTION

GPs should assess the suicide risk at each visit or phone call until the young person is stable. They should also proactively work out with the adolescent a strategy (preferably one that has been written down) that they can follow if they begin feeling distressed, or if they develop ideas of self-harm and anywhere in between these two states (for example, write a diary, go to school co-ordinator, call a friend, talk to their parent, ring the GP, ring the Kids Help Line, Lifeline or a crisis team, or go to the accident and emergency department at the hospital).

PSYCHOEDUCATION AND OTHER SUPPORT

Apart from counselling, treatment or referral, the GP has a role to play in helping families and peers better understand the young person's condition and the ways in which they can help. Families or friends may also need support, and self-help groups in addition to psychoeducation can be helpful. Self-help materials or strategies may be useful as part of a planned package of care, along with advice about the benefits of regular exercise, good sleep hygiene and a balanced diet.[33] In addition, environmental stressors may be ameliorated by a GP intervention. For example, GPs can speak to school co-ordinators, with the young person's permission, and ensure there is support or consideration of disadvantage in school exams. Similarly, a working patient who cannot cope with work demands may temporarily need sickness benefits. Whenever GPs are talking to others about the young person's illness, they must have the young person's permission and preferably have rehearsed with the young person what they will say so that personal details are not unnecessarily divulged.

RECOGNISING SIGNS OF POSSIBLE RELAPSE AND ONGOING MONITORING

Finally, when the young person has recovered, the GP can check that they understand what to do if they start to feel troubled again and how important it is that they seek help early. A GP is well placed to identify early signs of relapse, and each time the young person visits them for other reasons, they should enquire how life is going, bearing in mind that relapses tend to be more common in times of stress or transition.

CONCLUSION

In this chapter we have described some of the common and important mental health disorders occurring in adolescence as well as the key points that will aid GPs in the recognition and management of these disorders in primary care. These include understanding normal adolescent psychosocial and neurobiological development as well as excellent communication skills. In addition, we have detailed some practical approaches to screening young people for psychosocial problems and for handling the clinical encounter in order to reduce the barriers adolescents may perceive to discussing sensitive issues (for example, addressing confidentiality concerns and having time to talk with the adolescent on their own) and so that families can be involved, where appropriate. We have also highlighted where there are significant differences and similarities in presentation and management of these disorders compared to adults. There are no magic solutions to mental health problems in adolescence, but an aware and empathetic primary care provider is a major advantage. To complement the material in this chapter are some suggested resources for both professionals and young people (see below).

RESOURCES
RESOURCES THAT GPs CAN RECOMMEND TO YOUNG PEOPLE
WEBSITES
www.reachout.com.au
www.getontop.org
www.moodgym.anu.edu.au
www.adf.org.au
www.beyondblue.org.au
www.orygen.org.au

24-HOUR TELEPHONE HELP LINES
Over 18: Lifeline 131114
Under 18: Kids Help Line 1800 551800

RESOURCES FOR GPs IN ADOLESCENT MENTAL HEALTH

Chown P, Kang M, Sanci L, Bennett D. Adolescent Health: Enhancing the Skills of General Practitioners in Caring for Young People from Culturally Diverse Backgrounds. A Resource Kit for GPs. Sydney: Transcultural Mental Health Centre and NSW Centre for the Advancement of Adolescent Health, 2004. Download for free on: www.caah.chw.edu.au/resources/#03 (has even more resources for GPs in it)

Drlink: www.drlink.com.au (resources for young people and GPs working with youth)

Eating Disorders for Health Professionals: A Manual to Promote Early Identification, Assessment and Treatment of Eating Disorders. Contact Victorian Centre for Excellence in Eating Disorders, Level 1, North Main Hospital Block, Royal Melbourne Hospital, Royal Parade, Parkville Vic 3050
Phone: +61 3 9342 8184; fax: +61 3 9342 8216
Email: ceed@mh.org.au
Web: www.ceed.org.au

National Divisions Youth Alliance: http://ndya.adgp.com.au/site/index.cfm (resources for GPs working with youth)

Orygen Youth: www.orygen.org.au (has fact sheets for young people and professionals on the different mental disorders, and other information and resources on mental health and services available, advocacy and education)

REFERENCES

1. Rapp CJ. The adolescent patient. Annals of Internal Medicine 1983;99(1):52–60.
2. Goldenring J, Cohen E. Getting into adolescents' heads. Contemporary Pediatrics 1988;July:75–90.
3. Moon L, Meyer P, Grau J. Australia's Young People: Their Health and Wellbeing. Canberra: Australian Institute of Health and Welfare, 1999.
4. Sawyer M, Arney F, Baghurst P, Clark J, Graetz B, Kosky R, Nurcombe B, Patton GC, Prior MR, Raphael B, Rey J, Whaites LC, Zubrick SR. Child and Adolescent Component of the National Survey of Mental Health and Well-Being. Canberra: Mental Health and Special Programs Branch, Commonwealth Department of Health and Aged Care, 2000. http://www.health.gov.au/internet/wcms/Publishing.nsf/Content/mentalhealth-resources-young-index.htm/$FILE/young.pdf (last accessed October 2005)
5. Lewinsohn P, Hops H, Roberts R, Seely J, Andrews J. Adolescent psychopathology: I. Prevalence and incidence of depression and other DSM-III-R disorders in high school students. Journal of Abnormal Psychology 1993;102:133–44.
6. Costello E, Mustillo S, Erkanli A, Keeler G, Angold A. Prevalence and development of psychiatric disorders in childhood and adolescence. Archives of General Psychiatry 2003;60:837–44.
7. Steinhausen H, Metzke C, Meier M, Kannenberg R. Prevalence of child and adolescent psychiatric disorders: the Zurich Epidemiological Study. Acta Psychiatrica Scandinavica 1998;98(4):262–71.
8. National Health and Medical Research Council (NHMRC). Clinical Practice Guidelines: Depression in Young People. Canberra: Australian Government Publishing Service, 1997.
9. Australian Institute of Health and Welfare (AIHW). Australia's Young People: Their Health and Well-Being 2003. Canberra: Australian Institute of Health and Welfare (AIHW), 2003.
10. Bonomo Y. Adolescent substance use. In: Hamilton M, King T, Ritter A, eds. Drug Use in Australia: Preventing Harm. South Melbourne: Oxford University Press, 2004:116–28.

11. Shiers D, Lester H. Early intervention for first episode psychosis. British Medical Journal 2004;328:1451–52.
12. Schulz CS, Bass D, Vrabel CS. First episode psychosis: a clinical approach. Journal of the American Board of Family Practice 2000;13(6):430–9.
13. McKelvey R, Pfaff J, Acres J. The relationship between chief complaints, psychological distress and suicidal ideation in 15–24-year-old patients presenting to general practitioners. Medical Journal of Australia 2001;175:550–2.
14. Kramer T, Garralda E. Psychiatric disorders in adolescents in primary care. British Journal of Psychiatry 1998;173:508–13.
15. Booth M, Bernard D, Quine S, Kang M, Usherwood T, Aplerstein G, Bennett DL. Access to health care among Australian adolescents: young people's perspectives and their sociodemographic distribution. Journal of Adolescent Health 2004;34:97–103.
16. Michaud P-A, Fombonne E. ABC of adolescence: common mental health problems. British Medical Journal 2005;330:835–8.
17. Feldman SS, Elliot GR. At the Threshold: The Developing Adolescent. Cambridge MA: Harvard University Press, 1990.
18. World Health Organization. Young People's Health: a Challenge for Society. Geneva: WHO, 1986.
19. Heaven P. General introduction: developmental tasks. In: Contemporary Adolescence. A Social Psychological Approach. 1st edn. South Melbourne: Macmillan Education Australia, 1994:4–5.
20. Goldman-Rakic PS, Brown RM. Postnatal development of monoamine content and synthesis in the cerebral cortex of rhesus monkeys. Brain Research 1982;256:339–49.
21. Kaufman J, Martin A, King RA, Charney D. Are child-, adolescent- and adult-depression one and the same disorder? Biological Psychiatry 2001;49:980–1001.
22. Lidow MS, Rakic P. Scheduling of monoaminergic neurotransmitter receptor expression in primate neocortex during postnatal development. Cerebral Cortex 1992;2:401–16.
23. Rosenberg DR, Lewis DA. Postnatal maturation of the dopaminergic innervation of monkey prefrontal and motor cortices: a tyrosine hydroxylase immunohisto-chemical analysis. Journal of Comparative Neurology 1995;358:383–400.
24. De Bellis MD, Keshavan MS, Clark DB. Developmental traumatology. Part II: brain development. Biological Psychiatry 1999;45:1271–84.
25. Sheline YI, Wang PW, Gado MH, Csernansky JG, Vannier MW. Hippocampal atrophy in recurrent major depression. Proceedings of the National Academy of Sciences of the USA 1996; 93:3908–13.
26. Rechtschaffen A, Siegel J. Sleep and dreaming. In: Kandel ER, Shwartz JH, Jessell TM, eds. Principles of Neural Science. 4th edn. New York: McGraw-Hill, 2000.
27. Goldenring J, Rosen D. Getting into adolescent heads: an essential update. Contemporary Pediatrics 2004;July:75–90.
28. Chown P, Kang M, Sanci L, Bennett D. Adolescent Health: Enhancing the Skills of General Practitioners in Caring for Young People from Culturally Diverse Backgrounds. A Resource Kit for GPs. Sydney: Transcultural Mental Health Centre and NSW Centre for the Advancement of Adolescent Health, 2004.
29. American Psychiatric Association. Diagnostic and Statistical Manual of Mental Disorders. 4th edn. Washington DC: American Psychiatric Association, 1994.
30. Bernstein G, Borchardt C, Perwien A. Anxiety disorders in children and adolescents: a review of the past 10 years. Journal of the American Academy of Child and Adolescent Psychiatry 1996;35(9):1110–19.
31. Belsher G, Costello C. Relapse after recovery from unipolar depression: a critical review. Psychological Bulletin 1988;104(1):84–96.
32. U.S. Preventive Services Task Force. Screening for Depression: Recommendations and Rationale. Annals of Internal Medicine 2002;136:760–4.
33. National Institute for Health and Clinical Excellence. Depression in children and young people: identification and management in primary, community and secondary care. Clinical Guideline 28

by National Collaborating Centre for Mental Health. London: National Institute for Health and Clinical Excellence, 2005.

34. The Kessler Psychological Distress Scale (K-10). Brief Reports: Department of Human Services, Centre for Population Studies in Epidemiology, 2002. http://www.dh.sa.gov.au/pehs/PROS/br-kessler-scale02-14.pdf (last accessed November 2005)

35. Christensen H, Griffiths KM, Jorm AF. Delivering interventions for depression by using the internet: randomised controlled trial. British Medical Journal 2004;328:265–70.

36. Proudfoot J, Ryden C, Everitt B, Shapiro DA, Goldberg D, Mann A, Tylee A, Marks I, Gray JA. Clinical efficacy of computerised cognitive-behavioural therapy for anxiety and depression in primary care: randomised controlled trial. British Journal of Psychiatry 2004;185:46–54.

37. Chan R, Rey J, Hazell P. Clinical practice guidelines for depression in young people: are the treatment recommendations outdated? Medical Journal of Australia 2002;177:448–51.

38. Whittington CJ, Kendall T, Fonagy P, Cottrell D, Cotsgrove A, Boddington E. Selective serotonin reuptake inhibitors in childhood depression: systematic review of published versus unpublished data. Lancet 2004;363(9418):1341–52.

39. Jureidini JN, Doecke CJ, Mansfield PR, Haby MM, Menkes DB, Tonkin AL. Efficacy and safety of antidepressants for children and adolescents. British Medical Journal 2004;328:879–83.

40. March J, Silva S, Petrycki S, Curry J, Wells K, Fairbank J, Burns B, Domino M, McNulty S, Vitiello B, Severe J. Fluoxetine, cognitive-behavioural therapy, and their combination for adolescents with depression: treatment for adolescents with depression study (TADS) randomized controlled trial. Journal of the American Medical Association 2004;292:807–20.

41. Australia's Adverse Drug Reactions Advisory Committee (ADRAC) Guidelines. Selective serotonin re-uptake inhibitors in child and adolescent depression. In: Guidelines ADRAC, ed. National Prescribing Service, Rational Assessment of Drugs and Research, 2005. http://www.tga.gov.au/adr/adrac_ssri.htm (last accessed June 2005)

42. Patton G, Selzer R, Carlin J, Wolfe R. Onset of adolescent eating disorders: population based cohort study over 3 years. British Medical Journal 1999;318:765–8.

43. Marks P, Beumont P, Birmingham C. GPs managing patients with eating disorders: a tiered approach. Australian Family Physician 2003;32(7):509–12.

44. Wilson K, Harry S, Blaney S, Bruere T. Eating Disorders Resource for Health Professionals: A Manual to Promote Early Identification, Assessment and Treatment of Eating Disorders. Melbourne: The Victorian Centre of Excellence in Eating Disorders, 2005.

45. Freund KM, Graham SM, Lesky LG, Moskowitz MA. Detection of bulimia in a primary care setting. Journal of General Internal Medicine 1993;8(5):236–42.

46. Grilo CM, McGlashan TH, Quinlan DM, Walker ML, Greenfeld D, Edell WS. Frequency of personality disorders in two age cohorts of psychiatric inpatients. American Journal of Psychiatry 1998;155(1):140–2.

47. Westen D, Shedler J, Durrett C, Glass S, Martens A. Personality diagnoses in adolescence: DSM-IV Axis II diagnoses and an empirically derived alternative. American Journal of Psychiatry 2003;160(5):952–66.

48. Levy KN, Becker DF, Grilo CM, Mattanah JJF, Garnet KE, Quinlan DM, Edell WS, McGlashan TH. Concurrent and predictive validity of the personality disorder diagnosis in adolescent patients. American Journal of Psychiatry 1999;156(10):1522–8.

49. Bernstein DP, Cohen P, Velez CN, Schwab-Stone M, Siever LJ, Shinsato L. Prevalence and stability of the DSM-III-R personality disorders in a community-based survey of adolescents. American Journal of Psychiatry 1993;150(8):1237–43.

50. Kasen S, Cohen P, Skodol AE, Johnson JG, Brook JS. Influence of child and adolescent psychiatric disorders on young adult personality disorder. American Journal of Psychiatry 1999;156(10):1529–35.

51. Work Group on Borderline Personality Disorder. Practice guideline for the treatment of patients with borderline personality disorder. American Journal of Psychiatry 2001;158(Suppl:10):1–52.

52. Tyrer P, Gunderson J, Lyons M, Tohen M. Extent of comorbidity between mental state and

personality disorders. Journal of Personality Disorders 1997;11(3):242–59.

53. Westen D, Dutra L, Shedler J. Assessing adolescent personality pathology. British Journal of Psychiatry 2005;186(3):227–38.

54. Chanen A, Jackson HJ, McGorry PD, Allot KA, Clarkson V, Yuen HP. Two-year stability of personality disorder in older adolescent outpatients. Journal of Personality Disorders 2004;18(6):526–41.

55. Crawford TN, Cohen P, Brook JS. Dramatic-erratic personality disorder symptoms: I. Continuity from early adolescence into adulthood. Journal of Personality Disorders 2001;15(4):315–35.

56. Johnson JG, Cohen P, Skodol AE, Oldham JM, Kasen S, Brook JS. Personality disorders in adolescence and risk of major mental disorders and suicidality during adulthood. Archives of General Psychiatry 1999;56(9):805–11.

57. Rothschild L, Zimmerman M. Borderline personality disorder and age of onset in major depression. Journal of Personality Disorders 2002;16(2):189–99.

58. Lewinsohn PM, Rohde P, Seeley JR, Klein DN. Axis II psychopathology as a function of Axis I disorders in childhood and adolescence. Journal of the American Academy of Child & Adolescent Psychiatry 1997;36(12):1752–9.

59. Samuels J, Eaton WW, Bienvenu O, Brown C, Costa PT, Nestadt G. Prevalence and correlates of personality disorders in a community sample. British Journal of Psychiatry 2002;180(6):536–42.

60. Torgersen S, Kringlen E, Cramer V. The prevalence of personality disorders in a community sample. Archives of General Psychiatry 2001;58(6):590–6.

61. Bateman A, Fonagy P. Effectiveness of partial hospitalization in the treatment of borderline personality disorder: A randomized controlled trial. [Comment]. American Journal of Psychiatry 1999;156(10):1563–9.

62. Linehan MM, Armstrong HE, Suarez A, Allmon D, Heard HL. Cognitive-behavioral treatment of chronically parasuicidal borderline patients. Archives of General Psychiatry 1991;48(12):1060–4.

63. Mulder RT. Personality pathology and treatment outcome in major depression: A review. American Journal of Psychiatry 2002;159(3):359–71.

64. Chanen A, Jackson HJ, McGorry PD, McCutcheon L, Berkovitch C, McDougall E, Yuen HP, Clarkson V, Germano D, Nistico, H. A randomised controlled trial of psychotherapy for early intervention for borderline personality disorder. Mar del Plata: IX International Congress On Personality Disorders, 2005..

65. Phillips L. Prodromal Psychosis and the First Episode. Check Program of Self-Assessment, Adolescent Health II. South Melbourne: The Royal Australian College of General Practitioners, 1998:19–21.

66. Rey J. Is My Teenager in Trouble? Sydney: Simon & Schuster Australia, 1995.

67. Bloch S, Singh BS. Understanding troubled minds: a guide to mental illness and its treatment. Melbourne: Melbourne University Press, 1998.

68. McGorry PD, Yung AR. Early intervention in psychosis: an overdue reform. Australian and New Zealand Journal of Psychiatry 2003;37:393–8.

69. Pavluri MN, Birmaher B, Naylor MW. Pediatric bipolar disorder: a review of the past 10 years. Journal of the American Academy of Child and Adolescent Psychiatry 2005;44(9):846–71.

70. Orygen. Fact sheets. Melbourne, 2005. www.orygen.org.au (last accessed October 2005)

71. Loxley WM, Toumbourou JW, Stockwell TR. A new integrated vision of how to prevent harmful drug use. Medical Journal of Australia 2005;182:54–5.

72. Sellman D, Deering D. Adolescence. In: Hulse G, White J, Cape G, eds. Management of Alcohol and Drug Problems. South Melbourne: Oxford University Press, 2002:273–87.

CHAPTER 16

COMMON MENTAL HEALTH PROBLEMS IN THE ELDERLY

D O'Connor, L Piterman and L Darvall

Old age is the most unexpected of all things that happen to a man.

LEON TROTSKY, 1879–1940

CASE STUDY

Edith is a 75-year-old widow who was an infrequent attendee at the clinic until the death of her husband two months ago. She has a son who lives interstate. During her visits she complains of recurrent abdominal and chest pains, but investigations do not reveal any significant pathology. Although she misses her husband, she denies having difficulty in coping without him. On occasions she misses appointments, or attends when she does not have an appointment. Her son calls the clinic on one of his visits. It has been three months since the death of his father and since he last saw his mother. He is concerned about the state of the house and about her personal hygiene. He found soiled underwear in the cupboards. He decides to take her interstate to stay with him and feels that she should sell the house. He wants power of attorney to look after her affairs as he believes that she is no longer able to care for herself. In your discussions with Edith she indicates that she does not mind having a holiday at her son's place but wants to return home. On arrival at her son's house, she becomes confused and disoriented, and is admitted two days later to the local hospital in a delirious state.

KEY FACTS

While most of the information presented elsewhere in this book relates equally to older people, certain situations become more common in older people:

- Dementia rises steadily in frequency in this age group.
- Mental disorders—for example, dementia complicated by delirium—often coexist.
- Mental disorders are precipitated or exacerbated by physical illness—for example, depression triggered by chronic, painful illness.

continued overleaf

KEY FACTS *continued*

As a result, good clinical practice requires that general practitioners (GPs):

- have a high index of suspicion for dementia and delirium;
- optimise the physical health of a patient with a mental disorder in order to prevent comorbid illness;
- be sensitive to the feelings of patients who lack insight into their disability;
- work closely with the family and professional carers to maximise the patient's mental and physical health, social wellbeing and autonomy, and to reduce the strain on carers;
- are aware of the potential for elder abuse both in family and institutional settings, and appreciate the legal rights of the elderly and the application of guardianship laws designed to protect those rights;
- have the clinical skills to diagnose common mental health problems and are familiar with the local specialist facilities designed to assist in assessment and management; and
- keep abreast of the growing body of knowledge related to pharmacotherapeutic interventions used in the management of Alzheimer's disease.

Among Australians aged 65 years and over:

- 15% of men and 49% of women are widowed.
- 13% of men and 31% of women live alone.
- 7% live in an aged residential facility.
- 18% of those born overseas speak little, if any, useful English.
- 17% have a severe or profound disability.
- 30% have consulted a doctor in the last two weeks.
- 71% have taken a prescribed medication in the last two days.

INTRODUCTION

Old age is often associated with bereavement, social isolation and physical, sensory and mental disability. All these factors can impact on mental health. GPs know many of their elderly patients very well and are ideally placed to both note the onset of mental disorders and manage these disorders effectively.

The case of Edith illustrates this well. While her husband was alive, she was able to cope, possibly because he carried out many of the essential tasks around the house and looked after her needs. With a patient such as Edith, who presents with a multitude of physical problems, the role of the GP is complex, and initially it is focused on excluding physical causes while being conscious that the underlying problem may be depression, prolonged grief reaction or dementia.

Patients with multiple disabilities, and especially those with dementia, are often perceived negatively; however, no problem is beyond help, and disentangling the complex medical, psychological, social and cultural constituents of the difficulties encountered in old age can prove most satisfying. This chapter highlights ways in which GPs can provide high quality mental health care to ageing patients.

DEMENTIA

Dementia refers to a permanent, usually progressive impairment of memory, thinking, behaviour and self-care. Its prevalence rises exponentially with age from 1% at 65 years to 25% at 85 years (see Figure 16.1)[1]. In developed countries, Alzheimer's disease accounts for roughly 60% of cases, followed by cerebrovascular disease (10%), Lewy body dementia (10%), frontal lobe dementias, also known as frontotemporal dementia or Pick's disease (5%), and other rarer causes, such as alcohol abuse and head trauma.

FIGURE 16.1 Prevalence of dementia with age

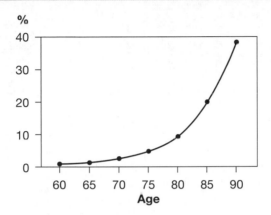

Dementias arising in the fifth and sixth decades of life typically have a single cause. By contrast, very old people with dementia often have multiple pathologies with combinations of amyloid plaques and neurofibrillary tangles due to Alzheimer's disease, infarctions and haemorrhages due to cerebrovascular disease, and cortical Lewy bodies.

CLINICAL FEATURES

The clinical features of the four most common conditions are summarised in Table 16.1 and amplified by means of examples in Figure 16.2. These distinguishing features blur with time: eventually all dementias result in profound disability. It helps if patients present early when profiles are distinct and treatments for Alzheimer's disease and Lewy body dementia can be offered at an opportune time.

A GP's concern may typically be triggered when a patient forgets appointments, muddles prescriptions, shows self-neglect or develops delirium in response to minor physical illness. Factors that impede recognition include a youthful onset, a relatively well preserved memory, and the presence of a spouse who compensates for the patient's deficits. This is illustrated in Edith's case. She hardly attended the GP while her husband was alive, but after his death she either missed appointments or attended, thinking that she had an appointment. Such occurrences should make GPs suspicious that memory loss is a problem and that formal assessment of memory should be carried out at this early stage. Patients with dementia develop coping strategies, and well educated, articulate patients, who nonetheless lack insight into their condition, can escape attention for years.

TABLE 16.1 Types of dementia

TYPE	PATTERN OF ONSET	COGNITIVE DEFICITS	OTHER FEATURES	IMAGING CHANGES	TREATMENT
Alzheimer's disease	Gradual	Global	Insight lost early, rapid forgetting of new information	Initially none, later widespread cortical atrophy	Cholinesterase inhibitors
Vascular dementia	Sudden or gradual	Patchy, variable	Insight often retained, greater risk of depression	Cortical and/or subcortical infarcts, deep white matter ischaemia, seen best on MRI	None
Lewy body dementia	Gradual	Slowed thinking, impaired attention, impaired memory	Visual hallucinations, Parkinsonism, extreme sensitivity to traditional high potency antipsychotic medications (e.g. haloperidol)	Initially none	Cholinesterase inhibitors
Frontal lobe dementia	Gradual	Highly variable, memory often well preserved	Marked changes in personality, mood and behaviour. May exhibit striking language changes	Frontal and/or temporal atrophy, often asymmetrical	None

Most patients lose insight into their condition at an early stage and fail to report lapses in memory and behaviour. This will change in the future as knowledge of dementia becomes widespread. In the meantime, doctors are often alerted to a patient's decline by the spouse and children, whose reports correlate well with objective measures. It is important not to dismiss concerns about cognitive and behavioural change without making further enquiries. By the time family members seek help, dementia is typically well established and easy to diagnose. The visit of Edith's son serves to illustrate this point.

Most dementias worsen slowly. In middle and late stage conditions, patients often show mood disorders, delusions and hallucinations, disturbed behaviours and altered personality.

FIGURE 16.2 Early symptoms of dementia

ALZHEIMER'S DISEASE

Mrs Anderson's memory of recent events is slowly worsening. She forgets messages, misplaces objects, muddles her medications and repeats herself. Her insight is limited, but she is content when left to her own devices. A computerised tomograph (CT) brain scan is normal.

VASCULAR DEMENTIA

Mr Belenki has mild, patchy memory loss after a cortical stroke and two transient ischaemic attacks. He recalls matters of personal significance but muddles details and time sequences. He acknowledges his lapses and is distressed by them. A CT brain scan shows strokes and deep white matter ischaemia.

LEWY BODY DEMENTIA

Mrs Chen has vivid visual hallucinations (not due to delirium) of visitors to her home. She converses with the visitors and offers them food. Her memory varies from day to day, sometimes to the point of confusion. She has limited insight. A CT brain scan is normal.

FRONTOTEMPORAL DEMENTIA

Mr Drew's personality is slowly changing. He is now demanding and abusive, and he collects useless objects. His memory is generally intact. He lacks insight and becomes angry when his behaviour is questioned. A CT brain scan shows frontal atrophy.

DIFFERENTIAL DIAGNOSIS

The following conditions must be distinguished from dementia.

SEVERE DEPRESSION This can lead to such withdrawal and inactivity that to the untrained eye the patient seems to have dementia. This so-called 'pseudodementia' responds to treatment with antidepressant medication or electroconvulsive therapy (ECT) and must never be missed. Pointers include: a past history of depression; recent onset; an obviously lowered mood with anxiety and agitation; disturbed appetite and sleep; and 'I don't know' responses to cognitive tests. These cases are complex, and referral to a specialist is warranted. Depression is occasionally the first pointer to dementia and some patients with well established dementia also become depressed (see 'Depression' on page 269).

LATE ONSET PSYCHOSES Dementia with secondary delusions and hallucinations must be distinguished from the relatively uncommon late onset psychoses, which present with persecutory delusions and auditory hallucinations (see 'Bipolar disorder, delusional disorder and schizophrenia' on page 273 and Chapters 8 and 12). About half of all dementing illnesses are complicated by delusions and hallucinations at some stage. Cognitive impairment is usually obvious in these cases, except in people with early Lewy body dementia who report striking visual hallucinations with only minimal, variable intellectual deficits (see Table 16.1 and Figure 16.2).

DELIRIUM Delirium is an acute condition—secondary to physical illness, drug toxicity or drug withdrawal—that results either in a quietly obtunded mental state or else florid confusion, agitation, persecutory delusions and visual hallucinations. People with dementia are especially vulnerable to delirium, sometimes in response to minor medical conditions, such as urinary tract infections. Delirium is sometimes the first pointer to an underlying dementia. When this happens, improvement is sometimes incomplete: each episode of delirium results in a further downward step. It is important, therefore, to prevent delirium and to treat new episodes as quickly as possible. The onset of delirium when Edith moved interstate occurred against a background of change in her environment that is well known to cause confusion in patients with dementia; however, confusion is not synonymous with delirium. In Edith's case delirium was in fact triggered by a chest infection with minimal respiratory symptoms.

NORMAL OLDER PEOPLE Some normal older people seek reassurance that they are not dementing. They are typically high achievers who are distressed by age related changes in cognitive speed, concentration and memory. Some have a family history of dementia. Most have experienced major upsets in their lives that tax their cognitive resources. They respond best when their concerns are taken seriously by means of baseline cognitive testing and a medical review. Refer the patient for a detailed neuropsychological assessment if there is still reason for concern.

COMORBIDITY

Patients with dementia are vulnerable to the following conditions:

- depression, especially in cases of vascular dementia;
- psychotic symptoms in the form of complex, persistent visual hallucinations in Lewy body disease; or simple, fleeting hallucinations in most other forms of dementia; or as delusions that are typically simple (for example, a missing purse has been stolen), but can be complex (for example, a spouse is an imposter); and
- delirium resulting in an abrupt worsening of confusion, incapacity, behavioural disturbance, delusions and hallucinations. An abrupt worsening of mental state and behaviour in a person with dementia points to delirium until proven otherwise.

ASSESSMENT

Assessment of people with possible dementia encompasses diagnostic, medical, psychiatric, carer and safety issues. These require a history, mental state examination, cognitive testing, physical check-up and a family and safety review. (See Figure 16.3.)

> **FIGURE 16.3** Key facts for dementia assessment
>
> - Establish the presence, severity and likely cause of dementia.
> - Exclude delirium, depression and psychosis as primary diagnoses.
> - Check for comorbid delirium, depression and psychosis.
> - Check physical health.
> - Record a baseline MMSE score (see 'Cognitive testing' on page 264).

HISTORY Since the patient's account is often inaccurate, questions must be directed to a knowledgeable person about the duration and speed of symptom onset. If the patient lives alone, it is helpful (if the patient consents) to contact a family member to check basic information. Informants' accounts of cognitive and behavioural change correlate well with objective measures.

The history should cover risk factors for Alzheimer's disease (family history), vascular dementia (stroke, hypertension, smoking, diabetes mellitus, hypercholesterolaemia) and other causes of dementia, such as head trauma and alcohol abuse.

Distinguishing between cognitive changes that develop slowly, usually as the result of dementia, and those that develop acutely because of delirium, is crucial. Since delirium may be superimposed on dementia, it is helpful to ask, for example, 'Did your relative have memory problems before she became physically unwell and very confused three days ago?'

MENTAL STATE EXAMINATION Appearances can be deceptive. People with advanced dementia who live alone often look neglected. By contrast, those living with a family member are often neatly groomed and well nourished; deficits can be concealed for years. Consultations with a trusted GP often follow an established format that even moderately confused people negotiate successfully. In most research studies, GPs recognise only half the cases of dementia in their practice.[?]

Demands that exceed a patient's capacity to cope can lead to anxiety, agitation and even 'catastrophic reactions' at any time. In the later stages of dementia, a patient becomes agitated without clear triggers in the late afternoon and evening (a syndrome known as 'sundowning').

About 5% of people with dementia have a comorbid major depressive disorder. This figure is doubled in dementias due to cerebrovascular disease, Parkinson's disease and other neurological conditions. Pointers to comorbid depression include social withdrawal, agitation, tearfulness, calling out, insomnia and anorexia. Special care is required as some of these features are also part of uncomplicated dementia. Depressed, confused old people look anxious and unhappy and, when asked, admit to feelings of sadness and despair.

Disorientation to time is common. Patients often attribute it to a lack of interest in current events—'The news is so depressing now'—or to poor vision or hearing but, in reality, most cognitively intact old people are aware of the day, month and year. Orientation to place is less revealing for people who have lived in the same home for many decades, but it should be checked nonetheless.

Language abnormalities range from word-finding difficulty to profound aphasia. Thinking becomes simple in content, rambling and repetitive.

In the middle stages, half of all dementias are accompanied by misinterpretations, delusions and hallucinations. When a dementia patient misplaces a purse or wallet, they accuse others of stealing it. These misinterpretations usually settle once the item is found. In more complex cases, a patient may accuse their spouse of being an imposter; think their long deceased parents are alive; and accuse neighbours of interfering with possessions. Hallucinations can occur in all modalities but visual ones are more common; they are usually of children and animals. Florid, bizarre visual hallucinations suggest delirium or Lewy body dementia.

Loss of insight is often evident early. Patients insist that they are coping well when clearly they are not.

COGNITIVE TESTING Cognitive testing is an essential element of assessment. Mildly affected people who are articulate and socially skilled conceal their deficits easily. Cognitive tests provide a definitive check and help track changes over time. Testing rarely causes offence if it is conducted sensitively.

The Mini Mental State Examination (MMSE) is used widely in aged care services and provides a baseline reference for all professionals involved in a patient's care; however, it should not be used to confirm a diagnosis without additional information, since a poor performance might actually be due to deafness, limited vision, depression, lack of co-operation or limited education. Patients from non-English speaking backgrounds require special care. Generally speaking, however, a score of 23 or less suggests significant cognitive impairment (see Table 16.2).

The tone of answers to cognitive tests is often revealing. Glib responses—for example, 'One day seems much like another' or 'I don't follow the news any more'—often conceal gaps in knowledge. Incorrect answers need not be exposed. Tact and sensitivity are essential. Test results should be recorded in detail. Useful supplementary tests include clock drawing, which is highly sensitive to early cognitive decline, and knowledge of recent news events and the names of political leaders.

MEDICAL EXAMINATION Truly reversible dementias are rare in developed countries. Normal pressure hydrocephalus—which results in the triad of a rapidly progressive dementia, ataxia and urinary incontinence—can certainly be reversed if detected early by means of a brain scan. The 'pick-up' rate of the standard dementia screen is otherwise low. Laboratory batteries (FBC, glucose, thyroid and liver function tests, vitamin B12 and folate levels) are better viewed as a means of detecting common unreported conditions that complicate dementia and limit functional capacity. Correcting anaemia and hypothyroidism, for example, might not reverse a dementia but will still improve a patient's quality of life.

MANAGEMENT

Management might entail the following: treating Alzheimer's disease; reducing vascular risk factors; preventing and treating comorbid delirium, psychiatric symptoms and disturbed behaviours; educating and supporting family and professional carers; and helping co-ordinate medical, social and respite services (see Figure 16.4).

TREATMENT The cholinesterase inhibitors (donepezil, rivastigmine and galantamine) correct low acetylcholine levels in Alzheimer's disease, resulting in small but worthwhile

TABLE 16.2 Mini Mental State Examination (MMSE)

QUESTION/TASK	MAXIMUM SCORE	ACTUAL SCORE
Ask the patient what (year) (season) (date) (day) (month) it is.	5	
Ask the patient what (country) (state) (town) (street/hospital) (street number/floor of building) it is.	5	
Name three objects slowly. Ask the patient to repeat them. Repeat up to 5 times till all are learnt. Give 1 point for each correct answer at first attempt.	3	
Ask the patient to subtract 7 from 100, and keep subtracting 7 from what's left until you ask them to stop. Give 1 point for each correct subtraction.	5	
Ask the patient to name the three objects that you identified earlier.	3	
Ask the patient to name a pen and a watch.	2	
Ask the patient to repeat after you: 'No ifs, ands or buts.'	1	
Ask the patient to read this sentence and do what it says: 'Close your eyes'.	1	
Ask the patient to follow a three-stage command: 'Take this paper in your right/left hand, fold it in half, and put it in your lap.'	3	
Ask the patient to write a sentence.	1	
Ask the patient to copy a design of two overlapping pentagons.	1	
Total score	30	

FIGURE 16.4 Key facts about dementia management

- For Alzheimer's disease, consider prescribing cholinesterase inhibitors.
- For vascular dementia, reduce risk factors.
- Optimise physical health.
- Treat delirium urgently.
- Treat persistent major depression and psychosis.
- In Lewy body dementia, avoid traditional high potency antipsychotics such as haloperidol.
- Use psychotropics sparingly to relieve disturbed behaviours.
- Support and educate carers.

improvements in memory, energy and mood. They can reduce the burden on carers and postpone admission to residential care. Restrictions on their use apply in some countries. Currently in Australia, the diagnosis of mild to moderate Alzheimer's disease must be confirmed by a specialist (not necessarily in person) and the MMSE score must improve by 2 or more points over a six-month period. Common side effects include nausea, diarrhoea, vivid dreams and leg cramps. Bradycardia is almost invariable, especially when combined with beta blockers. There is generally little value in continuing treatment once a patient has entered a nursing home, although doses should be reduced slowly in case behavioural disturbance worsens.

Cholinesterase inhibitors can produce dramatic improvements in Lewy body dementia but are not yet approved for this condition in Australia. GPs should refer likely cases to a specialist for advice. Management of vascular dementia entails the reduction of risk factors. There is no treatment for frontal lobe dementia.

PSYCHIATRIC SYMPTOMS Comorbid depression warrants a trial of antidepressant medication if the patient is persistently low in mood, anxious and agitated, and is sleeping and eating poorly.

Fleeting beliefs by the patient, such as thinking a purse has been stolen when it has only been misplaced, respond well to reassurance. However, recurrent perturbing delusions warrant treatment with an antipsychotic medication. Newer, atypical antipsychotics are preferable if they are available locally. Patients with Lewy body dementia are sensitive to traditional, high potency antipsychotics such as haloperidol, small doses of which induce alarming Parkinsonism and confusion.

DISTURBED BEHAVIOURS Disturbed behaviours—for example, persistent wandering, resistiveness, 'sundowning', verbal and physical abusiveness, calling out and sleep–wake disruption—arise commonly in middle and late stage dementias. Family and professional carers find them stressful and often request assistance. Management is guided by the following questions:

- What is the behaviour? What form does it take? How frequent is it?
- Is it due to comorbid delirium, major depression or psychosis?
- What precedes the behaviour? Can these antecedents be modified?
- How do the caregivers respond? Do their responses inadvertently worsen the situation? If so, how can they behave differently?
- What risk does the behaviour present to the patient and carer? Do all staff in a residential facility perceive it as a problem or only some?
- Is psychotropic medication essential? What treatment is least hazardous? Is the treatment helpful? If not, is the dose too high or too low? Should it be stopped? What is the next best choice?
- Is help required from the Alzheimer's Society, aged psychiatry team or dementia nurse (if available)?

A behavioural analysis can generate strategies to minimise conflict. Consider these strategies, for example:

- Humour patients and avoid challenging them directly.
- Be flexible about when unpleasant tasks such as showering are scheduled.
- Use distraction, exercise, music and hand massage to reduce any tension the patient may be experiencing.
- Allow carers an opportunity to vent their frustration.

■ Organise practical supports such as dosette boxes for organising medications, home help, meals on wheels, day care and respite care.

Psychotropic medications play a limited role (with the exception of antidepressants and antipsychotics as treatments for comorbid major depression and psychosis, respectively). They help some patients to some extent for some of the time—but all can worsen confusion.

■ If all else fails, hypnotics such as temazepam can settle nocturnal disturbance.
■ Antipsychotic medications can reduce daytime anxiety, agitation, delusions and hallucinations, and most are less sedating than benzodiazepines. Atypical antipsychotics such as olanzapine and quetiapine are preferable to typical ones such as haloperidol.
■ Where they are not available or affordable, consider prescribing benzodiazepines with intermediate half-lives such as oxazepam.
■ Mood stabilisers—for example, sodium valproate—can also relieve agitation and irritability.

Since side effects are dose related, doses are kept to a minimum. Typical maximum total daily doses in confused elderly people are olanzapine 10 mg, quetiapine 200 mg, haloperidol 1 mg, oxazepam 45 mg and sodium valproate 800 mg; most patients require less.

Atypical neuroleptics may slightly increase the risk of cerebrovascular events, and regulatory authorities in the United Kingdom and the United States recommend against their use in people with dementia. This is controversial, as other medications have significant side effects too.

FAMILY AND CARER ISSUES People with dementia should participate as much as possible in decisions regarding their treatment and care. If diagnosed early, they can assign a power of attorney, make a will while still competent and talk with family members about future care arrangements.

An assessment of the patient's ability to perform everyday tasks is critical. Is help required with dressing, washing, toileting, bathing, cooking, housework, shopping and handling money? What services are in place and who will assist in a crisis?

Admission to a residential facility comes sooner for those who live alone or whose carer is frail. A move to new surroundings is disruptive and can temporarily worsen the patient's confusion. The nursing home must be informed in advance of the patient's needs, difficulties and personal preferences. It is helpful for new carers to know who started psychiatric medications as well as when, why and with what success.

LEGAL AND ETHICAL ISSUES See also the 'Legal issues' section at end of this chapter as well as Chapter 4.

People with dementia will insist that they drive safely and respond angrily to suggestions that they should stop. Emotions can run so high that GPs rightly ask specialists or hospitals to initiate a formal driving assessment. This is acceptable except where patients pose such a danger to the community that licensing authorities must be notified urgently.

Patients ask doctors to endorse their testamentary capacity when they suspect a challenge to their will. This points strongly to family discord and the need to proceed with caution. It is not enough to state that a person seems to be cognitively intact. Testamentary capacity requires knowledge of the nature and effect of a will as well as the nature and extent of assets, and likely claimants against the estate. Many mildly demented people are fully aware of these issues, especially where the estate and family circumstances are straightforward. The more advanced the dementia, and the more complex the estate, the greater is the need for specialist assessment by a geriatrician, psychiatrist or neuropsychologist before a will is written.

In Edith's case, the son may have appeared well meaning; however, as events unfolded, it emerged that he wanted her money to settle failed business debts, and so her affairs ultimately had to be put into the hands of the Public Trustee through the Office of the Public Advocate. GPs should be aware of the rights of patients with dementia and how those rights are administered (see Chapter 4 and Figure 16.5).

Elder abuse within families typically entails the theft of money from a frail, confused parent by a child with business or gambling difficulties. Where a patient with dementia is clearly at risk of financial disadvantage or abuse, GPs must ask an aged care agency to apply for an administration order or its local equivalent. In residential facilities, all instances of abusive behaviour by staff must be reported to the director. It is unethical to do nothing.

Medical and psychiatric conditions that are disabling but remediable—for example, major depression or fractured neck of femur—warrant treatment, but patients with severe dementia need not be treated aggressively for pneumonia or other immediately life-threatening illnesses. Palliative care is mandatory but attempts to postpone death when it is inevitable are cruel. Ask relatives if their spouse or parent had previously expressed a wish regarding medical care in the event that they became incompetent.

FIGURE 16.5 Key facts about legal and ethical issues

- Ensure patients with obvious dementia have a driving assessment.
- Do not witness wills or other legal documents if there is any reason to question the patient's competence.
- You must report all instances of financial, physical or emotional abuse.
- Talk with patients and families in advance about end-of-life care.

DELIRIUM

Delirium is an acute organic mental disorder that arises over hours or days in response to an acute physical illness or injury, drug toxicity or withdrawal from alcohol and benzodiazepines. In its most severe form, it is a frightening condition with high mortality. Even milder cases result in significant morbidity, such as longer hospital stays, falls and pressure sores.

Characteristic features include: rapid onset; reduced attention with consequent distractibility; confusion; anxiety, suspiciousness and agitation; visual hallucinations; and diurnal variation with a characteristic worsening at night.

As noted already, delirium arises most commonly in people with dementia, sometimes in response to minor illnesses. The underlying dementia is sometimes so mild that families have paid it no regard. The onset of delirium is therefore an alarming 'wake up call'. Other risk factors include physical frailty, sensory handicap, polypharmacy and pain. All psychotropic medications can precipitate or worsen delirium, as can narcotics and other medications with anticholingeric properties, such as digitalis and non-steroidal anti-inflammatory drugs.

Recovery can be prolonged and incomplete, especially when dementia is also present. Repeated delirium can therefore greatly reduce the quality of life of the patient, worsen carer burden and hasten admission to residential care. Rapid detection and treatment are therefore essential. Prevention is even better.

In nursing home practice, dementia is often so advanced that it blurs imperceptibly with delirium. Pointers to the latter include an abrupt shift to daytime drowsiness, worsened agitation and plucking at imaginary objects.

Management consists of treatment of the noxious precipitant and prompt functional rehabilitation. Psychiatric medications are occasionally required to treat extreme anxiety, agitation, insomnia, delusions and hallucinations. Daytime benzodiazepines worsen sleep–wake disruption and are best avoided. Neuroleptics—for example, haloperidol 0.5 mg bd, parenterally if necessary—are safer. If delirium stems from excessive psychotropic drugs, usually in patients with advanced dementia, the correct response is to reduce their use to a minimum.

DEPRESSION

About 20% of older people resident in the community report one or more depressive symptoms, but only 2% meet the criteria for major depressive disorder. Contrary to expectations, older people report less major depression than younger adults. They were often reared in tougher times and have learnt to withstand life's challenges. Major losses—illness, incapacity and bereavement—are often anticipated but are no less painful when they occur.

Risk factors for major depression include female gender; a past history of depression; an anxious, obsessive personality; chronic pain; physical or sensory handicap; recent adverse life events, such as bereavement; lack of a confiding relationship; and poverty. Depression can be precipitated by certain medications—for example, corticosteroids, L-dopa, methyldopa—and specific physical conditions—for example, occult carcinoma, stroke and degenerative neurological disorders. (See Figure 16.6.)

Previously, suicide rates were highest in very old men. Their risk of suicide is now dropping in many developed countries, perhaps because of greater confidence in social and medical supports. Older suicide victims typically live alone, have a serious physical illness and are depressed. Overdoses of medication as 'cries for help' are uncommon in old age. All threats of suicide must be taken seriously.

FIGURE 16.6 Key facts about depression

- Feelings of loneliness and grief are common.
- Major depression is uncommon (only 2–3%) but rates are higher in residential facilities (up to 25%).
- Risk factors include gender, health, isolation, past depression and personality.
- Talk of suicide must be taken seriously.

CLINICAL FEATURES

The usual features of major depression occur in older patients, and these include: a persistently lowered mood; anxiety and agitation; slowed thinking and movement; complaints of poor concentration and memory; fatigue; insomnia; anorexia and weight loss. These 'vegetative' depressive features predict a good response to biological treatments. Small numbers of patients also have delusions of poverty, sinfulness or disease.

Since depression often co-exists with serious physical illness and disability, complaints of worsening pain in a patient with rheumatoid arthritis, for example, might be due to physical relapse, depression or a combination of the two. To complicate matters, conditions such as heart failure, airways disease, renal failure and carcinoma also lead to anorexia, insomnia and fatigue. Pointers to depression as the major culprit include a persistently lowered mood, levels of pain out of keeping with physical signs and a poor response to medical treatments.

Depression impacts negatively on cognitive function. Despairing, helpless patients often respond with 'I don't know' when questioned about orientation, memory and thinking. With time and encouragement, they often complete tests correctly. Some patients conclude that they have dementia when clearly they do not. Their complaints are not in keeping with their function in everyday life. In extreme cases, patients sit mutely, wet and soil themselves, and to the untrained eye seem to have dementia. This condition, called depressive pseudodementia, is described on page 260 (see 'Severe depression').

To complicate matters, people with dementia often feel anxious and frustrated when the demands made on them exceed their capacity to cope. Dysphoria varies, depending on the circumstances, but 5–10% of dementias are complicated by major depression. This comorbid syndrome should not be confused with the apathy, inertia, social withdrawal and diminished self-care that stem directly from the underlying dementing process. Major depression results in a persistent lowering of mood, anxiety, agitation, irritability, insomnia, anorexia and weight loss. Because of their forgetfulness, patients (many of whom live in residential facilities) cannot report accurately on symptoms in recent days and weeks (this needs to be confirmed by an informant), but they can certainly describe their present feeling state. In advanced dementias, depression is revealed more in anxious and agitated behaviour than in words.

ASSESSMENT

Some patients believe that depression is a normal part of ageing and do not disclose it to their doctor. Others are concerned that endless complaints will antagonise family and friends, and so they keep their worries to themselves. In addition, patients from certain cultural backgrounds express emotional distress in somatic terms that do not fit with recognised syndromes and that have great emotional overlay. Direct questions about mood and related symptoms quickly uncover the true state of affairs. If patients find the term 'depression' offensive, there is no need to insist on using it.

A history and mental state examination are mandatory assessment tasks. Relevant questions to ask the patient concern the persistence and severity of depression and changes in appetite, sleep and energy. To detect self-neglect, ask about diet, exercise and social interaction. If dementia coexists, question an informant as the patient's own report might not be reliable. Other steps include a physical examination and laboratory screen—for example, full blood count, erythrocyte sedimentation rate (ESR) and thyroid function tests—to exclude physical causes. A chest X-ray should be ordered for current and ex-smokers. If depression is recurrent, it is important to know the timing of previous episodes and what past treatments were helpful (and unhelpful). (See Figure 16.7.)

FIGURE 16.7 Key facts about depression assessment

- You should enquire about the 'biological' depressive symptoms that respond well to medical treatments.
- Physical illness precipitates depression. Conversely, depression worsens complaints of pain and disability.
- Five to ten per cent of people with dementia have comorbid major depression.

MANAGEMENT

SOCIAL AND PSYCHOLOGICAL THERAPIES Many unhappy and distressed old people who do not have major depression, and are therefore not likely to respond to antidepressant medication, or benefit from psychological therapies. Sessions can be set aside to give them time to vent their fears of frailty, dependence, bereavement and family neglect. Banal reassurance is counterproductive. Listening is always helpful.

Older people were previously considered too set in their ways to benefit from counselling. This is untrue. Many are insightful and articulate, and welcome the opportunity to review their lives, take pleasure in their achievements and make amends for past hurts. These steps take courage. Cognitive behavioural therapy works best with practically minded people who wish to focus on tasks such as socialisation, exercise, self-care and nutrition. Family counselling can repair the damage inflicted by marital, parental and sibling disharmony in previous decades.

PHYSICAL TREATMENTS Antidepressant medications do not alleviate loneliness or grief (unless these trigger major depression). Distinguishing between life related distress and major depression is not straightforward in primary care. It may take a number of consultations to establish that a patient's mood, thinking, energy, appetite and sleep are worsening, despite efforts to optimise physical and emotional wellbeing.

Tricyclic antidepressants are effective but have unpleasant and possibly hazardous side effects (blurred vision, dry mouth, constipation and postural hypotension) and are dangerous in overdose. Despite this, patients who have taken them for many years without adverse effects are reluctant to shift to newer preparations. Novel medications such as serotonin specific and noradrenergic reuptake inhibitors are better tolerated and almost as effective. Starting doses are halved for old, frail people and for those who also have dementia. Fit, healthy, older people require standard adult doses.

PERSONALITY AND AGEING

Most querulous, suspicious or dependent behavioural traits in older people are due to underlying anxiety, depression or dementia; however, small numbers of old people have always been clinging, reclusive or antisocial. These traits are part of an enduring

> **FIGURE 16.8** Key facts about depression management
>
> ■ Antidepressant medications lift mood in major depression but not in cases of uncomplicated loneliness and grief.
> ■ Opportunities to vent distress are always helpful.
> ■ Counselling and psychotherapy are used increasingly with older people.

personality profile and have often led to dysfunctional relationships, abnormal illness behaviour or abusive behaviour over many decades (see Chapter 18).

Two examples will illustrate the difference. Mrs Alexander is an anxious, dependent widow who calls her children, friends and doctor many times a day. She makes unreasonable demands and threatens suicide when these demands are not met quickly. She previously relied on her husband, and has coped poorly since his death two years earlier. Her symptoms remit quickly when help is provided but her children are exhausted and angry.

Mr Brookes, on the other hand, is a reclusive, suspicious man who is alarmed by his admission to a medical ward. He finds enforced dependency and proximity to others threatening, and he responds with angry outbursts and demands to be discharged. His irritability is not due to major depression, psychosis or dementia, rather it is consistent with a life-long pattern of relating to others.

A detailed history is invaluable. Has the patient always been anxious, angry or suspicious? How did this manifest and how did family members respond? Have matters recently changed? Is this due to the death of a spouse, admission to residential care, physical illness or the onset of dementia or another mental disorder?

Management plans will stem from this analysis. Very anxious, dependent old people might benefit from practical and psychological supports coupled with reasonable, consistent limits on help-seeking behaviour. Angry, controlling people appreciate efforts to involve them in decision making (assuming they have capacity).

ANXIETY

While most anxious old people have always been 'nervy', anxiety disorders can arise acutely in response to physical illness, bereavement, family upheaval, crime and other adverse events. Symptoms include insomnia, headache, tremor, palpitations, gastric churning and hyperventilation. Patients and doctors can easily mistake panic attacks for myocardial infarction. Anxiety due to falls can lead to a refusal by the patient to leave home unaccompanied (agoraphobia) and to an unwarranted and dangerous insistence on grasping onto articles of furniture.

Anxious patients require time and reassurance. If possible, anxiolytic medications should be avoided to prevent falls and psychological dependence. Better options include encouragement, practical supports and graded exposure to walking unaided through referral to a rehabilitation centre. If this fails, small doses of a medium-acting benzodiazepine may be warranted for a few weeks—for example, oxazepam 7.5 mg bd. Most anxious older people comply with medical prescriptions (see Chapter 9).

SUBSTANCE ABUSE

There is a widespread perception that elderly people, and women in particular, do not drink alcohol to excess, and doctors often fail to recognise abuse when it is present. Some people have always consumed heavily, while others increase their intake in old age through loneliness, anxiety or depression. Those who live alone are at special risk: even housebound patients can obtain supplies surprisingly easily. Doctors are reluctant to enquire about drinking habits, and it may take a fall or withdrawal delirium to bring substance abuse to light.

Even long-term substance abusers can be persuaded to stop drinking if the adverse effects are spelt out clearly. Loneliness, anxiety and depression should be tackled directly through such measures as attendance at a day centre, bereavement counselling or antidepressants, as indicated. Intractable substance abuse, when it leads to an amnestic disorder or dementia, requires residential care (see Chapter 10).

BIPOLAR DISORDER, DELUSIONAL DISORDER AND SCHIZOPHRENIA

Bipolar disorder mostly arises earlier in life, but mania occasionally presents for the first time in old age, usually in the setting of cerebrovascular disease and other neuropathological conditions. Generally speaking, manic episodes lessen in severity over time but functional capacity worsens. Some older bipolar patients are a good deal more disabled than textbooks suggest. Mood stabilisers are effective, but breakthrough episodes sometimes make it necessary to change (and even combine) medications. Lithium carbonate and sodium valproate often prove effective at lower doses and blood levels than in younger adults; typical doses are 250 mg bd and 400 mg bd, respectively.

A few lonely, mistrustful old people have always believed that others take advantage of them. This personality pattern results in repeated arguments with family and neighbours as well as increasing social isolation. In extreme cases, patients live in squalor and steadfastly refuse help. Delusional disorder, by contrast, emerges in late life over a period of months or even years. Delusions are usually banal and unsystematised: neighbours are accused of banging on walls and throwing rubbish over the fence; less commonly, secret investigators tap the telephone and bombard the house with electricity. Neighbours are verbally abused and the police often summoned for protection. Risk factors include female gender, a suspicious personality and a family history of psychosis.

Bizarre visual, tactile or olfactory hallucinations, when coupled with delusions in a state of clear consciousness—for example, lights shining through windows, insects crawling beneath the skin and noxious smells—point to schizophrenia.

Most older people with schizophrenia have been unwell for many decades. Some remain actively psychotic but negative symptoms predominate with marked apathy, emotional blunting, poverty of thought and poor judgment. Issues in later life include a heightened susceptibility to the adverse effects of antipsychotic medications, polypharmacy and the loss through illness or death of carers. Isolation, poverty and sub-standard accommodation are common.

Schizophrenia occasionally arises for the first time in advanced old age. When it does, organic causes such as cerebral tumour treatment with corticosteroids or L-Dopa are considered. Delirium, dementia and affective disorder are important differential diagnoses, since all three can present with delusions, hallucinations and disturbed behaviour. Features characteristic of delirium include physical illness, altered arousal, impaired attention and confusion. Dementia is accompanied by forgetfulness and confusion. Depression and mania have characteristic signs and symptoms as outlined above.

Some acutely psychotic patients are so frightened that help is received gladly. Others are suspicious of doctors, refuse them entry and insist that treatment is unwarranted, even dangerous. Involuntary admission to hospital may be required to commence treatment.

Physical examination and pertinent laboratory tests are needed to exclude treatable precipitating conditions. Newer antipsychotics are preferred for treatment. Low potency drugs such as chlorpromazine are sedating, and postural hypotension leads to falls and fractures. Higher potency drugs such as haloperidol cause extrapyramidal side effects that also result in falls. Clozapine is an option in treatment resistant cases, although the risk of agranulocytosis increases with age. Depot preparations are used sparingly but have a role in patients who consistently refuse tablets, wafers or syrups. Treatment is long term. Doses of medication should be reviewed frequently and reduced if possible (see Chapter 12).

LEGAL ISSUES

See also Chapter 4. *Disclaimer*: This section states the law in a general manner and is not intended as a substitute for legal advice.

The laws dealing with elderly patients and others who lack decision-making capacity may vary from state to state and country to country. The information below, provided by Dr Leanna Darvall as an example, sets out the position in the state of Victoria.

STATUTORY PROVISIONS CONCERNING CONSENT TO MEDICAL TREATMENT

The *Victorian Guardianship Administration Act 1986* enables proxy decision makers to make legally valid treatment decisions on behalf of incompetent adults. A person is deemed incompetent—that is, unable to provide a valid legal consent to treatment—if she/he lacks a basic understanding of the nature and effect of the proposed treatment, or procedure, or cannot indicate whether or not he/she consents to the proposed treatment, or procedure.

The following persons are legally entitled to consent to treatment on behalf of incompetent adult patients:

GUARDIANS APPOINTED BY THE VCAT A Victorian Civil and Administrative Tribunal (VCAT) appointed plenary guardian may make health care, work and accommodation decisions in respect of a represented person, but cannot make decisions in respect of financial or civil legal matters.

ENDURING GUARDIANS A competent adult may appoint an adult person to act as an enduring guardian in the event that he/she becomes incompetent. A statutory form, obtainable from the Office of the Public Advocate (OPA), must be signed by both parties. An enduring guardian has identical powers to those of a plenary guardian, unless limited by the document of appointment. *Note*: The legislation excludes a person who provides professional care or services to an appointor from being appointed as an enduring guardian.

PERSON RESPONSIBLE Because few people appoint an enduring guardian, the legislation provides that 'a person responsible' may act as a proxy decision maker on their behalf. A 'person responsible' is the first person listed below who is responsible for the patient, and who is available and willing to make a decision in relation to medical treatment:

- an agent appointed by the patient under the *Medical Treatment Act 1988* (Vic);
- a VCAT appointed guardian;
- a person appointed by the patient as an enduring guardian, with power to make decisions about the proposed treatment;
- a person appointed by the patient in writing to make decisions about medical treatment, including the proposed treatment;
- the patient's spouse, including someone not legally married to the patient who lives with them in a marriage-like relationship;
- the patient's primary carer, including carers in receipt of a social security benefit but excluding paid carers or service providers; and
- the patient's 'nearest adult relative'.

IF THERE IS NO PERSON RESPONSIBLE, OR IF A PERSON RESPONSIBLE CANNOT BE LOCATED

Medical treatment without the consent of the 'person responsible' may be undertaken if a medical practitioner considers it to be in the patient's best interests, but only after giving a S.42K notice to the Public Advocate (the relevant form can be obtained from the OPA).

WHEN A PERSON RESPONSIBLE REFUSES CONSENT TO TREATMENT CONTRARY TO THE BEST INTERESTS OF THE PLAINTIFF

If a medical practitioner and a person responsible do not agree about the necessity and/or desirability of the proposed medical treatment, and the practitioner believes that the proposed treatment would be in the patient's best interests, he/she must give the responsible person and the Public Advocate a statutory prescribed (Section 42 M) notice. The notice, which can be obtained from the OPA, must be given within three days of the person responsible indicating to the medical practitioner that he/she does not consent.

WHEN CONSENT OF A PERSON RESPONSIBLE IS UNNECESSARY

MINOR TREATMENTS The legislation permits practitioners to carry out some minor or non-invasive treatments—such as a visual examination of the mouth, first aid or the administration of a prescribed drug—without first obtaining a substitute consent.

EMERGENCY TREATMENT Consent from the person responsible is not necessary in the case of urgent treatment that is required to save the patient's life, to prevent serious damage to health or to prevent the patient from suffering, or continuing to suffer, significant pain or distress.

SPECIAL PROCEDURES

'Special procedures' are particular procedures that may only proceed with VCAT consent. Those relevant to the elderly are:

- any procedure carried out for medical research; and
- tissue removal for the purposes of transplantation to another person.

STATUTORY PROTECTION FOR MEDICAL PRACTITIONERS

Statutory immunity from criminal prosecution for assault or battery, civil liability proceedings for assault or battery and from disciplinary proceedings before the Medical Practitioners Board of Victoria is granted in the following circumstances:

- where treatment was undertaken in reliance on consent given by a person whom the doctor reasonably believed was authorised to give consent when in fact this was not the case; and
- where medical treatment was provided in good faith in accordance with the legislation, without the consent of another person, in the belief on reasonable grounds that the relevant statutory requirements had been complied with.

CONCLUSION

As the proportion of elderly people making up the population of developed and developing countries continues to rise, the role of the GP in the biopsychosocial management of these people is vital. This requires GPs to diagnose mental health problems (in particular dementia, depression and delirium) often in the context of comorbid physical illness and concurrent polypharmacy. Sound clinical assessment, accompanied by Mini Mental State Examination and appreciation of the social dimensions of illness, will differentiate most presentations in the elderly. Management often requires a multidisciplinary team approach, so familiarisation with local aged care services is important. In cases where the rights of patients need to be protected, the role of the GP as the patient advocate is essential.

REFERENCES

1. Henderson AS, Jorm AF. Dementia in Australia: Aged and Community Care Service Development and Evaluation Report No 35. Canberra: Australian Government Printing Service, 1988.
2. O'Connor DW, Pollitt PA, Hyde JB, Brook CPB, Reiss BB, Roth M. Do general practitioners miss dementia in elderly patients? British Medical Journal 1988;297:1107–10.

CHAPTER 17

PSYCHOLOGICAL INTERVENTIONS

G Hodgins, K Wilhelm, C Hassed and D Pierce

'Evidence based medicine is the conscientious, explicit, and judicious use of current best evidence in making decisions about the care of individual patients. The practice of evidence based medicine means integrating individual clinical expertise with the best available external clinical evidence from systematic research...Good doctors use both individual clinical expertise and the best available external evidence, and neither alone is enough.'

DL SACKETT et al, 1996

CASE STUDY

Mary, a 45-year-old mother of two, has experienced anxiety for 'as long as I can remember'. She has been a long-standing patient of the clinic. At times she has been depressed, usually in response to crises in her life. Even when well, she is 'tense and stressed'. Various approaches have been tried in the past but despite these, she continues to struggle with her anxiety problems. She is reluctant to see a specialist as she feels embarrassed; it is also difficult for her to travel while caring for young children.

KEY FACTS

- Psychological interventions include stress management and relaxation strategies, focused psychological strategies and formal psychotherapies.

- There is a variety of models or schools of psychotherapy that differ in their conceptualisation of the cause of a patient's problems.

- Focused psychological strategies consist of a range of circumscribed techniques that can be applied to a variety of problem areas in a range of settings.

continued overleaf

KEY FACTS *continued*

■ The decision to use a psychological intervention should be informed by a comprehensive biopsychosocial assessment.

■ The type and level of psychological intervention is largely determined by the target for treatment.

■ Focused psychological strategies, stress management and relaxation techniques are particularly helpful for patients with anxiety and depressive disorders.

■ Psychological interventions require the active participation of patients.

■ When using brief interventions, the patient's willingness and commitment to change are vital factors in therapeutic progress.

■ The quality of the therapeutic relationship, and issues such as transference and countertransference, can have a powerful influence on treatment.

■ The provision of psychological interventions may constitute a departure from the usual role for the general practitioner (GP); both the GP and the patient may experience difficulties adapting to such change.

INTRODUCTION

Psychological interventions include stress management and relaxation strategies, focused psychological strategies and formal psychotherapies. While they encompass many different procedures and techniques, they share important common elements. Each type:

■ has a rationale that contains an explanation of the patient's distress;
■ provides information about the nature and origins of the patient's problems and ways of dealing with them;
■ offers hope to the patient, who expects help from the therapy; and
■ provides the patient with an opportunity to experience success during the course of therapy and thus gain a sense of mastery over their problem.

However, psychological interventions do differ in their conceptualisation of the causes of a patient's problems and whether they lie in the remote past, the immediate past or the present. For example, psychodynamic psychotherapy, and other therapies derived from psychoanalysis, view symptoms and difficulties in social functioning as derivative of deeper or fundamental unresolved personality difficulties or character problems. By contrast, interpersonal psychotherapy and cognitive behavioural therapy respect past history, but focus on the more immediate past and present interpersonal situations.

Therapies that focus more on the immediate past or present are effective for symptoms as well as for a range of social and interpersonal difficulties. However, there is little expectation that this treatment approach will have a marked impact upon the more enduring aspects of personality structure, which may underlie a patient's difficulties. While personality change is not a goal of such therapies, personality is an important consideration in therapy, because it may:

- predict treatment outcomes;
- influence the doctor–patient relationship; and
- be a determinant of the behaviours or symptoms that are the focus of treatment.

PSYCHOLOGICAL INTERVENTIONS

At a descriptive level, psychological interventions can be broadly categorised into three major groups: stress management and relaxation strategies, focused psychological strategies and formal psychotherapies.

Stress management and relaxation strategies—including muscle relaxation, imagery, meditation, mindfulness and relaxation using music, art, exercise and a range of other activities—are interventions where the aim is to reduce arousal or anxiety, focusing on the here-and-now feeling state. Often used to improve mental wellbeing, these strategies can be incorporated into cognitive interventions. They are also very useful as a first step in the management of patients with a variety of psychiatric disorders featuring prominent levels of anxiety. In the case of mindfulness based therapies, they are useful for preventing depression relapse.

Focused psychological strategies (FPS) are interventions that include behaviour modification, exposure techniques, activity scheduling, cognitive interventions, relaxation strategies, psychoeducation, problem solving, interpersonal counselling, assertiveness skills, anger management, stress management and motivational interviewing (see Chapter 10). This range of specific or circumscribed therapeutic strategies can be applied to a wide range of problem areas in a variety of settings, including primary care. They are mainly focused on the present—that is, the here-and-now problems rather than past issues— and can be distinguished from formal therapies in a number of ways:

- They select and target discrete aspects of a problem area—for example, sleep difficulties due to depression.
- They do not require extensive formal training.
- They are generally applied with, but are not necessarily restricted to, less complex presentations.
- They are well suited to primary care settings, including general practice and community health.
- They are frequently used in combination with other therapeutic interventions as part of a 'package of treatment' rather than as a complete therapeutic intervention.

Formal psychotherapies are therapies that are practised within particular models and have well developed bodies of theory and protocols of practice. Some examples include cognitive behavioural therapy (CBT), interpersonal therapy (IPT), systemic therapy and psychodynamic therapy. These therapies are undertaken by, or are conducted under the supervision of, a specialist practitioner trained in the particular school of psychotherapeutic work. Typically, practitioners will have received training (at a postgraduate level) in a range of psychological theories, later specialising in a formal psychotherapeutic approach—for example, the training routes for clinical psychologists and psychiatrists.

Formal psychotherapies are complete therapeutic interventions rather than specific components of a broader integrated program, and are usually offered in the form of a series of set sessions, after a management plan has been generated by an assessment. These interventions require extensive training and ongoing professional development, including regular clinical supervision, and are regulated by relevant professional bodies. They are often practised in specialist mental health services for people who present with more complex and severe mental health problems. Consequently, they are generally relatively long and intensive interventions and, as such, are not compatible with routine general practice.

Formal psychotherapies vary along a number of dimensions—for example, they may be:

- offered to individuals, couples, families or groups—that is, these interventions have different targets;
- open-ended or unstructured—that is, they are not limited by the number of sessions so they can address issues as they arise;
- brief, time limited and structured—that is, they identify and target a specific area for change and restrict therapy, in terms of time and number of sessions, to that problem;
- active, in the sense that the patient and therapist are working towards clearly defined goals for change; and
- supportive, in that the aim is to stabilise the patient's clinical status and reduce the likelihood of deterioration.

GPs can provide one or more of these psychological interventions for the benefit of patients they treat. However, a specialist mental health practitioner, such as a psychiatrist or clinical psychologist, will usually provide formal psychotherapies. By contrast, many GPs provide FPS and stress management and relaxation strategies, so they will be the focus of this chapter. The following is a brief synopsis of commonly used psychological interventions. Training for GPs so they can develop skills in delivering stress management and relaxation strategies and FPS is now widely available in Australia, and recent changes to the Medicare Benefits Schedule support GPs in delivering these interventions.[2]

STRESS MANAGEMENT AND RELAXATION STRATEGIES

Occasional activation of the fight or flight response is a natural, necessary and appropriate adaptation to challenging situations. However, when this response is activated unnecessarily and chronically, it places a significant physiological (allostatic) load on the body, which predisposes to illnesses as diverse as cardiovascular disease, osteoporosis, immunosuppression and depression.[3]

A lot of stress is caused by distortions in perception, the replaying of the past and the anticipation of the future, so techniques that help to ground attention on the here and now have the ability to not only produce direct physiological benefits but also to help people consciously change unhelpful cognitive patterns. One of the main mechanisms of the operation of relaxation based forms of stress management may be their ability to reduce the levels of emotional and physiological reactivity to daily events and thoughts while enhancing the mind's ability to focus and therefore deal with daily life.

Relaxation and meditation techniques have a range of therapeutic benefits;[3,4] however, it takes time and sustained effort for the benefits of these strategies to accrue, and it also takes insight and motivation for a person to engage in them in the first place. Although these strategies can potentially help the majority of patients, some patients will choose not to use them for personal or cultural reasons and others may simply not find them helpful. There are various reasons for this: the strategies were not applied consistently over a sufficient duration of time; some patients may not present their questions or difficulties to their practitioner in order to receive guidance; or, occasionally, patients may not have been well instructed in how to apply them (some therapists think that these strategies are best taught by therapists who have practised them personally).

Many patients—especially those for whom stress or anxiety is the prime motivator, as it is associated with achievement and performance—will resist using relaxation therapies. For these people, stress management and relaxation therapies will have connotations of lowering performance. However, as the stress–performance curve indicates (see Figure 17.1), significant stress can have a detrimental effect, actually impeding performance. In order to engage these patients, the GP needs to help them understand that relaxation therapies have the potential to enhance performance because they can reduce the inhibiting effects of mental and physical tension as well as improve focus and concentration.

FIGURE 17.1 The relationship between anxiety and performance

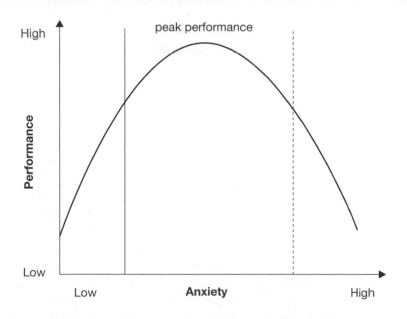

PROGRESSIVE MUSCLE RELAXATION

Not only is progressive muscle relaxation (PMR) useful in itself, but it is also a first step in learning many other relaxation techniques. It works primarily by bringing awareness to each part of the body in sequence and helping it to relax by letting go of tension. For example, patients can start with their feet and then move to their legs, hands and arms, stomach and chest, and then to their shoulders, head and face. For patients who have lost awareness of physical tension, it can be helpful to get them to tense muscle groups first and then relax them. In addition, asking them to take deep breaths, then slowly release them, can also help to deepen the relaxation response. PMR can significantly reduce levels of physiological and mental arousal and provide profound relief.

IMAGERY AND VISUALISATION

Imagery and visualisation techniques were among the first to be used therapeutically and are still among the most widely used, although there is far less evidence on the efficacy of these techniques in comparison to some of the others discussed in this chapter. Many people associate these exercises with meditation, although they are quite different to the meditative practices mentioned below.

Imagery and visualisation exercises are often guided, in person, then using the recording on a tape or CD. In the practice setting, while in a relaxed state, the person might be slowly drawn into a visualisation of a scene that is assumed to be restful, safe and pleasant, thus eliciting the relaxation response. Variations on the theme are also used—for example, a person may visualise healing, such as cancer cells being destroyed by immune cells, or visualise a successful outcome in an upcoming event. More esoteric forms of visualisation and imagery, hoping to tap into more subconscious thought processes, may involve having an imagined 'conversation' with an 'inner guide' to help resolve some conflict or decision.

MEDITATION

Meditation techniques have a long history; some have been the subject of a considerable amount of contemporary research. Although meditation is often perceived as an Eastern practice, it would be true to say that every culture has its own meditative traditions and practices. Traditionally they have been used as spiritual disciplines, but in the contemporary setting most patients use them to cope with physical or psychological illness and to maintain health. It is important that a person uses them in a way that is philosophically and culturally congruent with their own background.

The most widely known and studied meditative practice—apart from mindfulness based strategies that will be discussed separately below—is Transcendental Meditation (TM™), which utilises a mantra that is mentally repeated, rhythmically and silently. A mantra is a sound, word or even a short phrase. Many forms of prayer overlap significantly with mantra meditation—for example, in the Christian tradition, Aramaic mantras were used. The person meditating focuses on the mantra and whenever they digress onto distracting thoughts, they gently bring their attention back to the mantra. The mantra is a vehicle for helping one transcend from activity to stillness or simple being. Herbert Benson[5] suggested the use of simple words such as 'one' or 'peace'. Every meditative practice has a particular focus of attention; others may focus on the breath, 'candle-gazing' or an image.

MINDFULNESS BASED INTERVENTIONS

Mindfulness is a very ancient practice, with elements that can be found in many philosophical and religious traditions. It is not a simple stress management technique, rather it encompasses a broad approach. Today it is increasingly the subject of research, and it can be applied to contemporary psychology and psychiatry. Here is one definition: 'Mindfulness is characterised by dispassionate, non-evaluative and sustained moment-to-moment awareness of perceptible mental states and processes.'[6] Kabat-Zinn[7] describes mindfulness even more simply as 'a way of being'. Grossman et al[6] describes a number of basic assumptions associated with mindfulness and these, along with some of the language often used in descriptions of mindfulness, will be expanded in the following discussion:

- People generally operate on automatic pilot and are unaware of moment to moment experience.
- People are capable of developing sustained attention.
- Development of this ability is gradual and progressive, and requires practice.
- Awareness makes life richer and more vivid and replaces unconscious reactiveness.
- Awareness gives rise to veridicality (ability to discern the accuracy) of perceptions.
- Awareness enhances perceptiveness.

Recent studies on the efficacy of mindfulness have been very promising.[6] Researchers have found it to be helpful in the management of stress, anxiety and panic disorder,[8] eating disorders,[9] chronic pain,[10] immune modulation,[11] and sleep and coping, particularly in people with serious illness.[12] Probably the area of application that has stimulated more interest than any other has been the effect of mindfulness in significantly reducing the relapse rate for people with severe relapsing depression.[13, 14]

Crucial to the mindfulness approach is the emphasis on the present moment; the past is only relevant in that it is revealed through the patterns it has laid down in our thought and actions *now*, and what is practised *now* is the foundation for future experience and behaviour. Thus, in mindfulness, emphasis is always placed on moment by moment experience and not resolving the past, unless it is relevant to what is happening in life now. Analogies often assist in explaining the simple principles of mindfulness to patients. For example, one analogy relates to 'trains of thought': 'They will come and go by themselves if allowed. They will not move us in the process, if we do not get on the trains. In time, if we are consistent, various "trains of thought" become far less frequent visitors.' Experienced teachers of mindfulness tend to advise proceeding slowly. Audio tapes and CDs can be useful, at least in the initial stages, although the ultimate aim of mindfulness is for patients to be able to practise independently.

A related approach is mindfulness based CBT, which, in its various forms, has some important points of difference with conventional CBT,[15–17] notably: it is non-evaluative, involves 'non-doing' and places value on present moment experience.

Many other stress management interventions have various features in common with the mindfulness approach. Music and physical exercise are two commonly used methods, but traditional approaches such as tai chi and yoga are also extremely effective. It is also worth noting that many people will describe feeling very focused and in the present moment when they are engaged in their hobbies. There is also some overlap of mindfulness with other approaches, such as acceptance-commitment therapy (ACT), hypnosis, biofeedback, artistic therapies, focused communication and effective time management.

REVISITING THE CASE STUDY While seeing her GP for a repeat prescription of her antihypertensive medication, Mary mentions that she has heard that meditation can be helpful in managing stress and would like to try this approach. The following exercise (adapted from Hassed, 2002[17]) is explained to her.

> Sit in a chair so that your spine is upright and balanced but relaxed. Have your body symmetrical and allow your eyes to gently close. Now, move your attention gently through each step. Be conscious of your body and its connection with the chair. Feel your feet on the floor. Notice if your feet are tense. If so, allow them to relax if they want to. Similarly, be aware of your legs and allow them to relax if they wish. And so gently move up through each part of your body—your stomach, hands, arms, shoulders, neck and face. If tension or discomfort remains, just notice the presence of tension or discomfort without judgment.
>
> Now take in a deep breath, and slowly and gently let the breath out. Repeat this twice more, then just allow the breathing to settle into its own natural rhythm without having to control it in any way. If you observe a tendency to try and control the breath, just impartially notice that. Simply be conscious of the breath as the air flows in and out of your nose. If thoughts come to your awareness, allow them to come and go without judgment and let your attention return to the breathing. There is no need to struggle with the activity of your mind, nor even to wish that it was not there. Like 'trains of thought', just let them come and go.
>
> After a time, let your attention move to the listening. Hear whatever sounds there are to hear without having to analyse the sounds. Once again, if thoughts come, let them pass. If your mind becomes distracted—for example, by listening to some mental commentary or chatter—simply notice and return to the sounds as a gentle way of returning to the present moment.
>
> At the end of this exercise simply be aware of your body again, and then slowly allow your eyes to open. After a few moments quietly move into whatever activities await you.

FOCUSED PSYCHOLOGICAL STRATEGIES WITH A COGNITIVE BEHAVIOURAL FOCUS

Cognitive behavioural therapy (CBT) has proven to be effective in the treatment of mood and anxiety disorders,[18] and there is growing evidence of its applicability to both psychotic[19] and personality disorders.[20] CBT can be seen as a combination of behavioural therapy and cognitive therapy:

- Behavioural therapy is based on learning theory. The focus of treatment is on changing behaviour rather than feelings and thoughts. The primary aim is symptom relief. Behavioural therapy is commonly used for treating patients with obsessive-compulsive disorder and phobic disorders.
- Cognitive therapy is concerned with the way in which maladaptive behaviour or feelings may be reinforced by thoughts. For example, a depressed person may

interpret or misinterpret many things in their environment in a negative way, and so undermine their self-esteem. The cognitive therapist will challenge this thinking and ask the patient to identify the thoughts that are maintaining the depressed mood, and to re-evaluate the assumptions they are making. Cognitive therapy is used for the treatment of patients with depression and various anxiety disorders.

Adequate professional training in CBT involves hundreds of hours of didactic and supervised clinical work, and often necessitates seeing patients weekly. However, there are circumscribed elements of the CBT approach that can be readily learnt and applied within a GP's normal working time frame.

Cognitive behavioural strategies have been developed as a brief form of psychological intervention for working with particular symptoms. These cognitive behavioural strategies include breathing retraining; identifying and challenging dysfunctional thoughts; exposure work; and activity scheduling.[21] Such cognitive behavioural strategies are primarily directed at the amelioration of anxiety and mood symptoms and, as they are 'problem focused', they can be used in patients with a variety of diagnoses.

BEHAVIOURAL ASSESSMENT

Conducting a thorough psychiatric assessment is covered in Chapter 7. When using a cognitive behavioural intervention, this assessment should be supplemented to enhance the measurement of change in patients, and for tailoring the use of appropriate strategies. By helping the patient to think of what may be achieved, rather than dwelling continually on problems, cognitive behavioural assessment emphasises the possibility of change and sets reasonable limits on what might be achieved through treatment. It also allows the patient to see that variations in the intensity of distress are predictable in terms of internal and external events, and are therefore controllable.

A successful behavioural assessment includes the following steps:

1   Generate a formulation of the problem with the patient by finding out the answers to the following questions:
    — What?
    — When?
    — Where?
    — How often?
    — With whom?
    — How distressing?
    — How disruptive?

2   Describe the contexts, antecedents and maintaining factors for the problem behaviour, including the following factors:
    — Situational
    — Behavioural
    — Cognitive
    — Affective
    — Interpersonal
    — Physiological

3   Assess the coping resources, strengths and other assets of the patient.
4   Explore the patient's beliefs about the problem and their readiness to change.
5   Devise a treatment plan according to the problem formulation.
6   Set 'homework' tasks for the patient.

BREATHING CONTROL

Acute anxiety is a common component of all the anxiety disorders; it is common in patients with depression and may also occur in many other situations. One of the features of the alarm reaction is a change in breathing. When patients become tense or anxious, their breathing tends to be rapid and shallow, occurring high in the chest. When shallow breathing becomes rapid, it can lead to hyperventilation, resulting in physical symptoms much like those found in panic attacks. Indeed, many of the features of panic appear to be due to the physiology of anxious breathing. One of the most effective ways to reverse this psychophysiological pattern is to consciously adopt a more relaxed breathing style. More relaxed breathing occurs when the breath is full and deeper, hence the term 'abdominal breathing'. There are two elements to abdominal breathing: the rate of breathing should be relatively slow; and the breath should be drawn from the abdomen rather than the chest. It is also better to inhale through the nose than through the mouth.

In acute anxiety management, breathing control includes:

- introducing the notion of the alarm reaction, and its four components (cognition, action, physiology and emotion);
- describing the abdominal breathing technique and comparing its effects with shallow breathing;
- demonstrating the technique and asking the patient to practise in front of you;
- prescribing practising of the skill and setting homework exercises; and
- reviewing the homework exercises.

Abdominal breathing is just one of the techniques for managing acute anxiety. Others include isometric relaxation, positive self-statements and active relaxation.

SLEEP HYGIENE

Difficulty sleeping is a problem confronted by everyone at various times in their life. Not surprisingly, there is a strong association between sleep disturbances and mood, anxiety and other problems. There are a few simple procedures, and some important information, which together can be very effective in improving sleep management. These include: learning about the sleep cycle; creating good conditions for sleep; and dealing with sleep problems when they arise using behavioural and cognitive strategies.

ASSERTION AND ANGER MANAGEMENT

ASSERTION MANAGEMENT Assertion is the ability to communicate your opinions, thoughts, needs and feelings in a direct, honest and appropriate manner. It involves:

- believing you have the right to express yourself and meet your needs, and feeling okay about it;
- having a willingness to share yourself with others;

■ respecting the rights and needs of others; and
■ choosing how to respond in different situations.

The assertiveness spectrum ranges from passive to assertive to aggressive. Effective assertiveness training involves:

■ explaining to patients that assertion is the ability to communicate opinions, thoughts, needs and feelings in a direct, honest and appropriate manner;
■ reviewing the rules of assertion with the patient;
■ identifying obstacles to healthy assertion;
■ helping the patient to develop protective skills, which are sometimes needed when people react unreasonably to someone else's assertive behaviour; and
■ encouraging the patient in making a decision to become more assertive.

ANGER MANAGEMENT Anger is a natural human emotion. Sometimes you can respond with anger to a situation, and this can lead to behaviours that include lashing out, yelling and physical abuse. When anger gets out of control and starts to dictate your life, it is important to learn skills that manage the emotion, and in some instances, to understand the thinking and beliefs that are leading to the anger response.

Successful anger management can include reminding the patient that anger is a natural emotion and then proceeding through the following steps for controlling anger, as follows:

1 Recognise and acknowledge the anger.
2 Accept responsibility.
3 Recognise the early warning signs.
4 Decide what to do.
5 (a) Express anger directly (when appropriate).
  (b) Express anger indirectly (when direct expression is inappropriate).
6 Analyse the anger management.

STRUCTURED PROBLEM SOLVING

Structured problem solving is a valuable, evidence based, focused psychological strategy, often seen as part of a CBT approach, which is readily applicable in the day to day clinical practice of many GPs. It is variously known as problem-solving therapy (PST) or structured problem solving. The word 'structured' is central to this technique. It is a structured approach, with a well established format, which allows the patient, supported by their GP, to develop and implement solutions to problems in their life that are at the basis of significant health problems, especially depression and anxiety disorders. It is of particular value when a patient is overwhelmed by a number of problems related to their life circumstances.

In understanding and using problem solving, it is important to recognise what it is not—it is not the provision of advice to the patient by the GP. In many other areas of general practice the provision of advice may be common, often evolving from the clinical knowledge and experience of the GP. With problem solving as a psychological therapy, the aim is to assist the patient in recognising the link between specific life problems and their symptoms, to encourage the patient in the recognition of potential solutions and support them in the choice and implementation of the solution they feel is most appropriate. If required, continuing review, support and dealing with further symptom-causing problems completes the process.[22] This approach allows the patient to develop a new skill that is applicable to future situations: they are empowered to have greater control of their lives in the future.

As a focused psychological strategy, problem solving is divided into a number of stages.[23] These may be implemented over a few sessions, or a series of sessions, depending on the complexity of the problems and the patient's circumstances. The stages are as follows:

- Establish the link between the patient's problems and symptoms.
- Define the problem and solution goals.
- Decide upon a solution as well as actions to implement the solution.
- If necessary, review and consider other problems.

While this is essentially a cognitive approach, problem solving will frequently be applied using worksheets. These may be formally prepared, or based on a blank page, on which the patient notes their thoughts. It is important that worksheets are utilised in the appropriate circumstances; it is not a suitable approach for all patients. If the predominant problem relates to a distorted view of the world or is not realistically solvable, alternative approaches, such as cognitive interventions, are more applicable.

As a psychological approach in general practice, problem solving is not a complex technique; it has been referred to as 'structured commonsense'. If it is appropriately utilised, following the structure upon which its evidence base is formed, it will satisfy the desire of many patients to receive effective non-drug treatment for a range of mental health problems, especially depression.

REVISITING THE CASE STUDY Mary returns to your clinic three months later. At first she found meditation very useful, but over the months prior to seeing you this time, she has been confronted by a range of problems that have just overwhelmed her. She describes a plethora of problems, and is so overwhelmed by them she cannot see where to start. This presentation is not dissimilar to previous ones, which led to her become quite depressed. Mary's inability to see how to tackle the problems, coupled with the obvious effect on her mood, leads you to adopt a problem-solving approach with her.

ACTIVITY SCHEDULING

In the early stages of treatment, particularly with more severely depressed patients, the GP will attempt to induce patients to counteract their withdrawal and to become involved in more constructive activities. Severely depressed patients often believe that they are no longer capable of carrying out their role related activities, and furthermore they see no hope of gaining satisfaction from activities that had previously brought them pleasure. These patients are caught in a vicious cycle, in which the reduced level of functioning leads to feelings of being ineffectual, which in turn leads to discouragement and further immobility.

There is no easy way to 'talk the patient out' of their conclusions that they are 'weak' or 'inept'. However, by facilitating a change in patient behaviour, the therapist can demonstrate to the patient that their negative, overgeneralised conclusions are incorrect.

As a result of specific behaviour changes, the GP can show the patient that their ability to function at previous levels has not been lost. The patient thereby comes to the conclusion that it is their discouragement and pessimism that makes it difficult to mobilise their resources. Behavioural techniques can therefore be regarded as a series of small experiments designed to test the validity of the patient's hypotheses about themselves.

The use of activity schedules serves to counteract the patient's loss of motivation, inactivity and preoccupation with depressive ideas. This approach aims to improve mood and self-esteem by exploring, monitoring and increasing rewarding behaviours—both pleasurable and masterful.

If the patient's time is scheduled on an hour by hour basis, there is less likelihood of them slipping back into immobility. In addition, the focus on specific goal oriented tasks provides the patient and GP with concrete data on which to base realistic evaluations of the patient's functional capacity.

Effective activity scheduling involves:

- remembering the importance of presenting the rationale of activity scheduling to the patient;
- asking the patient to record daily activities, with particular reference to pleasure and mastery activities;
- leading into changing activities, again focusing on pleasure and mastery activities; and
- utilising strategies to assist in maintaining the new activities.

EXPOSURE

Despite its effectiveness, exposure is not a comfortable process to undergo. This strategy involves applying avoidance theory and exposure principles to anxiety problems. Not all patients are willing to tolerate the unpleasantness of facing fear-provoking situations, nor to persist with exposure therapy on a regular basis. Patients must be willing to:

- take the risk of facing long-avoided situations;
- tolerate the initial discomfort of entering phobic situations, even when exposure occurs in small increments; and
- persist in practising exposure on a consistent basis, despite probable setbacks, over a long period (six months to two years).

Severe levels of anxiety rarely last more than 90 minutes, so if an individual with a phobia stays in a phobic situation for this length of time, the fear will eventually dissipate and the situation will be less threatening next time. However, few people are prepared to remain in a fearful situation for this length of time. As a result, the key to exposure therapy is to encourage the patient to face their fears in incremental steps so that they can build up their tolerance to these situations.

A well constructed exposure hierarchy allows the patient to gradually approach a phobic situation through a sequence of steps. Patients can rank their anticipated anxiety using the Subjective Units of Discomfort Scale (SUDS). Using this scale, patients rank phobia related situations in ascending order between two extremes already defined.

A successful exposure program involves the following components:

- confronting fear-provoking situations 3–4 times a week at first;
- monitoring progress;
- using relaxation exercises before exposure;
- mentally rehearsing exposure activities;
- monitoring breathing rate if circumstances allow;
- using coping statements during exposure;
- remaining in situations for as long as possible, and not leaving until the anxiety starts to diminish; and
- recognising successes.

COGNITIVE RESTRUCTURING

It is not a situation in and of itself that determines what a person feels, but rather the way in which they construe a situation. Cognitive restructuring helps patients to notice and challenge distorted automatic thoughts. It is particularly aimed at the level of thinking that operates simultaneously with the more obvious, surface level of thinking. These thoughts are called automatic thoughts and are not the result of deliberation or reasoning. Rather, these thoughts seem to spring up automatically; they are often quite rapid and brief. People may be barely aware of these thoughts, and are far more likely to be aware of the emotion that follows. As a result, they are likely to uncritically accept their automatic thoughts as true.

The relationship between thoughts and emotions can be illustrated as follows:

situation → automatic thought → emotion

Cognitive restructuring initially focuses on the identification of automatic thoughts, then evaluates the validity of these thoughts. If the patient finds their interpretations erroneous and then subjects them to rational reflection, a mood change generally follows.

Successful cognitive restructuring involves:

- educating the patient that it is not a situation in and of itself that determines what they feel, but rather the way they construe or think about the situation;
- demonstrating to the patient that therefore it is important to identify automatic thoughts that lead to certain emotions;
- assisting the patient to evaluate the validity of these automatic thoughts by questioning them;
- demonstrating that such automatic thoughts can make up cognitive distortions or thinking errors; these should also be identified by and with the patient;
- subjecting automatic thoughts and thinking errors that are found to be erroneous to rational reflection—from this a mood change should follow; and
- using tools such as 'thought records' that can be used to assist the patient in achieving the above steps.

SCHEMA MODIFICATION

The term 'schema' is used to describe those mental structures that integrate and attach meaning to events. Schema modification aims to address psychological vulnerability by identifying and working with a patient's core schemas.

The content of the schemas may deal with personal relationships, such as attitudes towards the self or others, or impersonal categories—for example, inanimate objects. An individual's cognitive schemas contain deeper, often unarticulated ideas or understandings that they have about themselves, others and their personal worlds, which give rise to specific automatic thoughts. Their most central or core beliefs are understandings that are so fundamental and deep that they often do not articulate them, even to themselves. The individual regards these ideas as absolute truths—just the way things are.

When activated, these idiosyncratic schemas displace and probably inhibit other schemas that may be more adaptive or more appropriate for a given situation. They consequently introduce a systematic bias into information processing. For example, in clinical depression, negative schemas are in ascendancy, resulting in a systematic negative bias in the interpretation and recall of experiences as well as in short-term and long-term predictions, whereas the positive schemas become less accessible.

Schemas are the most fundamental levels of belief; they are global, rigid and overgeneralised. Such beliefs develop in childhood as the child interacts with significant others and encounters a series of situations (see Figure 17.2). For most of their lives most people maintain relatively positive core beliefs—for example, 'I am worthwhile'—and negative schemas may only surface during times of psychological stress. It is important for the therapist to emphasise that such beliefs are not innate, and so they can be revised.

FIGURE 17.2 The relationship between schemas, thoughts and emotions

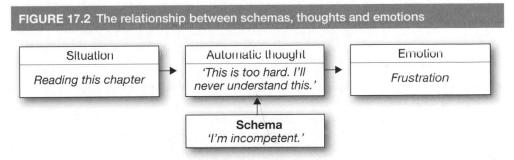

Effective schema modification involves:

- introducing the concept of schemas, and how they fit into the cognitive model of automatic thoughts leading to emotions; and
- identifying and modifying schemas (using cognitive tools as well as handouts).

FOCUSED PSYCHOLOGICAL STRATEGIES WITH AN INTERPERSONAL FOCUS
INTERPERSONAL THERAPY AND INTERPERSONAL COUNSELLING

Interpersonal therapy (IPT) is a structured psychotherapy developed in the United States in the 1970s, based on the interpersonal approaches of Myer,[24] Sullivan[25] and attachment theory.[26] While most psychotherapies have developed from 'clinical observations which gradually coalesced into more or less coherently articulated theories explaining how the treatments *worked*', IPT was specifically developed as a model, structured, short-term therapy to be delivered as a structured manualised program for a study of psychotherapy and antidepressants.[27] The therapy was designed for use in a treatment arm, to be compared to CBT and antidepressants. It therefore had to present an approach that was demonstrably different to CBT.

The developers[28] had a strong track record in the psychosocial aspects of depression, and sought out experts in the four identified interpersonal domains (grief, role transition, interpersonal disputes, interpersonal deficits) to advise on suitable psychotherapeutic approaches for each. Originally, IPT was designed to be used by psychiatrists and psychologists over 8–15 sessions. The therapy has evolved since then and is used on an individual or group basis in the treatment of bulimia, substance abuse and somatisation. It retains the interpersonal focus, with the use of an interpersonal inventory and formulation; some authors have increased the focus on attachment and the concentration on affect.[29]

Interpersonal counselling (IPC) was developed as a brief form of IPT, using the same structure of psychoeducation and identification of key problem areas, with a clear agenda for the number of sessions and the termination of therapy.[30, 31] It was envisaged as six 30-minute sessions focusing on the patient's current psychosocial issues, for use in a primary care setting (see Figure 17.3). It was originally designed to be used for patients who did not have a significant psychiatric diagnosis rather than for patients with acute stress related problems.

FIGURE 17.3 Interpersonal counselling: structure of sessions

VISIT 1

Discussion of diagnosis, context, risk assessment:

- Education about need for psychological and pharmacological treatment
- Interpersonal inventory and formulation
- Identifying key relationships and problem areas from the four domains: grief, interpersonal disputes, role transitions, social isolation and loneliness

VISITS 2–5

Working on the problem area by encouraging coping, exploring new strategies. See Table 17.1.

VISIT 6

Tidying up, planning for the future, including possible sessions for review.

REVISITING THE CASE STUDY Mary re-presents two weeks later. Together you review the problem-solving activities she's been trying. Although she understands the techniques and has been applying them, she reports her mood is no better and she is still very anxious. Talking with her more, you both realise that although there are many problems, there is an important one that had escaped attention. Mary's son left home twelve months ago, and in retrospect, she did have trouble dealing with this. However, her second son moved out to live in shared student accommodation two months ago. Now, there are no children at home, and Mary is obviously having difficulty adjusting to

TABLE 17.1 Specific stress area and treatment goals

PROBLEM AREA	GOALS OF TREATMENT	STRATEGIES
Grief or loss	■ Facilitate the mourning process ■ Help the patient re-establish interests and relationships that can act as substitutes for what has been lost	■ Relate symptom onset or exacerbation to death/loss of significant other ■ Talk about the deceased—the type of person he/she was, relationship with them, circumstances of illness and death **Homework** ■ Look over old photographs, see old friends and discuss at subsequent sessions ■ Encourage involvement in new social activities
Interpersonal disputes	■ Identify the dispute ■ Guide the patient in making choices about a plan of action ■ Encourage the patient to reassess expectations or poor communication in order to bring about satisfactory resolution of the dispute	■ Relate symptom onset to overt or covert dispute with significant other **Key questions** ■ What are the issues in the dispute? ■ How likely is change to occur? ■ How do the patient and the person with whom they are in dispute usually work on differences? ■ Is there a pattern—has this happened before in other relationships? **Homework** ■ For example, more direct expression of wishes to family/ friends ■ For example, in work relationships, seek opportunities to talk and explain point of view and see the other person's point of view

continued overleaf

TABLE 17.1 *continued*

PROBLEM AREA	GOALS OF TREATMENT	STRATEGIES
Role transitions	■ Mourn, accept loss of old role ■ Enable the patient to regard the new role in a more positive, less restricted manner, or see it as an opportunity for growth ■ Restore self-esteem by developing in the patient a sense of mastery in relation to the demands of the new role related attitudes and behaviours	■ Relate symptoms to difficulty in coping with recent life changes ■ Similar to those for grief (giving up old role)—facilitate evaluation of what has been lost, encourage release of affect and develop social support system **Homework** ■ To assist the transition, seek transitional objects—for example, transform an old picture, furniture from former place in life into new role ■ Make new contacts—for example, prescribe a social outing with new neighbour, work colleague
Loneliness and social isolation	■ Reduce the patient's social isolation ■ Find examples of relationships that have been meaningful in the past ■ Help the patient to form new relationships	■ Relate symptoms of problems to social isolation or lack of fulfilment ■ Review past relationships, identify the best and worst part of each ■ Identify difficulties in past relationships: — Role play a social situation — Identify any correctable deficits in patient's communication skills **Homework** ■ Make contact with old friends ■ Seek out social situations, for example, clubs, sports, church

Source: Judd, Weissman, Davis, et al, 2004.[30]

this change; previously much of her time was devoted to 'running around' after her son. Dealing with this role transition, and the losses inherent in it, will be an important focus of ongoing work.

PSYCHODYNAMIC INTERPERSONAL THERAPY

Psychodynamic interpersonal therapy is based on a 'conversational mode', where the therapist aims to discuss identified interpersonal issues with a 'mutual feeling language'. This means that the therapist uses statements rather than questions; adopts a negotiating style; uses pronouns such as 'we' and 'I'; and introduces metaphors and understanding, and explanatory and linking hypotheses.[32] The therapy has been successfully used in a randomised control trial of 119 adults who presented with deliberate self-poisoning.[33] Four sessions of brief psychodynamic interpersonal therapy (BPIPT) were offered soon after the index presentation, with the aim of resolving the interpersonal difficulties that were precipitating distress. In each case, the sessions were delivered by a nurse therapist in the patient's home, and each session also involved a risk assessment and liaison with the patient's GP. It has also been useful in patients with somatisation, functional medical problems—for example, irritable bowel, dyspepsia—and depression.

COGNITIVE ANALYTIC THERAPY

Cognitive analytic therapy (CAT) was developed to provide a contained brief therapy for anxiety and depression for use in the British public health system. As the name implies, it uses cognitive techniques (identifying problems, thoughts and behaviours, and encouraging understanding and change) but also uses psychoanalytic ideas to consider the feelings of both the patient and therapist. These concepts are brought together in a reformulation letter that is given to the patient and discussed. A 'procedural sequence model' is used to evaluate the patient's aims, their environmental context, a plan, actions and remedial actions. The patient is very much involved, both in identifying their faulty thinking and its effect on themselves and others. The patient receives a written reformulation letter, laying out their life history and making links to assist in understanding the psychological issues, followed at the end by a 'goodbye letter' that gives a summary of the therapy. The initial reformulation[34] may also be diagrammatic, demonstrating the current dilemmas and the effect on significant others. This therapy has also been applied to deliberate self-harmers, delivered in a structured format by psychiatric trainees. The various elements of the reformulation letter and diagram can be used independently. The diagram is very helpful in demonstrating patterns of maladaptive behaviour and a possible exit strategy for new, more adaptive behaviour (as illustrated in Figure 17.4).

CHOOSING AND USING A PSYCHOLOGICAL INTERVENTION
WHEN TO USE A PSYCHOLOGICAL INTERVENTION

In all cases, the choice of treatment should be guided by a thorough assessment, leading to a diagnosis and formulation of the presenting problems. The formulation should

FIGURE 17.4 Diagrammatic formulation based on CAT principles

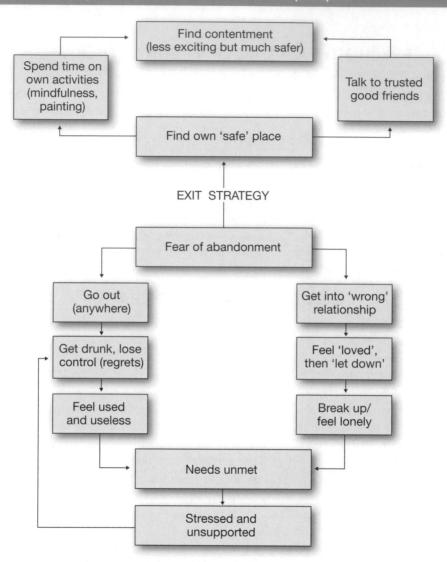

describe how and why the problems arose in terms of predisposing, precipitating, maintaining and protective factors, and so lay the framework for planning the treatment. As was highlighted in Chapter 7, comprehensive mental health assessment and problem formulation requires that information be obtained at a number of levels, using the biopsychosocial model. Thus, psychological interventions may be used alone or in combination with a range of social interventions and/or pharmacotherapy.

WHICH PSYCHOLOGICAL INTERVENTION?

The decision to use a psychological intervention—and which one—and the level of intervention (stress management and relaxation, FPS or formal psychotherapy) is determined largely by the target for treatment. These consist of symptoms, problem behaviours, interpersonal relationships or a combination of these. Thus, in patients with mild to moderate severity disorders, for example, the particular FPS may be chosen as follows:

- Exposure techniques may be used for phobic avoidance.
- Breathing retraining may be used for hyperventilation.
- Cognitive interventions may be used for obsessions.
- Activity scheduling may be used for socially avoidant behaviour.
- IPC may be used for depression secondary to role transition problems.

Generally, it is useful to decide whether to use a predominantly interpersonal or cognitive behavioural approach to treatment. Where there are clear interpersonal issues that appear to have precipitated, or to be acting as, maintaining factors for mood disturbance, an interpersonal focus is favoured. However, often a mix of FPS will be required to address the combination of problems experienced by patients (see Figures 17.5 and 17.6 over the page). These figures depict a systematic approach to treatment, commencing with general strategies and then adding additional FPS according to the patient's most prominent problem and needs.

WHO SHOULD PROVIDE TREATMENT?

Stepped collaborative care is an approach that defines different types of intervention based on patient need. As described in Chapter 1, it advocates the treatment of patients with mild disorders by primary care clinicians, and the provision of opportunities for referral for patients with complex presentations or who do not respond to usual care to specialist services (see Figure 17.7).

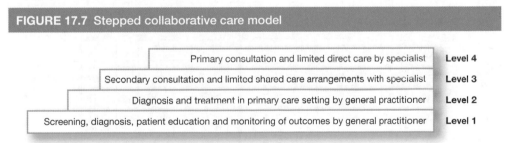

FIGURE 17.7 Stepped collaborative care model

Primary consultation and limited direct care by specialist	Level 4
Secondary consultation and limited shared care arrangements with specialist	Level 3
Diagnosis and treatment in primary care setting by general practitioner	Level 2
Screening, diagnosis, patient education and monitoring of outcomes by general practitioner	Level 1

Taking a stepped care approach allows us to readily identify those patients who will be appropriately treated using psychological interventions in the primary care setting (those with mild to moderate problems that can be managed by primary care clinicians, with or without support from clinical psychologists or psychiatrists) and those who require formal psychotherapy (and so referral to and treatment by psychiatrists or clinical psychologists) (see Table 17.2).

In the model illustrated in Table 17.2, FPS are applied mainly at level 2 in primary care settings. FPS may also be applied at level 3, where collaborative links between primary care and specialist mental health providers allow for secondary consultation, shared care arrangements and support/supervision. With more severe and/or complex disorders, formal psychotherapies are often indicated and care is provided directly by skilled specialists (level 4).

FIGURE 17.5 GP use of FPS for mood disorders

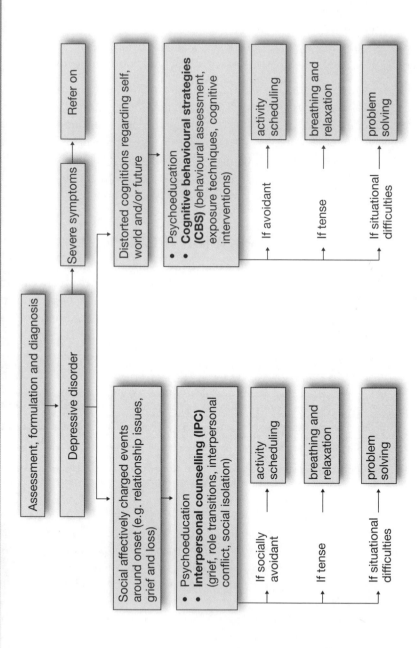

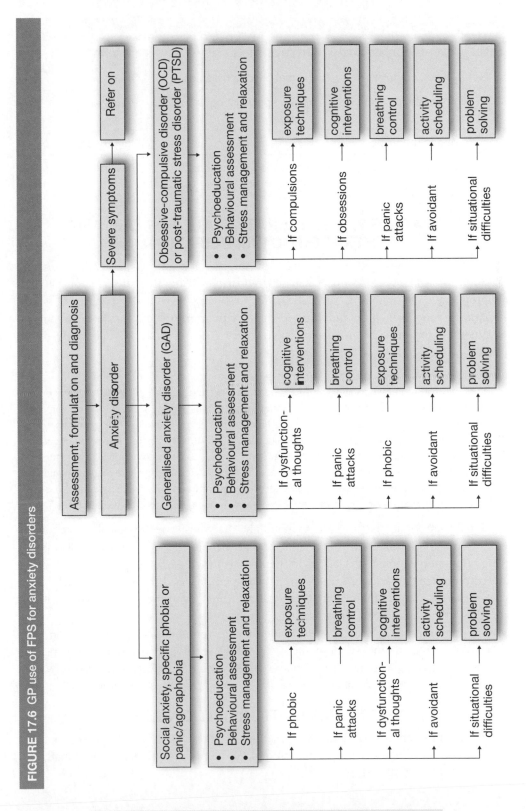

FIGURE 17.6 GP use of FPS for anxiety disorders

TABLE 17.2 Intervention levels, types and settings, and problem severity or complexity

LEVEL	SEVERITY/COMPLEXITY	INTERVENTION	SETTING
4	Severe, complex	Formal psychotherapies	Specialist
3	Moderate to severe	FPS ± specialist consultation/ support	Primary care
2	Mild to moderate	FPS	Primary care
1	Mild to moderate	Stress management and relaxation strategies	Primary care

PREPARING PATIENTS: RATIONALE FOR USE AND THERAPEUTIC PARTICIPATION

An important feature of all the psychological intervention approaches is the rationale. This may be defined as: 'a conceptual scheme that explains the cause of the patient's symptoms and prescribes a…procedure for resolving them'.[35] A vital part of the preparation process involves providing patients with appropriate information about the reasons for recommending the use of one or more FPS and what, in practical terms, is involved. An example of a rationale is given below:

> From the information obtained so far, it seems that you are suffering from a type of anxiety disorder known as agoraphobia. The anxiety related to this condition seems to be associated with avoidance of a range of situations, such as leaving home alone or going into busy shopping centres, where you fear that you might be unable to get to somewhere safe in the event that something terrible—such as a panic attack—should happen. Graded exposure, a technique through which you learn to reduce these avoidance behaviours through a graduated program, is a proven method for breaking that cycle of anxiety, which is reinforced by your avoidance and associated negative thinking. It has been shown to be a highly effective way of both reducing anxiety and increasing levels of functioning.

Equally important is the need to highlight that most psychological interventions require the active participation of patients through out-of-session homework tasks. When using brief interventions, vital factors in therapeutic progress are the patient's willingness and commitment to change, and this needs to be emphasised from the outset. In cases where patients appear ambivalent about change, it may be appropriate to use strategies such as motivational interviewing (see Chapter 10).

Another important factor in psychological interventions is the need for ongoing evaluation and measurement of outcomes. This process serves not only to provide clinicians with an objective indication of the patient's response to therapy but may also provide a useful means by which the patient can view their own progress (see Chapter 21).

THE THERAPEUTIC RELATIONSHIP

Perhaps the most appropriate relationship adopted by the GP using FPS with patients is one of active collaboration, where patient and GP identify target areas for change, and work in a kind of partnership.

Although it is difficult to assess the relative contributions of the many factors that result in the therapeutic outcome, studies have consistently found that the quality of the therapeutic relationship has a powerful influence on change (most estimates are around 30%). While it is important that GPs develop competence and an adequate level of technical proficiency in using psychological interventions, it is also vital that they remain cognisant of the critical role of therapeutic alliance. Being oneself within the boundaries of the professional role can facilitate communication. Emphasising the positive and reminding patients of the gains they have made can be reassuring and also increase self-efficacy.

Regardless of the attitude and approach that one brings to psychotherapeutic work, all clinicians have blind spots, which affect their perception of patients and their problems. These unconscious aspects of the therapeutic relationship, referred to as transference and countertransference, affect both clinician and patient. As it is generally applied in the clinical context, transference refers to the situation in which patients tend to develop (usually) intense feelings towards the treating clinician. Frequently, such feelings really belong to someone in the patient's past, from whom they have been transferred—hence the term transference. This term has gradually become more loosely used for any feelings that the patient may have about the clinician. In the clinical situation, it is important that transference situations are understood and handled sensitively.

Perhaps of greater importance is the situation in which the clinician transfers intense feelings from his or her past (or from other situations) on to the patient. In these cases, referred to as countertransference, it is important that the clinician addresses their own emotional responses to a patient outside of the therapeutic relationship (for example, in clinical supervision) in order to minimise their potentially adverse influence (see Chapter 18).

PRACTICAL ISSUES FOR PRIMARY CARE MENTAL HEALTH PROVIDERS

In some settings, the provision of psychological interventions may constitute a departure from the usual role of the GP. For example, this is likely to be the case in general practice where the GP provides care for patients with a range of problems of varying levels of acuity. This may affect the GP–patient relationship, the consultation structure and the level of patient acceptance. In some instances, practice wide changes may be needed. The degree of change required is greatest when formal psychotherapies are used, but will nevertheless be significant if the delivery of FPS becomes part of a GP's approach. This is illustrated in Figure 17.8.

The impact of any changes necessitated by the delivery of psychological care in the GP setting needs to be carefully considered. As treatment becomes more structured, time limited and focused, patients will need to adapt to an altered consultation structure that may be less acceptable to them. One important, and often difficult aspect for patients, is the realisation that the FPS session cannot also include the opportunity to deal with intercurrent or unexpected physical health problems. For the GP used to delivering routine care and addressing clinical issues as they arise, the shift in relationship associated with a more structured approach may be difficult to maintain. Partly for this reason, it is essential that the GP highlight this change and its emphasis on structure and active collaboration.

FIGURE 17.8 The spectrum of GP psychological care

	Stress management and relaxation strategies	Focused psychological strategies (FPS)	Formal psychotherapies (including CBT and IPT)
GP–patient relationship	Unstructured Open ended Undirected Empathic		Structured Limited Focused Socratic

Consultation structure	Not contracted
	Not time limited
	Incorporated into
	  routine care
			Contracted
			Time limited
			Separate from
			  routine care

Patient acceptance	High
	No need to redefine
	  GP role
			Low
			Explicit explanation
			  of change in GP's
			  role essential

Source: Adapted from Blashki et al, 2003[1]

CONCLUSION

This chapter has introduced psychological interventions in the general practice context. It has focused on stress management and relaxation strategies, focused psychological strategies with cognitive behavioural and interpersonal foci as well as on how to choose and use psychological interventions. However, this chapter is not a substitute for training and supervision in the interventions. GPs who are interested in this are encouraged to access their local training providers, both profession based and government.

REFERENCES

1. Sackett DL, Rosenberg WMC, Gray JAM, Haynes RB, Richardson WS. Evidence based medicine: what it is and what it isn't. British Medical Journal 1996;312:71–2.
2. Blashki G, Hickie IB, Davenport TA. Providing psychological treatments in general practice: how will it work? Medical Journal of Australia 2003;179:23–5.
3. McEwen BS. Protection and damage from acute and chronic stress: allostasis and allostatic overload and relevance to the pathophysiology of psychiatric disorders. Annals of the New York Academy of Sciences 2004;1032:1–7.
4. Baer RA. Mindfulness training as a clinical intervention: a conceptual and empirical review. Clinical Psychology: Science and Practice 2003;10:125–43.
5. Benson H. The Relaxation Response. New York: William Morrow, 1975.
6. Grossman P, Niemann L, Schmidt S, Walach H. Mindfulness-based stress reduction and health benefits: a meta-analysis. Journal of Psychosomatic Research 2004;57:35–43.
7. Kabat-Zinn J. Wherever You Go, There You Are: Mindfulness Meditation in Everyday Life. New York: Hyperion, 1994.
8. Kabat-Zinn J, Massion AO, Kristeller J, Peterson LG, Fletcher K, Pbert L, Linderking W, Santorelli SF. Effectiveness of a meditation-based stress reduction program in the treatment of anxiety disorders. American Journal of Psychiatry 1992;149:936–43.
9. Kristeller JL, Hallett CB. An exploratory study of a meditation-based intervention for binge eating disorder. Journal of Health Psychology 1999;4:357–63.

10. Kabat-Zinn J, Lipworth L, Burney R. The clinical use of mindfulness meditation for the self-regulation of chronic pain. Journal of Behavioral Medicine 1985;8:163–90.
11. Davidson RJ, Kabat-Zinn J, Schumacher J, Rosenkranz M, Muller D, Santorelli SF, Urbanowski F, Harrington A, Bonus K, Sheridan JF. Alterations in brain and immune function produced by mindfulness meditation. Psychosomatic Medicine 2003;65:564–70.
12. Speca M, Carlson LE, Goodey E, Angen M. A randomized, wait-list controlled clinical trial: the effect of a mindfulness meditation-based stress reduction program on mood and symptoms of stress in cancer outpatients. Psychosomatic Medicine 2000;62:613–22.
13. Teasdale JD, Segal ZV, Williams JMG, Ridgeway VA, Soulsby JM, Lau MA. Prevention of relapse/recurrence in major depression by mindfulness-based cognitive therapy. Journal of Consulting and Clinical Psychology 2000;68:615–23.
14. Ma SH, Teasdale JD. Mindfulness-based cognitive therapy for depression: replication and exploration of differential relapse prevention effects. Journal of Consulting and Clinical Psychology 2004;72:31–40.
15. Segal ZV, Williams JMG, Teasdale J. Mindfulness-Based Cognitive Therapy for Depression: A New Approach to Preventing Relapse. New York: Guilford, 2002.
16. Kabat-Zinn J. Full Catastophe Living: Using the Wisdom of Your Body and Mind to Face Stress, Pain and Illness. New York: Delacorte, 1990.
17 Hassed C. Know Thyself: The Stress Release Programme. Melbourne: Hill of Content Publishing, 2002.
18. Nathan PE, Gorman JM. A Guide to Treatments that Work. New York: Oxford University Press, 1988.
19. Gould RA, Mueser KT, Bolton E, Mays V, Goff D. Cognitive therapy for psychosis in schizophrenia: an effect size analysis. Schizophrenia Research 2001;48(2–3):335–42.
20. Sperry L. Handbook of Diagnosis and Treatment of the DSM-IV Personality Disorders. New York: Brunner/Mazel, 1995.
21. Dattilio DM. Cognitive-behavioral strategies. In: Carlson J, Sperry L, eds. Brief Therapy with Individuals and Couples. Phoenix, AZ: Zeig, Tucker & Theisen, 2000;33–70.
22. Blashki G, Morgan H, Hickie IB, Sunich H, Davenport TA. Structured problem solving in general practice. Australian Family Physician 2003;32(10):836–42.
23. Mynors-Wallis L. Problem-solving treatment in general psychiatric practice. Advances in Psychiatric Treatment 2001;7:417–25.
24. Meyer A. Psychobiology: A Science of Man. Oxford: Charles C Thomas, 1957.
25. Sullivan HS. The Interpersonal Theory of Psychiatry. Oxford: Norton & Co., 1953.
26. Bowlby J. Attachment and Loss. New York: Basic Books, Inc., 1980.
27. Elkin I, Parloff M, Hadley S, Autry J. NIMH Treatment of Depression Collaborative Research Program: background and research plan. Archives of General Psychiatry 1995;42:305–16.
28. Klerman G, Weissman M, Rounsaville B, Chevron E. Interpersonal Psychotherapy of Depression: A Brief, Focused, Specific Strategy. New York: Jason Aronson, 1994.
29. Stuart S, Robertson M. Interpersonal Psychotherapy: A Clinician's Guide. London: Arnold, 2003.
30. Judd F, Weissman M, Davis J, Hodgins G, Piterman L. Interpersonal counselling in general practice. Australian Family Physician, 2004;33:332–7.
31. Weissman M, Klerman G. Interpersonal counselling for stress and distress in primary care settings. In: New Applications of Interpersonal Therapy. Washington: American Psychiatric Press, 1993.
32. Guthrie E. Psychodynamic interpersonal therapy. Advances in Psychiatric Treatment 1999;5:135–46.
33. Guthrie E, Kapur N, Mackway-Jones K, Chew-Graham C, Moorey J, Mendel E, Marino-Francis F, Sanderson S, Turpin C, Boddy G, Tomenson B, Patton G. Randomised controlled trial of brief psychological intervention after deliberate self poisoning. British Medical Journal 2001;323:135–8.
34. Beard H, Marlowe M, Ryle A. The management and treatment of personality-disordered patients: the use of sequential diagrammatic reformulation. British Journal of Psychiatry 1990;156:541–5.
35. Frank J. What is psychotherapy? In: Bloch S, ed. An Introduction to the Psychotherapies. Oxford: Oxford University Press, 1996;1–20.

CHAPTER 18

MANAGING DIFFICULT BEHAVIOURS

C Hulbert and N Carr

It is absurd to divide people into good and bad. People are either charming or tedious.

OSCAR WILDE, *1854–1900*

CASE STUDY

Jamie is a 28-year-old unemployed man who has presented to the practice for the first time seeking prescriptions for diazepam. He tells you that he recently moved to Melbourne from country Victoria after losing his job and ending a relationship, and that he is experiencing 'panic and high anxiety' and having difficulty sleeping. He adds that the general practitioner (GP) he attended previously gave him these scripts 'from time to time as I needed them'. When encouraged to discuss other options for managing his problems, he becomes insistent that he be given a prescription.

KEY FACTS

■ Disputes and disturbances related to substance abuse problems and/or personality disorder (PD) are the most common difficult behaviours encountered in general practice.

■ Personality disorders are underpinned by traits that are enduring, inflexible and pervasive across life domains, and that cause clinically significant distress and impairment.

■ In Australia the prevalence of PD is estimated at about 7%, with base rates for individual PDs varying from about 0.5% to 3%.

■ Genetic influences contribute significantly to PD, including to the co-occurrence of particular traits—for example, neuroticism and impulsivity in borderline PD.

KEY FACTS *continued*

- Severe childhood adversity is generally predictive of PD in adulthood, with PD usually being evident by late adolescence or early adulthood.

- PD, particularly borderline PD, is associated with poorer physical health, high levels of psychiatric comorbidity and impaired social and occupational functioning.

- Antisocial and borderline traits are associated with more confronting behaviours, including threats to self or others, and tend to evoke stronger countertransference reactions in health professionals.

- Deliberate self-injury, typically linked to borderline PD, is seen in a range of psychiatric disorders, including depression and schizophrenia.

- A clear understanding of appropriate interpersonal and behavioural boundaries, and how to maintain them in a challenging situation, improves the likelihood of a therapeutic outcome.

- Monitoring one's own emotional and behavioural responses during and following challenging interactions provides a vital source of clinically relevant information; not the least of these relates to the need for informal or formal debriefing.

INTRODUCTION

Little research exists on the range of difficult behaviours and their relative frequencies encountered in general practice. A recent survey of Australian GPs identified disputes about refused prescriptions and behavioural disturbance in substance affected patients as most problematic.[1] Other commonly cited problem behaviours include inappropriate sexualised behaviour or sexual advances by patients and actual or threatened harm to self or others.

A variety of factors may contribute to the development and presentation of difficult behaviours with some, but by no means all, being the result of mental disorders. In this chapter the focus is on the management of acute behavioural disturbance and patterns of difficult behaviour attributable to maladaptive personality traits or personality disorder (PD). Some examples of the difficult behaviours considered in this chapter are:

- drug-using patient requesting a prescription, or other document;
- patient engaging in or threatening deliberate self-harm;
- patient engaging in inappropriate sexualised behaviour;
- patient engaging in aggressive or threatening behaviour directed against staff;
- patient creating a disturbance in the waiting room and/or refusing to leave; and
- patient who has been difficult in the past re-presents, asking for a consultation.

DEFINING PERSONALITY AND PERSONALITY DISORDER

Personality has been defined as 'a complex pattern of deeply embedded psychological characteristics that are largely non-conscious and not easily altered, expressing themselves automatically in almost every facet of functioning'.[2] Personality serves an explicitly integrative function and, importantly, allows for a degree of predicability in human behaviour. There is considerable evidence from cross-cultural studies that personality can be reliably described in terms of five factors or traits that are dimensional in nature. These factors or traits are neuroticism, extroversion, openness to experience, conscientiousness and agreeableness. Personality disorders are defined as enduring patterns of perceiving, relating to and thinking about the environment and oneself that are exhibited in a wide range of social and personal contexts, and that cause clinically significant distress.[3]

Typically, although not invariably, individuals with either high or low levels of particular traits are seen as more likely to exhibit disordered behaviours or maladaptive functioning, particularly when experiencing a significant stressor and/or a mental or physical illness. The presence of any of the latter may further constrain already compromised adaptive coping responses increasing the likelihood of difficult behaviours, including those seen as problematic in general practice. Disordered personality functioning typically manifests itself in late adolescence or early adulthood.

CLASSIFICATION OF PERSONALITY DISORDER

Robust research findings indicate that personality exists on a continuum with no sharp distinction between normality and pathology.[4] In general, personality functioning is regarded as 'normal' when a person participates in behaviours and customs that are acceptable to their social group, and as 'pathological' when observed behaviours are uncommon, irrelevant or self-defeating.[2] Four of the five traits making up the five-factor model have been found to characterise disordered personality functioning, with both normal and disorder traits being normally distributed in the community. Openness to experience has been shown to have few pathological correlates.

While recent evidence clearly indicates that PD may be better represented using a dimensional model, the addition in DSM-III of a separate axis comprising eleven categories of PD represented a major advance, stimulating research and the development of effective treatments. There is empirical support for DSM-1V's grouping of the PDs according to descriptive similarities into the following three clusters:[3]

- Cluster A comprises paranoid, schizoid and schizotypal PDs, seen as characterised by odd or eccentric traits and behaviours.
- Cluster B comprises antisocial, borderline, histrionic and narcissistic PDs, defined by dramatic, emotional or erratic traits and behaviours.
- Cluster C comprises avoidant, dependent and obsessive-compulsive PDs, defined in terms of anxious and fearful traits and behaviours.

Major problems for GPs and other clinicians using the current DSM-IV categorisation of the PDs are diagnostic heterogeneity (for example, there are 151 ways to meet the criteria for a diagnosis of borderline PD) and the high level of comorbidity within Axis II. Not surprisingly, 'PD not otherwise specified' remains the most frequently assigned Axis II diagnosis. Planned revisions for DSM-V include a dimensional approach to the assessment of PD that will allow clinicians to more accurately and flexibly assess and diagnose personality dysfunction.[5]

EPIDEMIOLOGY

Australian community prevalence rates for PD have been estimated at about 6%, with rates for borderline PD being given as about 1% for males and 2% for females.[6] Studies showing a normal distribution for many PD diagnostic criterion behaviours as well as PD traits are an important reminder that personality dysfunction, as it informs disordered behaviour in clinical settings, may well have much higher base rates. The finding in usually well functioning individuals of personality dysfunction during phases of acute illness—including depression, anxiety disorders and early psychosis—is also relevant in general practice settings.[7]

AETIOLOGY

The development of personality and PD is understood to reflect a significant genetic influence, including a distinct genetic contribution to individual traits as well as to the combination or clustering of some traits—for example, neuroticism and impulsivity in borderline PD.[4, 8] Genetic predispositions encouraging the selection of particular environmental options may contribute to the accumulation of genetic influences across the life span.[9] Major environmental factors implicated in the aetiology of PD include disrupted attachment experience, and trauma, neglect and deprivation in childhood. While the experience of significant childhood adversity has been shown to be generally predictive of PD in adulthood, severity of childhood sexual abuse and neglect has been directly related to severity of clinical presentation in borderline PD.[10] There is evidence, also, of a more specific link between neglect in childhood and the later development of avoidant PD.[11]

CLINICAL PRESENTATION

The clinical features for DSM-IV Axis II PDs cover a wide range of dispositions and behaviours. Using Axis II PD clusters, some broad prediction can be made in terms of likely presenting problems and clinical management difficulties in general practice. For example, individuals with Cluster A traits may present with odd, eccentric or erratic behaviours, anxiety features or persistent complaints, or may question your treatment approach and motives. Those with Cluster C traits may present as anxious and/or dependent and perhaps unwilling to relinquish the sick role. However, the behaviours identified by GPs as problematic are seen most frequently in those with Cluster B personality traits. These behaviours include verbal aggression, inappropriate demands, angry behaviour, drug seeking, repeated self-harm, and inappropriate flirtation and/or sexual advances.

MANAGEMENT OF DIFFICULT BEHAVIOURS

Approaches to the management of the diverse challenging behaviours referred to above have some common, as well as some specific, elements. This chapter will first consider general principles in the management of difficult behaviours—including the maintenance of a professional approach—and the management of boundary issues. We will then detail specific issues relating to the management of the drug-seeking patient, deliberate self-harm (DSH) and sexually inappropriate behaviour. Finally, we will present guidelines relating to whole of practice issues, such as maintenance of a safe work environment, including management of aggression and debriefing.

MAINTENANCE OF PROFESSIONAL RELATIONSHIPS

Maintaining the professional working relationship between GP and patient provides the most effective basis for the management of difficult behaviours. Most challenging situations involve an implicit or explicit invitation to step outside the professional relationship. This is most obvious in the example of sexually inappropriate behaviour. It is also very much the case when, for example, a patient with dependent or borderline traits requests the type of assistance that would be more appropriate from a family member or partner. The aim in such situations is to maintain a focus on therapeutic outcomes, including assisting the patient's learning about what is realistic and appropriate in the doctor–patient relationship. Clear thinking and skilled communication remains the GP's most effective tools in such instances. Some practical communication strategies for the management of challenging situations are set out in Figure 18.1.

FIGURE 18.1 Strategies for working with patients with challenging behaviours

- Convey a sense of warmth and respect for the patient.
- Try to sound calm and speak moderately, keeping your statements clear and brief.
- Be clear in your own mind about what your position is.
- Avoid being drawn into problem solving, prescribing and so on before you have established an understanding of the patient's situation and resources.
- Stick with your agenda (use 'I' statements) and avoid being sidetracked into peripheral issues.
- Be *very* clear about role boundaries and behavioural limits.
- In a matter of fact way, inform the patient of relevant constraints in relation to your role, available time, facilities and treatment options.
- Be prepared to calmly restate your position.
- Do your best to avoid power struggles by 'stepping out of the battle'.
- If necessary, take time out to think and/or to consult or debrief with others.
- Rehearse in advance how to respond to key situations that you can anticipate.

Patients with a diagnosis of borderline PD or other significant personality pathology often evoke a range of intense emotional reactions in treating GPs. Referred to as countertransference phenomena, these responses may include frustration, anxiety, hopelessness and the strong desire to either help or to dismiss the patient. In such cases it is helpful to try to characterise and to reflect on your own behaviour and emotional responses. Thus, phrases from the patient such as, 'You're the best doctor I've seen; no one's tried to help me like you have…', while potentially heartening and perhaps even seductive, may need to be interpreted as a reflection of emotional need rather than of objective reality. Interactions involving inappropriate demands or threatening or self-harming behaviour may quite understandably evoke anxiety, frustration or anger in the treating doctor. In all such interactions, it is important to maintain your usual professional boundaries and to be cautious about offering more, or indeed less, help than you can reasonably provide.

The concept of boundaries can be applied to further clarify major issues and realistic options. Most difficulties arise when patients challenge boundaries of one kind or another, and the successful resolution of those difficulties requires a clear understanding of what the boundary issue is and where the appropriate boundary should be. The next step, after you have established the boundary, is to maintain it. This requires translating the general principles into words, which can be difficult in the heat of the moment. Examples of the type of responses that may be useful are given in Table 18.1.

DRUG-SEEKING BEHAVIOUR

A detailed description of the presentation and management of drug-seeking behaviour is beyond the scope of this chapter, but is well described elsewhere.[12] What follows is a summary of some of the main points as well as a suggested management approach.[13] The formal definition of drug-seeking behaviour by a patient is one who has:

- a history of obtaining prescriptions for 'target drugs', such as the benzodiazepines and codeine-containing compounds: and
- seen 15 or more different doctors in the calendar year.

The most common difficulty arises with a new patient who presents to the GP with either a direct request for a drug of addiction, or with a story that strongly implies the need for one. According to Prochaska and DiClemente's[14] Stages of Addiction model, someone who attends a new GP seeking a supply of their preferred drug is almost by definition in the 'precontemplative' stage of addiction. People at the precontemplative stage are not yet ready to question their substance use and are relatively immune to offers of help. The most effective strategy for managing a drug-seeking consultation is to not facilitate access to their drug of choice, so that the uncomfortable realities of their addiction may jog the patient into realising they have a problem, and to remain open as an avenue for help.

When seeing a new patient, a usual first step is to listen to the patient's story and ask open-ended questions. With a patient who is seeking drugs, the difficulty is that this approach takes the doctor deep into the patient's agenda, from whence extrication can be difficult. *As soon as the possibility of drug-seeking behaviour is considered*, the focus should move from seeking more broadly relevant information to attempting to elicit a specific request for the drug (Stage 1). Phrases such as 'In what way did you think I might be able to help?' are respectful and appropriate for any patient, but in this context will often immediately result in a request for a drug by name. Sometimes a follow-up question such as 'Was there anything specific you had in mind?' may be needed. If neither of these produces a request for a drug, the suspicion of drug-seeking behaviour may be wrong, and it may be appropriate to go back to ask about the patient's history in more detail.

If the patient does request a drug, the next step is to refuse the request in simple but respectful terms (Stage 2). Again, this is appropriate for any patient, although on the few occasions when the patient turns out not to be drug-seeking, it can be temporarily disarming. This is usually apparent from the patient's genuine bewilderment, and can lead into a discussion about the appropriate management of their problem.

TABLE 18.1 Definition and management of boundary violations

BEHAVIOUR	ACCEPTABLE SIDE OF BOUNDARY	UNACCEPTABLE SIDE OF BOUNDARY	INTERPRETATION OF BOUNDARY ISSUE	RESPONSE OPTIONS
Patient requests a certificate because they 'want to take a "sicky"'	Compliance with the request is acceptable if patient actually has some illness	Giving way to pressure from the patient—'Just this once' or 'C'mon, Doc, at least I didn't lie to you' etc.	While the patient has been honest about their intentions, asking you to lie on their behalf is not acceptable	'I'm sorry, but I can't give you a certificate if you're not unwell.' 'I appreciate your honesty with me, but you're asking me to lie for you – that's not reasonable.' 'Yes, if you'd lied to me and said you were sick I'd have given you the certificate, but how can I treat you properly if you lie to me?'
Patient getting angry; shouting, swearing or threatening	Very occasional outbursts in context of known stressor(s)	Persistence noisy unpleasantness and bad language; any kind of threat	Patient is responsible for their behaviour and is expected to comply with accepted standard of behaviour	'Please stop shouting and swearing at me.' 'I realise you're angry, but if you don't stop behaving like this I'll have to ask you to leave.' 'I'm not going to put up with being threatened. Please leave, or I'll have to call the police.'
Patient (usually male with female doctor) requests/requires a genital examination	Reasonable medical indication and appropriate patient behaviour	Doctor feels uncomfortable; patient behaviour inappropriate +/- erection	Both doctor and patient can expect to feel personally safe and respected	'I'm not comfortable continuing this consultation.' 'I'll get one of the other doctors to see you.' [If patient aroused]: 'This isn't appropriate.' 'Please put your clothes back on. You'll have to see someone else.'

What happens next varies, but usually there will be some form of query or persistence (Stage 3). At this point, many patients realise that they are not going to get the prescription they want, and choose to leave. However, some patients persist in the hope of persuading the doctor (Stages 4 and 5). The appropriate response here is to restate the practice position and then move on to an offer of other forms of assistance. This is an essential part of the process. The goal is not simply to get the patient out of the surgery but also to ensure that they are aware of your willingness to help and to leave the door open should they have a genuine interest in non-drug strategies at a later date.

If the patient is persistent or becomes aggressive, a helpful tactic is to depersonalise what you are saying (Stage 6). This often seems to help defuse the situation, as it reinforces for the patient that you are not refusing them just because you suspect they are addicted, but because it is your usual practice not to prescribe. By this point the majority of people who just want a *drug*, as opposed to *help*, choose to leave.

MANAGING THE DRUG-SEEKING PATIENT Using the case study cited at the beginning of this chapter, the following dialogue demonstrates the application of the key stages in the effective management of a drug-seeking patient.

STAGE 1
[Elicit request for drug *early*.]
    Jamie: 'I've just come down from the country and I'm staying in a terribly noisy place and finding it all very stressful. I've only been here for two days, but I've hardly slept at all and I'm getting very nervous. If I don't get some sleep soon...'
    GP: 'In what way did you think I might be able to help?'
    Jamie: 'Oh, I just wondered if I could get some more Valium...'

STAGE 2
[Respectfully refuse the patient's request with minimal explanation.]
    GP: 'I don't prescribe drugs like Valium.'

STAGE 3
[Avoid being drawn into extended discussion around the patient's drug-seeking agenda.]
    Jamie: 'Oh, why is that?'
    GP: 'Because they're addictive drugs that cause a lot of problems, and I choose not to prescribe them.'
    or
    Jamie: 'Well, how about some Serepax then?'
    GP: 'I've already said we don't prescribe Valium or any of those kinds of tablets, and that includes Serepax.'
    Jamie: 'But why is that?'
    GP: 'Both these drugs are addictive and can be dangerous, so I don't prescribe them.'

STAGE 4
[Be prepared to repeat your refusal to prescribe.]
    Jamie: 'Well, I think your practice is @#$%^&! You're supposed to help people and I need my tablets. What kind of a doctor are you anyway?'

GP: 'I'm sorry if you find my practice unhelpful, but that's the way I work. I'm happy to try and help any other way I can, but not with those sorts of tablets.'

STAGE 5
[Offer alternative help.]

Jamie: 'What sort of help are you suggesting?'

GP: 'There are various options we could talk about, and I'm more than happy to do so, but they don't involve medication. Do you want to talk some more about them?'

STAGE 6
[Depersonalise your refusal.]

Jamie: 'Listen, I need those tablets, I CAN GET REALLY VIOLENT IF I DON'T HAVE THEM!

GP [trying to sound calm]: 'Look, there's no point in shouting at me, this is nothing to do with you personally, I don't prescribe these things for anyone and yelling at me isn't going to change that. As I said, I'm happy to help you some other way, but I'm not going to write you a prescription.'

DELIBERATE SELF-HARM

Patients who present to their GP threatening self-harm or suicide, or who have a self-inflicted injury demanding immediate attention, represent a major challenge in a general practice setting. Self-harm, defined as a self-destructive act with a non-fatal outcome, aimed at bringing about change in the patient's life situation, may or may not be accompanied by suicidal ideation. The most frequently seen forms of self-harm are cutting of the arms and overdose of prescribed or over the counter medications. Self-injury, a relatively common feature in the clinical presentation of borderline PD (see Figure 18.2), has been found to be associated with a range of psychiatric disorders, including mood disorders, schizophrenia and the substance use disorders. Importantly, investigations into the motivations and functions of self-harm in patients with and without PD reveal no significant differences between the two groups.[15] Patients from both groups identified the need to escape painful affect as the key motive while loneliness, interpersonal difficulties and the presence of psychiatric symptoms were the main precipitating factors. Paris[16] however, reported that about 10% of patients with a diagnosis of borderline PD complete suicide.

Assessment of acute risk for suicide represents a major challenge in the general practice setting. Figure 18.3 presents the key principles relevant to the assessment and management of acute suicidality. In situations where initial assessment confirms a high likelihood of significant risk for suicide, referral for additional psychiatric assessment should follow. Referral options may include a consultant psychiatrist, a local hospital emergency department and/or a specialist acute mental health service, such as a Crisis Assessment and Treatment Team. For a more comprehensive account of the assessment and management of risk for suicide see Shea.[17]

For those patients presenting with recurrent self-injury and suicidal ideation, a useful distinction can be made between acute and chronic suicidality.[18] Acute suicidality, typically seen in mostly well functioning individuals, is characterised as

---

FIGURE 18.2 DSM-IV Diagnostic Criteria for borderline PD[3]

According to DSM-IV, borderline PD is characterised by a pattern of unstable interpersonal relationships, self-image and affects as well as marked impulsivity beginning in early adulthood and present in a variety of situations, indicated by five (or more) of the following:

- frantic efforts to avoid real or imagined abandonment;
- a pattern of unstable intense interpersonal relationships characterised by alternating between extremes of idealisation and devaluation;
- identity disturbance: markedly and persistently unstable self-image;
- impulsivity in at least two areas that are potentially self-damaging (for example, spending, substance abuse, reckless driving, binge eating);
- recurrent suicidal behaviour, gestures or threats, or self-mutilating behaviour;
- affective instability due to marked reactivity of mood;
- chronic feelings of emptiness;
- inappropriate, intense anger, or difficulty controlling anger; and
- transient, stress related paranoid ideation or severe dissociative symptoms.

FIGURE 18.3 Assessment and management of acute risk for suicide

- Assess mental state and psychiatric competence.
- Determine if the patient has a clear intent to attempt suicide, a considered plan and access to means.
- Assess likely lethality of method, considering factors known to enhance lethality, such as current substance use/intoxication and/or current clinical depression or psychotic episode.
- Determine level of current recent stressors, taking particular note of recent losses.
- Assess the patient's 'attachment to life' and availability of social supports.
- Question the patient regarding their willingness to contract to attend for further treatment or accept referral to specialist mental health service.
- If necessary, attempt to persuade the patient to accept immediate psychiatric assessment.
- Fully document the consultation and all related contacts.
- If necessary, seek debriefing for yourself and other staff involved.

---

having a clear precipitant and sudden onset as well as a good response to treatment. Chronic suicidality is associated with ongoing crises, preoccupation with self-harm and suicide, and a slow treatment response. Periods of greatest risk of suicide for those with patterns of recurrent self-harm are identifiable as 'acute on chronic' crises, being defined by a marked change in behaviour and or clinical presentation. Examples include the presence of severe and sustained depressive symptoms in a chronically dysphoric and self-harming patient with borderline PD, with an associated change in the type and lethality of self-harm behaviour.

Treatment options in the latter instances should parallel those for any patients deemed to be at risk for suicide and should include ongoing monitoring of risk alongside interventions such as hospitalisation and encouragement of appropriate family involvement. Patients presenting to you who require treatment for self-injury in the absence of suicidal ideation should be offered medical treatment only if you have the time and appropriate facilities. Otherwise, treat and/or refer the patient for emergency medical treatment as you would any other injured patient.

A practitioner providing medical treatment following DSH should aim to provide high standard medical intervention in a manner that neither reinforces the self-harming behaviour nor punishes it. There should be no unnecessary discussion of the details of the self-harm behaviour with the patient. Any counselling provided in relation to the instance should be formally scheduled to another time. In most cases, it is not advisable for medical treatment and counselling to be provided by the same person. Psychotherapeutic treatment of patients with recurrent DSH requires the long-term involvement of trained, well supervised clinicians.[18] Other key components of the treatment of such patients include the provision of continuity in care and support, monitoring of mental state and medical management of comorbid physical and psychiatric conditions. The latter may include anxiety disorders, eating disorders, depression and post-traumatic stress disorder. The key principles for the management of self-harming patients in a general practice setting are summarised in Figure 18.4.

FIGURE 18.4 Principles for managing patients with recurrent DSH

- Be cautious of offering more, or less, to patients with DSH than you would for other patients.
- If appropriate, medically treat self-injury, utilising a non-reinforcing, matter of fact manner.
- Take careful note of marked changes in mental state or in the pattern of DSH.
- Monitor your countertransference responses to the patient by noting your emotional reactions during or after consultations.
- Consider seeking supervision or secondary consultation with seriously 'at risk' or personally challenging patients.
- Maintain communication with key members of the treating teams of long-term patients presenting with recurrent DSH.
- Carefully document consultations, clinical liaison contacts and secondary consultations.

INAPPROPRIATE SEXUAL ADVANCES

Inevitably, at times sexual attraction occurs between the GP and their patient, which may or may not be reciprocated. If the GP is attracted to the patient, it is a standard principle of medical ethics that it is inappropriate for the GP to act on that attraction. Further discussion of this situation is outside the scope of this chapter. For an example of published guidelines see *A Guide for Medical Practitioners*.[19]

A difficulty arises when the patient becomes sexually attracted to the GP and begins to act on this attraction. In contrast to most of the difficult behaviours considered in this chapter, which usually involve a patient whom the GP does not know well, sexual advances tend to come from someone whom the GP does know well.

Sometimes the patient's behaviour may be overt, with a direct physical or verbal approach, but more commonly there is a gradual and subtle change in behaviour—

for example, the patient behaves in a flirtatious manner, asking personal questions, or making appointment times when the GP is more likely to be alone. This is an area where the GP's own behaviour can be a large determinant of the likelihood of a problem developing. If the GP consistently maintains professional boundaries, then they may reduce the risk of the patient acting on the attraction.

If the GP begins to sense that the patient is becoming sexually attracted, it is important to recognise this and deal with it proactively. In a counselling relationship, this form of transference may be recognised and become part of the basis for the therapeutic work. However, in everyday general practice there may be other appropriate measures. GPs in this situation should consider:

- advising staff that this particular patient should not be given appointments at times when the GP is likely to be isolated;
- avoiding getting caught in flirtatious talk or touching, but steer the consultation back to a more clinical direction;
- insisting on a chaperone for physical examinations, particularly intimate examinations;
- if necessary, directly addressing the patient's behaviour, stating clearly that it is inappropriate; and
- referring a patient who makes persistent inappropriate advances to another doctor.

WHOLE PRACTICE APPROACH TO MANAGING CHALLENGING SITUATIONS

In this context, the maintenance of safe and congenial work environments requires a whole practice approach that may include training staff as well as regularly auditing the physical space. It is important to plan in advance how the practice and staff will respond when challenging situations arise. This will vary with the individual practice, but certain underlying principles apply:

- Put in place a system—such as panic buttons—to alert staff when there is a problem.
- Clarify staff roles for given situations, detailing who is supposed to respond and in what manner.
- Check if there are any heavy or sharp objects, either in the waiting room or consulting rooms, that an angry patient could easily grab and throw or use as a weapon. If so, are these essential to the practice or could they be moved to another location?
- Check the layout of the consulting room. Is the patient's chair between the GP and the door, making a quick exit in case of threat difficult for the GP? Ideally, the GP should be nearest the door.
- Have a system in place to ensure that staff involved in critical incidents undergo debriefing.

MANAGING AGGRESSIVE OR THREATENING BEHAVIOUR

Incidents involving aggressive or threatening behaviour are a relatively rare part of general practice, with most being settled with a few firm but calming words from the receptionist or medical staff; however, there are some situations when this is not enough, and more specific intervention by a GP might be required. Below are some examples of how to effectively manage four such situations.

1 A STAFF MEMBER IS A TARGET OF ANGER

This situation is usually immediately apparent— the patient directs their abusive behaviour at one person: 'She says I missed my appointment but it's her bloody fault, she told me the wrong time—and she keeps smirking at me as if I'm an idiot—there, she's doing it again!'

In this situation it is often effective to instruct the staff member to leave: 'Sharon, will you go down the back, please, and I'll sort this out.'

If the shouting continues, make it clear that this is unacceptable: 'Mr Smith, will you please stop shouting and tell me what the problem is?'

Allow the patient to explain and complain; do not bother trying to argue too much unless there is clearly a point of fact that needs to be corrected, and state clearly that you will not tolerate shouting or abuse. Do not bring the staff member back into the argument, but if the patient is justified in being upset, tell them you will speak to your staff member later.

2 THE PATIENT IS PERSISTENTLY ANGRY

When calm words and reason have failed with an angry patient, who may be intoxicated or drug affected, there comes a point when the main objective is to get the patient out of the surgery. Politely but firmly request that the patient leave. Hold the door open, but do not attempt to physically usher the patient out; any physical contact is likely to be interpreted negatively and increase the risk of violence. If you feel the police are necessary, give a calm, clear instruction to this effect to another member of staff and remain with the patient. Rarely will the patient wait for the police to arrive.

3 RE-PRESENTATION OF A DIFFICULT PATIENT

If a patient has been known to be a problem in the past and re-presents for a consultation, consider the following points:

- Should you see the patient again or would the dynamic shift if a different doctor were involved? Should that patient not be seen by a female doctor?
- Decide whether you should alert your colleagues to a potential problem so they can 'keep an ear out'.
- Leave the consulting room door ajar during the consultation.
- Address the problem upfront in the consultation. For example, it may be appropriate to begin by saying, 'Before we start, we need to get something clear. Last time you were here, you became quite unpleasant and swore at me. If it happens again, I'll have to ask you to leave.'
- Role play the anticipated consultation with a colleague, but it's important that you take the role of the patient while a colleague takes your role—that of the GP. Usually you will find no difficulty anticipating how the patient would respond. Even a brief

role play can often provide a remarkably accurate simulation of the forthcoming consultation and help clarify exactly which words to use.

4 BANNING DIFFICULT PATIENTS

After an unpleasant consultation, some practices mark a patient's file with something like 'not to be seen again'. Unfortunately this rarely works. There may be a long delay until the patient presents again, and the patient has not been informed that they are 'banned'. The receptionist dealing with the patient is in an almost impossible position unless he or she is given very clear advice about how to respond.

Practices are entitled to refuse to see someone on reasonable grounds.[20] If the decision is made not to see a particular patient again, it is essential to have a procedure in place. The patient should be informed in writing of the practice's decision, and a copy of the letter kept in the notes. A system must be in place so that if the patient rings in the future, the receptionist knows that the patient is not to be given an appointment.

Most of these situations arise where a patient is not well known to the practice, minimising the practice's responsibility for ongoing care; however, it is always appropriate, particularly if the patient has a significant history with the practice, to offer to forward a copy of the records to the practice of the patient's choice.

INDICATIONS FOR FORMAL DEBRIEFING

After dealing with any unpleasant or difficult situation, it is well worth taking a little time to discuss what has just occurred with any others who are immediately involved or with another colleague. Referred to as 'defusing', this may simply involve spending a few minutes talking through what happened or may include some education about likely responses and coping strategies. If other patients have witnessed the disturbance, it can also be reassuring to them that you acknowledge what has occurred and take the time to settle yourself.

While debate continues about the efficacy of formal debriefing, this step may be helpful in certain situations. Factors indicating the need for formal debriefing include the following:

- The incident was particularly distressing or traumatic.
- The person had experienced one or more quite similar events in the past.
- The person was already stressed or having personal difficulties.
- The person subsequently experiences depressive symptoms or post-trauma symptoms, such as anxiety or flashbacks.

CONCLUSION

This chapter outlined approaches to managing a range of challenging behaviours encountered not infrequently in general practice settings.

The range of challenging situations includes inappropriate requests for prescriptions by drug-using patients, threats of, or actual, DSH or regressive behaviour and inappropriate sexualised behaviour. Personality dysfunction, in conjunction with acute mental illness and/or substance misuse, often provides the context for these problematic presentations. Interventions aimed at addressing challenging presentations should be grounded in the professional relationship, with particular attention being paid to the maintenance of professional boundaries. Key principles for dealing with behaviours involving a risk of injury to the patient or GP staff include careful and regular monitoring of the mental state of the patient, non-reinforcement of DSH, thorough documentation, regular communication with members of the patient's treating team, and the implementation of a whole practice approach to safety in the workplace. All health professionals, including GPs, should monitor the range of their responses to challenging situations and make appropriate use of secondary consultation and/or debriefing interventions.

REFERENCES

1. Ferguson H. The danger out there. Australian Doctor 14/1/2005:17–18.
2. Millon T, with Davis RD. Disorders of Personality: DSM-IV and Beyond. 2nd edn. New York: Wiley, 1996.
3. American Psychiatric Association. Diagnostic and Statistical Manual. 4th edn. Washington DC: American Psychiatric Association, 1994.
4. Livesley JW, Jang KL, Vernon PA. Phenotypic and genotypic structure of traits delineating personality disorder. Archives of General Psychiatry 1998;55:941–8.
5. Widiger TA, Simonsen E. Alternative dimensional models of personality disorder. American Journal of Psychiatry 2005;19(2):110–30.
6. Jackson HJ, Burgess PM. Personality disorders in the community: results from the Australian National Survey of Mental Health and Wellbeing. Social Psychiatry and Psychiatric Epidemiology 2000;35:531–8.
7. Bronisch T, Klerman GL. Personality functioning: change and stability in relation to symptoms and psychopathology. Journal of Personality Disorders 1993;5(2):307–17.
8. Livesley, JW. Behavioral and molecular genetic contribution to a dimensional classification of personality disorder. Journal of Personality Disorders 2005;19(2):131–55.
9. Shiner RL. A developmental perspective: lessons from research on normal personality development in childhood and adolescence. Journal of Personality Disorders 2005;19(2):202–10.
10. Battle CL, Shea MT, Johnson DM, Yen S, Zlotnick C, Zanarini MC, Sanislow CA, Skodol AE, Gunderson JG, Grilo CM, McGlashan TH, Morey LC. Childhood maltreatment associated with adult personality disorders: findings from the Collaborative Longitudinal Personality Disorder Study. Journal of Personality Disorder 2004;18(2):193–211.
11. Joyce PR, McKenzie SE, Luty RT, Mulder RD, Sullivan P, Cloninger RC. Temperament, childhood environment and psychopathology as risk factors for avoidant and borderline personality disorders. Australian and New Zealand Journal of Psychiatry 2003;37:756–64.
12. Miller WR, Rollnick S. Motivational Interviewing. 2nd edn. New York: Guildford Press, 2002.
13. Carr N. I just want some Valium doctor. Australian Family Physician 1998;27:817–21.
14. Prochaska J, DiClemente C. Toward a comprehensive model of change. In: Miller W, Heather N, eds. Treating Addictive Behaviours: Processes of Change. New York: Plenum Press, 1986:327.
15. Soloff PH, Lynch KG, Kelly TM, Malone KM, Mann, J. Characteristics of suicide attempts of patients with major depressive episode and borderline personality disorder: a comparative study. American Journal of Psychiatry 157(4):601–8.
16. Paris J. Is hospitalization useful for suicidal patients with borderline personality disorder? Journal of Personality Disorders 2004;18(3):240–7.

17. Shea SC. The Practical Art of Suicide Assessment: A Guide for Mental Health Professionals and Substance Use Counsellors. Brisbane: John Wiley & Sons, 1999.

18. Krawitz R, Watson C. Borderline Personality Disorder: A Practical Guide. Oxford: Oxford University Press, 2003.

19. Medical Board of Practitioners of Victoria. A Guide for Medical Practitioners. Victoria: Medical Board of Practitioners, 1999.

20. Australian Medical Association Code of Ethics, Position Statement, 2004. http://www.ama.com.au/web.nsf/doc/WEEN-5ww598 (accessed October 2005)

CHAPTER 19

MANAGING GRIEF AND LOSS

A Love and L Kaminsky

Had we never lov'd sae kindly,
Had we never lov'd sae blindly,
Never met—or never parted—
We had ne'er been broken-hearted.

ROBERT BURNS, 'Ae Fond Kiss', 1791

CASE STUDY

Katrina is a smartly dressed woman in her fifties, with a warm smile that masks the depression she has felt since the death of her 97-year-old mother, two months ago. Katrina was her mother's sole carer, and that was a contributing factor to her own marital break-up. Her brother and sister were angered by what they perceived as the unnecessary transfer of their mother to a nursing home, a year ago. After her mother's death, Katrina feels alienated from her family, and describes her life as empty. She is having sleeping difficulties and presents to her general practitioner (GP), asking for sleeping tablets.

KEY FACTS

- Grief reactions to loss are a normal part of the human condition and cannot be avoided or cured in the conventional sense.

- Grieving involves coming to terms with loss and integrating the experience into our sense of self, the world and the future.

- Presentations vary, depending on factors such as personality and life history, the social context and cultural practices as well as the symbolic magnitude of the loss.

KEY FACTS *continued*

■ Individuals will often make faltering progress, sometimes going backwards, before resolving their grief reactions.

■ Although most people resolve their grief satisfactorily, there are factors that can improve the chances of successful resolution within a reasonable time.

■ GPs can contribute to the timely resolution of grief by employing clinical communication skills that facilitate the grieving process.

■ A range of psychiatric comorbidities—including depression, anxiety disorders and somatisation disorders—can be common complications in grief reactions.

■ Such grief reactions can be prolonged, intense or problematic. GPs can identify complicated grief reactions and ensure patients receive specialised treatment, including intensive grief therapy and medication.

INTRODUCTION

Human beings have a unique capacity to construct their worlds symbolically. We create meaning from our experience and invest our relationships with rich connections and emotional bonds. Human existence also inevitably involves loss. People close to us cannot be with us forever and our ever-changing worlds ensure that important relationships are often disrupted and reshaped. Disruption to or loss of a vital attachment is referred to as bereavement. It almost inevitably produces an intense, often overwhelming reaction, which is known as grief.[1]

While grief may feel like a catastrophic experience to those affected by it, it can be reassuring to know that it is a normal reaction to significant loss. No matter how terrible the experience feels, the waves of distress and despair will generally ease, both in intensity and frequency, as time unfolds. For most individuals, this process of mourning may persist for six months or more. Indeed, we now recognise that it may never remit fully.[2] With time, however, most people adjust to their new worlds, making sense of the loss and pain, and move forward with a reshaped understanding of their lives.

Whatever the depth of their current misery, most of those grieving will not require special assistance to undertake this journey. The majority of bereaved people neither need, nor benefit from, participation in a bereavement group or formal grief therapy.[3] Nonetheless, the availability and support of resourceful, sensitive others can assist this transition and facilitate a more productive resolution. Typical tasks of grieving can be identified and the support of a caring, informed practitioner can help facilitate their completion.

A sizeable minority, however, will be at risk of mental and physical complications following their loss. Complications can take many forms, including psychiatric comorbidities, such as major depression. Careful assessment can increase the likelihood of early identification and indicate when specialised intervention is warranted. Given their pivotal roles in people's health care, GPs can contribute to the management of typical grief reactions and ensure that additional professional assistance is provided whenever grief does not run its normal course.

GRIEF REACTIONS
NORMAL OR UNCOMPLICATED GRIEF

There are few essential features of grief—its presentation is as varied as the human condition. Nevertheless, we can identify five broad domains of grief reactions. These are outlined below and illustrated in Figure 19.1.

- **Emotional** Grief may involve feelings of sadness, anger, guilt, anxiety, fear, shame, relief, jealousy, hopelessness and powerlessness.
- **Cognitive** Changes to thinking may include obsessive preoccupation with former attachments, poor concentration, fantasising, apathy, disorientation and confusion, ruminating about the circumstances of the death, experiencing a sense of the presence of the deceased and trying to make sense of the loss.
- **Physical** Somatic symptoms may manifest as headaches, muscular aches, physical complaints including abdominal or chest pain, fatigue, nausea, menstrual irregularities, noise intolerance, tension and appetite and sleep disturbance. It can also have more subtle effects on health. These include the reduced activity of natural killer cells (immune system cells) and higher levels of the stress hormone cortisol compared with non-bereaved individuals. People may also neglect their usual diet, exercise and medication regimens.
- **Behavioural** The bereaved may report constant crying or agitated behaviour coupled with increasing illness behaviours, such as frequent visits to their GPs. They may also describe social withdrawal, increasing use of alcohol, searching for the deceased, avoiding reminders of the deceased, increasing physical activities, uncharacteristic behaviour and maintaining a sense of connectedness by, for instance, numerous visits to the cemetery.
- **Existential** Disruptions to people's life certainties, such as the death of a loved one, can precipitate searching for meaning in death and the questioning of spiritual beliefs and values, often resulting in a re-evaluation of core beliefs.

It is important to remember that because grief is a dynamic, cyclical process, each of the five domains will manifest in a variety of ways at different times, in different phases of the process. Even the most extreme reactions, seen after periods of relatively settled presentation, can be part of normal grief reactions. They do not, by themselves, indicate that the person is experiencing an atypical form of grief.

As indicated, phases of grief reactions can be identified, and it is instructive to consider these patterns. At first, in certain cases for periods lasting weeks, people can react to news of loss with shock and denial. They report disbelief and numbness as their initial responses. They are also likely to experience pining, yearning and a desire to be reunited with the loved one. After this initial reaction, a phase of acute anguish might be experienced. People report feeling waves of somatic distress, withdrawal behaviour, preoccupation with the loved one and feelings of anger, guilt and depression. They might be restless and agitated while reporting feeling aimless and unmotivated. Life can seem pretty meaningless and the purpose of living can be questioned. In time, a resolution phase will emerge. Individuals will report a sense of having grieved intensely but now feeling less overwhelmed by intense emotions. They might indicate a desire to return to

FIGURE 19.1 Multidimensional domains of grief reactions

Emotional	Cognitive	Physical	Behavioural	Existential
Sadness	Preoccupation	Somatic	Crying	Disruption
Anger	Ruminating	complaints	Agitation	to life's
Guilt	Fantasy	Lowered	Withdrawal	certainties
Anxiety	Confusion	immune	Searching	Questioning
		function	Avoidance	of core
				beliefs

Normal grief reactions

work and resume other roles. They will also express a wish to adopt new roles as they begin to re-experience pleasure from ordinary activities and social relationships.

COMPLICATIONS OF GRIEF

When grief does not resolve within a reasonable time, or individuals have extreme or exaggerated experiences, it is generally agreed that the process is no longer adaptive. These phenomena have been variously described as, for example, abnormal, unresolved, maladaptive and traumatic; but recently the term 'complicated grief reaction' has gained currency. Proponents argue that it represents a distinct diagnostic category requiring more complex, multimodal therapies, and they have prepared operational criteria for its inclusion in DSM-V[4] (see Figure 19.2). They maintain the syndrome can be differentiated from similar conditions, such as depression, that are often comorbid with grief.[4] Although not universally accepted, this perspective does highlight the importance of careful assessment, identifying the needs of and tailoring treatment interventions for people with more intractable problems stemming from a significant loss.

Symptoms characteristic of depression might include feelings of sadness, insomnia, poor appetite and so on. However, by DSM-IV[5] criteria, the diagnosis of major depressive disorder is not usually given within the first two months following the loss. In the early period, the symptoms tend to be transitory and self-limited. If they persist for longer, however, such a diagnosis might be warranted. Careful assessment can help distinguish depression and grief reactions. For example, in grief, guilt is usually restricted to events around the death of the loved one, and thoughts of death with wanting to be reunited. Depression is usually associated with more global feelings of worthlessness, and symptoms such as psychomotor retardation. About 20% of bereaved people will develop major depression,[6] although a follow-up study found that 70% of these were not depressed two years later. Symptoms may include:

- thoughts of worthlessness or hopelessness;
- thoughts of death or suicide;

- delusions;
- extreme weight loss;
- excessive and uncontrolled crying and psychomotor slowing;
- disbelief and inability to accept the loss;
- flashbacks and nightmares;
- fantasy relationships with the deceased;
- feeling the departed is always watching;
- withdrawing socially; and
- searching for the deceased.

There are risk factors for developing depression during bereavement. These include:

- a previous history of depression;
- high neuroticism scores on personality assessments;
- self-rated poor health or functional limitations and disability;
- male gender (but women have more severe symptoms); and
- less regularity in lifestyle patterns, such as sleeping and eating routines.

Grief related depression responds to psychotherapy and pharmacological interventions for major depression. Referral to specialist services is usually appropriate in these cases.

Anxiety symptoms may be prominent in grief reactions. A recent study revealed that 40% of people who lose a partner experience generalised anxiety or panic disorders in the first year.[7] Reminders of the deceased may be particularly associated with a panic attack. Social isolation and loneliness seem to exacerbate the pain of grief. Some researchers have described these features as a type of separation anxiety. Other anxiety disorders, such as obsessive-compulsive disorder, can be exacerbated when a person is grieving, and these may require careful consideration and management.

When loss is associated with trauma, or it is unanticipated, the ensuing grief reactions can be further complicated. It often overwhelms the coping capacity of individuals. They may be unable to comprehend the implications of the loss, they may see the world as particularly chaotic, and they may experience symptoms more usually seen in post-traumatic stress disorder, such as numbing and intrusive thoughts, as well as hyperarousal and avoidance.[8] Treatment strategies similar to those for post-traumatic stress disorder are recommended, with some experts arguing that they be undertaken before grief work is begun.

Grieving individuals often experience poorer physical health, or complain of physical concerns, as indicated earlier.[1] Studies have shown, for example, that recently bereaved widows and widowers present with a range of somatic complaints. There is some evidence that the use of health services increases following bereavement, although others have found that while health is poorer, health service use does not increase significantly. Increased service use, if it does occur, might be an opportunity to provide more appropriate support, and knowing that a recently bereaved patient is at risk of health deterioration can signal the need to inquire about recent changes in physical functioning.

Individuals can also develop conversion symptoms, with unexplained sensory loss and functional impairment. For example, a bereaved retired single woman, who had been very dependent on her aged mother, started using her mother's walking frame shortly after her loss; she reported experiencing weakness in her legs and difficulty walking, just as her mother had. She did not comprehend the connection between her symptoms and her feelings of still wanting to 'lean on her mother' even after death.

While grief increases in prevalence with age, young people in mourning have special needs. Bereaved children and adolescents often have a more difficult time adjusting to loss than adults do. They are less well equipped, emotionally or intellectually, to cope with the pain of separation or death of someone close to them. Thus, they are more at risk of developing complicated grief and so require careful assessment.

FIGURE 19.2 Proposed DSM-V diagnostic criteria for complicated grief reaction[4]

CRITERION A

Person has experienced the death of a significant other, and their response involves 3 or 4 of the following symptoms experienced at least daily or to a marked degree:

1 Intrusive thoughts about deceased
2 Yearning for deceased
3 Searching for deceased
4 Excessive loneliness since the death

CRITERION B

In response to the death, 6 of the following 11 symptoms experienced at least daily or to a marked degree:

1 Purposelessness, feelings of futility about future
2 Subjective sense of numbness, detachment, or absence of emotional responsiveness
3 Difficulty acknowledging the death (disbelief)
4 Feeling life is empty or meaningless
5 Feeling that part of oneself has died
6 Shattered world view (lost sense of security, trust, control)
7 Assumes symptoms or harmful behaviours of, or related to, the deceased
8 Excessive irritability, bitterness or anger related to the death
9 Avoidance of reminders of the loss
10 Stunned, shocked, dazed by the loss
11 Life is not fulfilling without the deceased

CRITERION C

Duration of disturbance (symptoms listed) is at least six months

CRITERION D

Disturbance causes clinically significant impairment in social, occupational or other important areas of functioning

EPIDEMIOLOGY

Grief becomes increasingly prevalent with age. At age 65, over 50% of women and 10% of men have experienced bereavment at least once. At age 85, the figures increase to 80% of women and 40% of men.[9] Many grief sufferers are at risk of mental and physical complications as a result of loss. Jacobs et al[8] has shown that 40% of people who lose a spouse experience anxiety disorders, such as panic syndromes, in the first year following the loss. Indeed, Prigerson et al[10] estimated that around 15% of all grieving individuals experience complications, such as comorbid depression, while others put the figure as high as 20%. As has been noted, children and adolescents are susceptible to complicated grief reactions. Around 4% of children in the US lose one or both parents by the age of 15, and this does not include losses from divorce and relationship breakdown.[11] Sibling death can also lead to complications requiring specialist intervention. (See Figure 19.3.)

FIGURE 19.3 Risk factors associated with complicated grief

PRE-LOSS

- Pre-existing mental health problems or few adequate coping mechanisms
- Current learning disabilities in children and adolescents
- Lack of knowledge and information about death
- Previous experience of trauma and loss
- Conflict between the person and the deceased
- Dependent or ambivalent relationships with the deceased
- Poor attachment in early life

WHEN LOSS OCCURS

- The loss is the result of violence, trauma or accident—for example, suicide, accident.
- Others are unable to offer support and comfort for whatever reason.
- The relationship with the deceased was overly close, intense or ambivalent.
- The death is associated with stigma, or shame—for example, AIDS.

POST-LOSS

- An unstable and inconsistent family environment
- Lack of adequate family or community supports
- Traumatic reminders
- Secondary stresses that seriously disrupt family functioning
- Inadequate physical and emotional care
- Anniversaries and other significant events
- Further losses or bereavements
- Relapse with depressive symptoms

ASSESSMENT

Information gathered from grieving individuals is critical to the assessment process. It may include standardised measures[10] but careful interviewing is often helpful. Some of the types of information a GP needs in order to assess a grieving individual are outlined in the following section. Information about pre-loss factors that needs to be obtained are listed in Figure 19.3. The mere presence of these risk factors—for example, having previously experienced severe traumas—does not inevitably lead to complicated grief symptoms. The quality of the relationship prior to the loss has to be established. Other possible reasons for various symptoms, such as loss of concentration, have to be considered—for example, have financial problems become an issue? The pre-loss characteristics of the deceased person can also be important. For example, the death of a child has a very different impact compared to that of an older relative who has been frail for some time. A parent might find it hard to let go of a relationship with a dead child and resent being told by well-meaning people that she should 'be strong' and that she will 'get over it'. A stigmatised death, such as one resulting from AIDS, is likely to produce additional complications.

The circumstances surrounding the bereavement have to be carefully considered. For example, an unexpected loss, or one resulting from an accident, can have a traumatic effect on the person. Feelings of numbness, unreality and disbelief can be magnified and combined with shock and even terror. Patients might benefit from appropriate referral if these reactions occur. The quality of relationships should be considered and the degree of support that survivors are able to offer each other assessed. Where the attachment to the lost one was overly close or intense, the person might initially feel overwhelmed by the prospect of having to live on alone. Low self-confidence and feelings of abandonment may accompany a sense of emptiness and despair. Where ambivalence has marked the relationship, the person might feel intense guilt, and become preoccupied with regret over things said and done, or not done. The positive aspects of the relationship might be denied or minimised, or the loved one idealised while the self is denigrated. Where death is associated with stigma, such as suicide, there might be overwhelming feelings of shame and social humiliation. The person might feel ostracised by friends and relatives, and avoid social contact. Such isolation can quickly become a self-fulfilling prophecy and patients can fail to take advantage of opportunities to seek social support.

Hence it is also important to assess the extent and quality of the person's social, cultural and spiritual support post-bereavement. Before the loss, the person might have enjoyed good social relations within a close family network. The event can lead to isolation and a reduction of social support, such as loss of income, straining the family functioning; this requires careful assessment, including the extent of practical resources, such as access to government services.

All the factors discussed have to be carefully assessed before any intervention is planned. A genogram can be a useful way of summarising the information gathered and of providing the person with a 'snapshot' of the issues assessed. The genogram can form the basis of further exploration and elaboration in counselling sessions; Figure 19.4 is a genogram summarising family related issues for Katrina in our case study.

One way to conceptualise the assessment of bereaved patients is to consider the framework provided by Maslow's hierarchy of needs, presented in Table 19.1, where example questions are used to illustrate how you can probe the various facets. The questions allow a GP to raise increasingly complex and abstract issues as the patient progresses, moving from crisis intervention to ensure physical safety in the early stages through to aspects such as existential questions that arise later in the process.

MANAGEMENT
HELPING PATIENTS WITH NORMAL OR UNCOMPLICATED GRIEF

Although grieving after loss is normal, the complexity of presentation and the uncertain course of resolution place extra demands on professionals facilitating the process. For

FIGURE 19.4 Katrina's genogram and related assessment notes

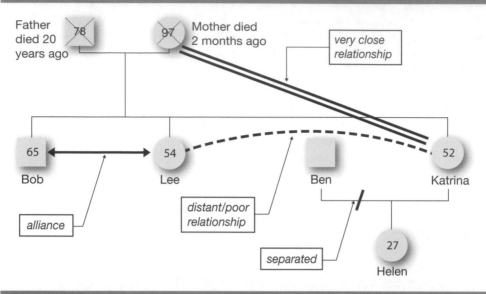

TABLE 19.1 Conceptualising bereavement assessment in terms of Maslow's hierarchy of needs

LEVEL OF NEED	THEMATIC QUESTION
Physiological needs	How are your eating, drinking, sleeping (etc.) patterns?
Safety needs	Are you in any way concerned about your own welfare (e.g. any thoughts about joining your loved one?)
Belongingness needs	How are things with your partner and children? With other family members?
Esteem needs	Are you still able to pursue your work roles, your hobbies etc., with the same interest?
Self-actualisation needs	How have these events affected your philosophy on life? Is it still worthwhile?

example, a surviving partner, burdened with her own grief, might feel overwhelmed by the responsibilities of managing the household, administering the estate and caring for others in the family who are grieving also. Problems that are subsequent to the death may appear easier to deal with, and apparently more pressing, than the unfinished business of grief. Feelings associated with the loss might go unacknowledged, and behaviour might swing from flat denial of the pain to strong experiences of anger and frustration. Effective facilitation therefore calls for advanced clinical communication skills (see Figure 19.5). The aim is to ensure that grieving individuals receive appropriate support as they experience and express their grief in their own ways, find ways of coping with the changes, transform their relationships with the departed person, regenerate existing relationships, develop new ones and ensure that their own health and wellbeing is maintained during the transition to a new view of self, the world and the future.

With uncomplicated grief, the clinical communication skills outlined in Figure 19.5 provide an excellent basis for facilitation of the grief process. Bear in mind that so many of the apparently helpful messages that others give a bereaved person are in fact wrong, and patients can benefit by learning to challenge the underlying assumptions. For example, it is not true that life prepares us adequately for loss. Nothing fully prepares us for separation from loved ones; only by experiencing grief can we truly come to terms with the impact of loss. A bereaved person needs to interact with others who are empathic and understanding. They might not find receptive people among their friends and family because they too might be grieving or might misunderstand how best to help. Exhortations from relatives to 'pull yourself together', or reassurances that 'you'll soon get over it', might be well meant but are not helpful to the bereaved. Professionals who are accepting and prepared to listen in a constructive manner can make an important contribution to patients' adjustment.

Placing a time limit on grieving is similarly counterproductive. While 6–12 months is the normal range in our society, many will grieve longer. They may need more time and

---

FIGURE 19.5 Effective clinical communication with patients experiencing grief

1 Remember that grieving involves pain and misery from which the bereaved cannot be protected. Help them identify and express these feelings by asking open-ended questions—for example, 'How has the death of…affected you?'

2 You may be troubled by your own sense of helplessness, but you can still provide support and encouragement as well as practical problem-solving contributions.

3 Be prepared to contain strong, often volatile, reactions that may be directed at you. You may feel frightened or angry when you feel maligned but a calm, assured, non-judgmental response can help the bereaved manage their reactions better.

4 Remember to take the perspective of the grieving person and maintain your empathic understanding. Even simple, well intended but disaffiliating questions can be counterproductive—for example, 'Surely you're feeling better today?'

5 Show your genuine concern and caring without being patronising. Avoid sounding as if you know best—for example, do not say 'You should be getting over this by now.'

6 Your personal needs can interfere with the process. Refer on if necessary.

7 Stay non-judgmental and reflect the person's feelings, especially early in the process, as attempts to explain the loss will usually be met with resentment or rejection.

8 Remarks about the person having to feel better 'for others' sake', or similar attempts to motivate change will usually be counterproductive.

9 Recognise and acknowledge the gravity of the situation for the person.

10 Nurture hope by normalising the process, while acknowledging the uniqueness of the person's response, and holding expectations that the person will ultimately accommodate the loss and that the pain will subside.

support to work through their feelings. Showing patience and tolerance is a critical part of management. Rather than needing encouragement to 'let go' or 'seek closure', they need support as they attempt to create new meaning in their lives. Grieving individuals will benefit from help in developing new interests and new friends as they seek to complete the task of transforming the former relationship and revising their world views.

ANTICIPATORY GRIEF

Most people will be familiar with the work of Elizabeth Kubler-Ross,[12] who proposed a five-stage model of anticipatory grief experienced by people facing death. She suggested that they first go through a period of denial, where shock and disbelief predominate. The second stage involves anger as the primary reaction, as the person struggles to answer the question 'Why me?' Next comes the stage of bargaining, where the person makes deals with fate, or a higher power, such as promising to be a better person in the future, if only a cure can be found. The fourth stage involves depression and despair as the person recognises that no miracles are going to occur and that the inevitability of death looms large. The final stage, acceptance, represents a period of relative serenity, where the person is accepting of their fate.

While this model was important in pioneering grief research, its limitations are known. It was developed for people with terminal illnesses, not for the grief reactions of survivors. What is more, the stage approach does not match people's experience. The process is not linear, as it suggests, and people do not attain higher stages and never again experience some of the supposedly lower level reactions, such as bouts of depressed mood. There is a danger that this descriptive model can become a prescription for how grief should progress, and patients can feel chastised or admonished because they have not moved to the next stage quickly enough. It has led to many common aspects of normal grieving, such as regression, being misidentified as evidence of complicated grief reactions.

Rather than consider grief as a process involving set stages, it is probably more useful to think of it as several broad, overlapping phases. These do not occur in a fixed order and progress through them is not a simple trajectory. People may edge forward in a faltering manner, typically with episodes of regression, outbursts of anger and other emotions, and loss of meaning. Grieving individuals must not be judged harshly for not 'getting on with their lives' in an orderly and predictable manner. The emphasis can be placed on the positive, adaptive aspects of grieving instead of concentrating solely on reducing or minimising loss oriented negative emotions.[13] Within these phases, four broad tasks of grieving can be identified.

ACCEPTING AND ACKNOWLEDGING THE LOSS Initially the person may wish to deny the importance of the loss. Events may seem unreal or dream-like, and they may report feeling numb and shocked. This may last a short time or as long as a few days. Common behaviour includes withdrawing, becoming non-communicative, crying or showing anger. For example, a woman who lost her daughter in an accident three months earlier still spent most nights awake, poring over family photographs and expecting her daughter to come home, bringing an end to the mother's living nightmare. The reality of the loss has to be absorbed and its meaning assimilated so that a sense of irreversibility emerges.

ASSIMILATING THE LOSS After the initial jolt has subsided, the person may be preoccupied with the loss and complain of intrusive thoughts, anxiety and restlessness, and difficulty sleeping, as well as physical symptoms, including loss of appetite, digestive problems and fatigue. They may feel anger, guilt and strong identification with the lost loved one to the point of reporting occasionally thinking they have seen the person or heard his or her voice. A possible depressive response on the anniversary of the loss can be anticipated. This phase cannot be hurried or closed prematurely. The individual has to get through it at their own rate.

ACCOMMODATING THE LOSS Resolution may begin any time from 3–12 months after the loss. Patients begin to recover by incorporating new habits and making lifestyle changes, and by planning for the future without the physical presence of the lost one. Gradually they will take charge of their lives and resolve the loss through activity, readjustment and education.

TRANSFORMING THE LOSS As the person starts to emerge from the preoccupation with the lost one and a past that is gone, an opportunity for revising their life philosophy may emerge. Questions about the meaning of life and spiritual understandings can come to the fore. Many people grow significantly as human beings after experiencing loss and grief. If the opportunity comes for them to explore these issues, they should be encouraged to grasp it.

COMPLICATED GRIEF REACTIONS

Aspects of complicated grief reactions were reviewed earlier. People experiencing complicated grief will often show other reactions, such as depression. Symptoms may include, but are not limited to:

- expressing a desire to commit suicide;
- a pattern of alcohol or drug abuse;
- inability to care for oneself (not getting sleep, not eating);
- uncontrolled rage directed at others;
- physical harm to self or others; and
- severe dysphoric mood.

Before grieving can be properly facilitated, treatment of the related problems should be considered. Treatment recommendations for depression accompanying complicated grief include the combination of tailored cognitive behavioural therapy, incorporating procedures such as counterfactual thinking, exposure techniques and activity scheduling, together with appropriate antidepressant medication. In some cases, inpatient care might be required. Specialist knowledge and advice is invaluable in these cases and referral should definitely be considered.

CASE STUDY REVISITED

Katrina was suffering from a grief reaction to her mother's death. The rift with her family, twelve months before, complicated her situation. Supportive grief counselling enabled her to confront various issues and improve her relationship with her siblings. At the suggestion of her GP, she was able to enrol in art therapy classes, which gave a creative outlet to her feelings of hopelessness. Over a period of six months, her depression lifted and she presented with a beaming smile to her GP, holding out an invitation to her first art exhibition.

CONCLUSION

Bereavement—the inevitable loss of, or disruption to, important relationships—usually produces intense grief reactions. Although most people's experience will be relatively uncomplicated and will resolve with time, they will usually benefit from appropriate support and encouragement. Effective clinical communication helps them assimilate and accommodate the loss. Some patients, however, will be at risk of complicated reactions and significant comorbidities, including major depression. General practitioners are uniquely positioned to monitor patients' adjustment and assess possible complications. Appropriate intervention and management, coupled where indicated with referral to specialised professional assistance, help patients achieve better resolution of their grief reactions and improve their quality of life.

REFERENCES

1. Parkes CM. Bereavement. In: Kendrick T, Tylee A, Freeling P, eds. The Prevention of Mental Illness in Primary Care. New York: Cambridge University Press, 1996;74–87.
2. Neimeyer R. Searching for the meaning of meaning: grief therapy and the process of reconstruction. Death Studies 2000;24:531–58.
3. Stroebe W, Schut H, Stroebe MS. Grief work, disclosure and counselling: do they help the bereaved? Clinical Psychology Review 2005;25:395–414.
4. Lichtenthal WG, Cruess DG, Prigerson HG. A case for establishing complicated grief as a distinct mental disorder in DSM-V. Clinical Psychology Review 2004;24: 637–62.
5. American Psychiatric Association. Diagnostic and Statistical Manual of Mental Disorders. 4th edn. Washington DC: American Psychiatric Associaiton, 1994.
6. Zisook S. Understanding and managing bereavement in palliative care. In: Chochinov HM, Breitbart W, eds. Handbook of Psychiatry in Palliative Medicine. Oxford: Oxford University Press, 2000;321–34.
7. Jacobs S, Prigerson H. Psychotherapy of traumatic grief: a review of evidence for psychotherapeutic treatments. Death Studies 2000;24:479–95.
8. Jacobs S, Mazure C, Prigerson H. Diagnostic criteria for traumatic grief. Death Studies 2000;24: 185–99.
9. Parkes C. Bereavement and mental health in the elderly. Review of Clinical Gerontology 1997;7: 47–53.
10. Prigerson H, Maciejewski P, Newsom J. The inventory of complicated grief: a scale to measure maladaptive symptoms of loss. Psychiatry Research 1995;59:65–79.
11. Weller RA, Weller EB, Fristod MA, Bowes, JM. Depression in recently bereaved prepubertal children. American Journal of Psychiatry 1991;148:1536–40.
12. Kubler-Ross E. Living with Death and Dying. New York: Macmillan, 1981.
13. Stroebe MS, Stroebe W, Hansson RO. Handbook of Bereavement, Theory, Research, and Intervention. New York, NY: Cambridge University Press, 1997.

CHAPTER 20

PSYCHOTROPIC MEDICATIONS IN GENERAL PRACTICE

SR Ellen and TR Norman

The desire to take medicine is perhaps the greatest feature which distinguishes man from animals.

SIR WILLIAM OSLER, *1849–1919*

KEY FACTS

■ A correct diagnosis ensures appropriate treatment.

■ Comorbidity of psychiatric conditions is common.

■ Consider a non-pharmacological approach to treatment.

■ Learn to use a few drugs well.

■ In group studies all psychotropic medications are equally effective for their indications, but individual patients may respond selectively.

■ To be effective, psychotropic medications need to be taken continuously.

■ Non-compliance with medications is a major cause of treatment failure.

■ Warn patients of the potential side effects of medications.

■ Be aware of potential drug–drug interactions.

■ Constantly assess the efficacy of treatment as poor response may indicate an incorrect diagnosis.

INTRODUCTION

General practitioners (GPs) provide the majority of professional care for psychological problems in the community, and pharmacological interventions are the most common treatments. Data from the Bettering the Evaluation and Care of Health program (BEACH), which is a continuous national study of general practice activity in Australia, shows that GPs treat psychological problems at a rate of 11.5 per 100 encounters.[1] Of these, depressive disorders are the most common individual disorders managed (3.8 per 100), with other common disorders being anxiety (1.7 per 100) and sleep disturbance (1.6 per 100).[1]

The most common treatments offered are pharmacological interventions. Medications are recommended in 70% of contacts for psychological problems and in 77% of cases of depression, and of these, 80% are antidepressants.[1] In anxiety disorders, medications are recommended in 56% of contacts (56% anxiolytics and 22% antidepressants), and in schizophrenia medications are recommended in 96% of contacts, with 74% being antipsychotics.[1]

GENERAL PRINCIPLES

The last forty years of psychiatric practice has seen an increasing emphasis placed on the role of pharmacotherapy in the treatment of psychiatric disorders. However, far from being a panacea, pharmacotherapy has its associated problems of lack of efficacy, unwanted side effects and problems of dependence and withdrawal. For example, there are some populations who are at high risk for drug–drug interactions: the medically ill who are being treated with several drugs; the elderly and debilitated; those with renal or hepatic disease; and those treated with drugs that are potent iso-enzyme inhibitors. The extent to which some of these problems can be surmounted by careful prescribing practices is addressed in this chapter. Figure 20.1 outlines the key issues to consider when prescribing a psychotropic.

FIGURE 20.1 Factors to consider when prescribing psychotropic drugs

- No objective tests predict an individual's response
- Single drug therapy is preferable
- Safety and tolerability of medication
- Likelihood of drug interactions
- Ease of administration
- Confidence in its use
- Cost effectiveness
- Previous positive response
- Predominant symptom pattern
- Concurrent medical illness

The single most important factor in ensuring a good outcome from medication is making the correct diagnosis (see Chapter 7). This may require more than one interview with the patient; it frequently requires some consultation with family members or significant others. Depression as an illness, for example, needs to be distinguished from the vicissitudes of life, while anxiety is often a symptom of many other disorders (for example, depression or schizophrenia).

Following diagnosis, the next biggest issue is the patient's attitude to medication. Does the patient have insight into their illness? Are they willing (and able) to take the medication as prescribed? One of the major reasons for a poor outcome from psychotropic medications is lack of compliance (either partial compliance or non-compliance). Up to 50% of patients may discontinue medication within three months of starting a drug, while a small number of patients never have the prescription filled. This may be brought about by a failure of communication between the doctor and the patient. Education about the illness, about the medication itself (side effects, necessity for continued medication, the possibility of therapeutic failure) as well as other treatment options (for example, psychological approaches) are all important in establishing a therapeutic alliance between the patient and GP. Even if the patient states that they will not take any medications, this is a useful transaction as further treatment decisions will not be based on the assumption that the patient has adhered to the drug regimen.

Where the decision to use medication is made, it is important to note that, with the possible exception of benzodiazepines, psychotropic drugs may take several weeks to produce significant clinical change. However, some changes should be apparent in the first week—for example, sleep is likely to improve in depressed and anxious patients. If there are no changes or significant worsening occurs after two weeks of treatment and compliance is not an issue, there are a number of factors that may work against achieving a good response. The most obvious is that the diagnosis is incorrect or that significant comorbidity has been overlooked. In particular, substance abuse problems, such as alcohol and illicit drug use, will need to be considered. Comorbidity is the rule rather than the exception. Problems arising in the context of significant psychosocial issues, such as marital breakdown and dysfunctional families, are not helped by medication alone and will require professional counselling. Where these issues have been considered or are not a significant factor in the illness, switching medication to another class of drug or even within members of the same class may be required. If a patient has failed to respond to two adequate courses of medication (that is, adequate with respect to dose and duration), a specialist opinion should be sought.

The emphasis on the use of medication in this review is not to demean the usefulness of non-pharmacological approaches to treatment. Indeed, the evidence suggests that psychological treatments may have better long-term outcomes than medication for some disorders (for example, various anxiety disorders). Furthermore, for the majority of cases, the combination of pharmacological and non-pharmacological approaches to treatment should be the norm rather than the exception.

ANTIDEPRESSANTS
CASE STUDY: DEPRESSION

Jack, a 32-year-old male, has recently been injured at work and he is now about to return part-time to limited duties. He is nervous about returning, and finds his mind preoccupied with how he will cope. He is concerned about the family finances, as he and his wife have a four-month-old baby and his wife is currently only working one day per week. He feels tired all day, cannot concentrate well, and finds he just cannot cheer up or enjoy himself any more. He looks teary as he tells you his problems.

After discussion, Jack acknowledges that he may well be depressed, and agrees to a trial of a medication. He is very concerned about being over-sedated, as he is determined to do his share of getting up to feed the baby. He is also anxious about side effects in general, never having been too keen on taking pills.

You elect a non-sedating selective serotonin reuptake inhibitors (SSRI) antidepressant, and suggest Jack start on half a tablet for the first four days in the morning, and then if he has no problems, he should increase that to a whole tablet, and return for review in about one week.

HISTORICAL DEVELOPMENT

The first antidepressants evolved from antituberculous therapy. Iproniazid, in contrast to isoniazid, was devoid of tuberculostatic effects but improved the mood of patients with tuberculosis. The monoamine oxidase-inhibiting properties were discovered at a later date. Iproniazid was introduced into clinical practice in 1957 as a 'psychic energiser', then later as an antidepressant. This class of drug lost popularity after the discovery of the so-called 'cheese effect'—the potentiation of the effects of tyramine present in some foods, and the emergence of significant hepato-toxicity with some members of the class.

Imipramine was synthesised by Ciba-Geigy in Switzerland as an antihistamine. The compound was introduced as an antidepressant in 1958, following observations by Roland Kuhn, who reported significant improvements in the mood of depressed patients. So began the era of the tricyclic antidepressants (TCAs).

A further development was that of the specific serotonin reuptake inhibitors (SSRIs). The first of these was zimelidine in 1982, followed by fluoxetine in 1987. Zimelidine was removed from the market because of the development of Guillian-Barre syndrome in some patients. Fortunately, this is not a class effect and other SSRIs soon followed; they are now among the most popular of antidepressants prescribed.

The majority of antidepressant prescriptions are written by GPs; a recent analysis of prescribing data showed that 86% of all antidepressant scripts were written by GPs and only 10% were written by psychiatrists.[2]

MECHANISM OF ACTION OF ANTIDEPRESSANTS

'You have a chemical imbalance in your brain!' This rather simplistic statement has become a catch-cry for the medical treatment of depression. While it is true that moods such as depression are associated with chemical changes at a cellular level in the brain and other organs, the causes of depression—and the mechanism of action of antidepressants—are far from understood.

Despite this, the classification of antidepressants is based on neuroreceptor profiles of the drugs. The key neuroreceptor systems implicated in depression are the serotonergic and noradrenergic. Pre-clinical and clinical data suggest that an underactivity of either or both of these systems is associated with depression (although cause and effect, or the direction of this association, has never been clearly established). Antidepressants are believed to act by increasing the activity of these systems by altering receptor numbers or increasing neurotransmitter flow. Despite fifty years of research, the exact mechanism of this action remains unknown. It may yet turn out that the mechanism of action is something entirely different, such as one of the many 'downstream' effects of receptors, including intra-neuronal and molecular actions of the drugs.

INDICATIONS

Antidepressants are clearly indicated as the first line treatment in severe depression, have approximately equal efficacy to the main psychotherapies in moderate depression, and are not indicated in mild depression, where supportive clinical care, psycho-education, problem solving and counselling are the appropriate strategies[3] (see Chapters 8 and 17).

Antidepressants have been studied and recommended for use in disorders other than depression, although this may differ between countries. Anxiety disorders are particularly responsive to antidepressants (panic disorder, obsessive-compulsive disorder, post-traumatic stress disorder, social anxiety disorder and generalised anxiety disorder), adding fuel to the theory that anxiety and depression represent different aspects of the same disorder. Antidepressants have also been shown to be effective in pain disorders (mainly tricyclic antidepressants), premenstrual syndrome (mainly SSRIs), insomnia and bulimia nervosa.

CHOICE OF ANTIDEPRESSANT

All antidepressants were created equal, but some were created more equal than others! They are all equally effective in treating depression, with approximately 65% responding, compared to a placebo response rate of 35%. Given this similar efficacy, choice is based on the preferred adverse effect profile, safety issues, drug interactions, costs and familiarity with the drugs.

In terms of safety, the newer antidepressants are far safer in overdose than the TCAs and MAOI antidepressants. Given the risk of suicide in mood disorders, this relegates the older antidepressants to second line drugs (unless the patient has had a good past response). Of the newer antidepressants, the costs are similar, and hence it comes down to preferred adverse effect profile, drug interactions and familiarity with the drug.

In the primary care setting, a clinician should be familiar with two or three drugs from different classes. This allows them to build enough expertise with each drug, while also giving a representative choice of the compounds available, and giving one or two options for change should the first choice prove ineffective. Two failed trials of an antidepressant should trigger reconsidering the diagnosis or referring for a specialist opinion.

When comparing adverse effect profiles, the tolerability of virtually all the antidepressants is similar. In clinical trials, patients drop out at similar rates, regardless of the antidepressant. Hence the choice of medication relates to which adverse events the patient would prefer, which is often related to the issue of sedating versus non-sedating drugs.

It is also worth remembering that the best predictor of future response is past response. Hence, always check for past use of antidepressants: if it has worked before, it will probably work again. Furthermore, there is some evidence to suggest that if it has worked in a family member, it is more likely to work for the patient.

SPECIAL ISSUES

STARTING AN ANTIDEPRESSANT As a general rule, many clinicians choose to start at half the recommended dose, at least for 4–7 days. This tends to minimise the adverse effects that are most prominent in the first two weeks. A benzodiazepine is often useful in the first two weeks to help with the initial agitation, especially if it is being used for an anxiety disorder.

THINGS TO TELL THE PATIENT Treating depression, especially when it is moderate or severe, may require a degree of salesmanship. By the very nature of the disorder, the patient is likely to believe there is nothing wrong with them (they are just 'weak' in some way), that they do not deserve help and that nothing will help anyway (so-called hopelessness and helplessness). Furthermore, many see medications for mood as a sign of weakness or 'surrendering' to one of life's challenges. Consequently, it is easy to fall into the trap of failing to adequately inform the patient regarding the medication issues simply to prevent scaring them away from treatment. The key issues to mention are these:

- The onset of action is at least two weeks, probably more like four weeks (otherwise patients may discontinue after a week, thinking the medication is not working);
- For the benefits to occur, the medications must be taken every day.
- The clinical course of improvement fluctuates ('three steps forward, one step backwards'). The patient should expect this, and not get disheartened and discontinue when these inevitable setbacks occur.
- The side effects profile: while not all patients want to know about side effects, it is important to tell them that they are common, mostly self-limiting, and that they should let you know about them. It is often helpful to point out that side effects are a good sign, as they are an indication that the drugs are having an effect, and with antidepressants the beneficial effects come after the side effects. Therefore you should reframe side effects as a path to improvement rather than a set back.
- The medications must be continued once the symptoms have resolved.

HOW AND WHEN TO INCREASE THE DOSE For most antidepressants there is a lack of evidence to guide dosing. As a general rule, the starting dose should be maintained for 2–4 weeks. If the patient is failing to respond, or the response is equivocal, try increasing by half to a whole tablet, and wait two weeks. Keep increasing the dose until a response is reported or the maximum dose is reached (or limited by adverse effects). If the maximum dose (or maximum dose tolerated) fails after two weeks, then the trial is considered to have failed, and switching to another class is the next step (after an appropriate withdrawal regimen and drug-free interval).

It should be noted that in anxiety disorders a higher dose is usually required, hence you should tend to increase the dose earlier.

The usual dose ranges and the common side effects for the newer agents are provided in Table 20.1. The quoted dose ranges represent usual practice, and for most of the drugs the manufacturer's recommended maximum dose is somewhat higher. Use of higher doses will depend on response, tolerability and the clinician's confidence and familiarity with the drug.

TABLE 20.1 Newer antidepressants, their dose ranges, and key adverse events*

DRUG	USUAL DAILY ORAL DOSE RANGE (MG) [NB1]	ELIMINATION HALF-LIVES OF DRUG AND ACTIVE METABOLITES (HOURS) [NB2]	INSOMNIA	SEDATION	SEXUAL DYS-FUNCTION [NB3]	AGITATION	GASTRO-INTESTINAL [NB4]	WEIGHT GAIN
SSRIs								
Citalopram	20–40	23–45	++	+	+++	+	++	+
Fluoxetine	20–40	24–144 (parent) 200–330 (metabolite)	++	++	+++	+	++	+
Fluvoxamine	100–200	9–28	++	+	+++	++	+++	+
Paroxetine	20–40	3–65	++	+–	+++	+	++	++
Sertraline	50–100	22–36 (parent) 62–104 (metabolite)	++	+–	+++	++	+++	+
OTHERS								
Mianserin	60–90	21–61	+	+++	++	+	+	0
Mirtazapine	30–45	20–40	+	+++	++	+	+	+++
Moclobemide	300–600	1–3	++	+	+	+–	++	0
Nefazodone	300–600	2–5 (parent) [NB5] 3–18 (metabolites)	+	+++	+	+	++	+
Reboxetine	8–10	12–13	+++	0	+	+	+	0
Venlafaxine	75–150	3–7 (parent) 9–13 (metabolite)	++	++	+++	++	+++	0

Approximate frequencies of adverse effects: 0 (< 2%) = negligible or absent; + (> 2%) = infrequent; ++ (> 10%) = moderately frequent; +++ (> 30%) = frequent.
NB1: Lower doses are usually sufficient to treat depression in most patients.
NB2: Where clinically significant.
NB3: May include decreased libido, anorgasmia and ejaculatory disturbance.

NB4: May include nausea, anorexia, diarrhoea and abdominal discomfort; taking the antidepressant after food may reduce nausea.
NB5: Dose dependent.
* *Note:* This is the frequency of occurrence of adverse effects, not the intensity with which they occur.

Source: Psychotropic Expert Group, 2003.[4]

WHEN TO CEASE There is a lack of evidence for guiding duration of treatment. Short-term studies suggest twelve months' treatment after the first episode of depression, and expert consensus supports treatment for three years for recurrent depression.[3] Most antidepressants are associated with withdrawal reactions and so gradual withdrawal is usually the safest option—for example, halving the dose each week. See Table 20.2.

TABLE 20.2 Withdrawal symptoms with antidepressant drugs	
SYMPTOM GROUP	**CHARACTERISTIC SIGNS**
General somatic symptoms	Fatigue, headache, sweating, myalgia, flu-like syndrome; anxiety, agitation, muscle tension, nervousness
Sleep	Insomnia, vivid dreams
Movement	Unsteady gait, abnormal involuntary movements, akathisia
Affect	Lowered mood, crying, irritability, lability
Miscellaneous	Dizziness, paraesthesias, electric shocks in arms and legs (most characteristic of SSRI withdrawal)

COMBINATION ANTIDEPRESSANTS Combinations of antidepressants are sometimes used in treatment resistant depression. While the evidence for the effectiveness of this strategy is hotly debated, it is agreed that the risks are increased for the patient, in particular the risks of adverse affects, and the lethality in overdose. As a consequence, this option should only be considered after all other strategies have been exhausted, and only in the specialist setting, if at all.

USE IN PREGNANCY AND BREASTFEEDING Antidepressants are generally reported to have low teratogenic potential, but studies do not tend to follow child development, and hence psychological treatments should be favoured in pregnant women.[3]

Most antidepressants are classed as either category B or C in Australia, indicating that caution should be taken when prescribing them in pregnancy. Paroxetine (an SSRI) has recently been upgraded to Category D, indicating it should not be used in pregnancy: studies suggest an increased risk of heart malformations if it is used in the first trimester. Further, as significant amounts of venlafaxine and SSRIs cross the placental barrier, late pregnancy exposure to antidepressants can be associated with neonatal withdrawl and/or toxicity syndromes.[5]

Antidepressants pass into breast milk in small amounts, and so care should be taken when treating breast-feeding women. As usual, the risks of treatment should be balanced against the risks of not treating and also the available alternative treatments. In the case of pregnancy and breastfeeding, consultation with an expert is advisable.

SEROTONIN SYNDROME The serotonin syndrome consists of abdominal cramps, diarrhoea and agitation, going on to myoclonus, hyponatraemia or hypernatraemia, confusion, fever and coma. It usually occurs secondary to a drug overdose, but can occur as a result of drug interactions and even as an idiosyncratic response to a single serotonin-increasing drug. It is often difficult to distinguish the serotonin syndrome from self-limiting adverse effects, discontinuation syndromes and drug interactions (in the context of ceasing one antidepressant and starting another) and even depression itself. If symptoms suggest a serotonin syndrome, urgent assessment in an emergency department is advisable.

TABLE 20.3 Some rarer adverse reactions with antidepressants	
ADVERSE EVENT	**DRUGS IMPLICATED**
Galactorrhea, amenorrhea	TCAs
Extrapyramidal syndrome (akathisia, acute dystonia, Parkinsonism)	SSRIs
Delirium (an anticholinergic effect)	TCAs
Cholestatic jaundice	TCAs, MAOIs
Switch to hypomania	All antidepressants
Teratogenicity	All antidepressants; check prescribing information for specifics
Seizures	TCAs

COMPLEMENTARY MEDICATIONS

A range of alternative or complementary medications for depression, none of which has been proven in well designed and replicated trials, are available as 'over the counter' preparations. St John's wort was initially supported in trials of mild to moderate depression, but more recent trials have found that it is not superior to placebo. It should be noted that St John's wort can be the source of drug–drug interactions due to its inhibition of liver enzymes. Omega-3 fatty acid levels are low in depression, but supplements have not been proven efficacious. Tryptophan and 5-hydroxytryptophan have been studied in many trials, but the evidence remains inconclusive, and given the adverse effect of the rare, but potentially fatal eosinophilia-myalgia syndrome, their use does not seem justified.[3]

ANTIPSYCHOTICS
CASE STUDY: ANTIPSYCHOTICS

Simon's parents report that over the last year he has been failing university subjects for the first time ever, and that he seems convinced his ex-girlfriend is telling others that he raped her. He has even gone to the police to tell them his side of the story, but the police told him they had no such complaint and he was imagining it. The parents have rung the ex-girlfriend, who also says Simon is imagining it, and says she stopped seeing him because he kept saying weird things and smoked too much marijuana.

Simon reluctantly agrees to see you, and during the consultation acknowledges that he may be overreacting about the rape, but is not sure whether the police are lying to him in order to keep their surveillance secret. He also has trouble sleeping, and does admit to daily marijuana use.

You prescribe olanzapine to be taken at night, which Simon agrees to take, as he is keen to get his sleeping pattern back. Simon also agrees to try and stop using marijuana.

For the first month the situation improves. Simon stops mentioning the rape, and seems to be attending university, only smoking marijuana occasionally. Two months later his parents attend and report his ex-girlfriend has rung to say he has been following her and asking her to stop telling people he raped her. When Simon attends for review, he reports he ceased the olanzapine as his weight had increased by 5 kg. He again seems preoccupied with the imagined rape and believes the police are taping his phone calls. His sleep has again deteriorated. This has occurred despite Simon's reduction in marijuana being maintained.

Simon agrees to go back on a medication, as long as it continues to help his sleep but causes less weight gain. The choices include aripiprazole, risperidone and quetiapine. Given the relapse, non-compliance and the likely diagnosis of schizophrenia, you also organise assessment at the local community mental health centre to consider engaging their early psychosis program to aid in the education and support of both Simon and his parents.

HISTORICAL DEVELOPMENT

Labroit first used chlorpromazine in 1951 as part of an anaesthetic cocktail for the prevention of shock following surgery. He noted the tendency of the drug to promote 'disinterest' without inducing sleep. He persuaded psychiatrists at the famed military hospital Val-de-Grâce in Paris to use the compound in psychiatric patients. Shortly afterwards, Delay and Deniker began to use the drug in psychotic patients and reported their results at a conference in 1952. Thus the credit for the discovery of the clinical use of chlorpromazine is generally attributed to Delay and Deniker. Within a few years, the use of chlorpromazine had spread to most countries of the developed world.

Chlorpromazine reached Australian hospitals in about 1954.[6] The beneficial effects were as dramatic as they were impressive. For the first time, patients with psychotic conditions in long-term hospital wards had a treatment option. Deaths from psychotic agitation rapidly fell, such that they are now largely forgotten. As more and more pharmacological options became available, psychosocial treatments improved and social movements emphasising patient rights gave patients and carers a voice. Schizophrenia became treatable in the community, and asylums began to close as psychosocial treatments improved.

Despite these improvements, the first wave of antipsychotics (now called typical antipsychotics) led to great dissatisfaction among patients, carers and clinicians due to the side effect burden, in particular the movement disorders that came with long-term use.

In the 1990s the next wave of antipsychotics became available. These were more tolerable and better for certain symptom clusters. Known as the atypical antipsychotics (atypical in that they had far fewer movement related side effects), they have now become the mainstay of the treatment of schizophrenia.

INDICATIONS

The primary indication for antipsychotic drugs is for the treatment of psychotic states arising from such disparate conditions as schizophrenia, schizophreniform disorder, schizoaffective disorder, affective disorder with psychotic symptoms and organic psychoses such as delirium (see Chapter 12). The drugs may also be used for the treatment of behavioural disturbance in the elderly (see Chapter 16). Schizophrenia, despite a prevalence of only 1%, is the more common of these conditions so the use of drugs in this condition is the focus of this section.

The main therapeutic effects of antipsychotic drugs are to ameliorate the core symptoms of the disorder, often referred to as the positive symptoms: thought disorder, hallucinations and delusions. The negative symptoms—flat affect, poverty of thought, emotional and social withdrawal—are also helped to varying degrees by the different classes of antipsychotic drugs.

EFFICACY OF ANTIPSYCHOTICS

There is clear evidence that antipsychotic drugs are superior to placebo in the treatment of acute and chronic schizophrenia. In terms of relative efficacy, there does not appear to be any difference between antipsychotic drugs, with the possible exception of clozapine being superior in the treatment of refractory cases. Nevertheless, clinicians consistently report that patients show much better responses to some agents than to others. The reason for this is not clear but may be related to genetic differences that determine response or perhaps to pharmacokinetic differences. Unfortunately, there are no a priori methods for determining who will, and who will not, respond to a particular medication.

PRESCRIBING ANTIPSYCHOTICS IN GENERAL PRACTICE

Schizophrenia is usually managed in conjunction with specialist services. Data from the BEACH program shows only 45 out of every 10 000 consultations in general practice are primarily related to the treatment of schizophrenia.[7] Medication prescription occurs in the vast majority of these consultations. The key issues are outlined below.

CHOICE OF DRUG The critical issue is the difference in adverse event profiles between drugs. The atypical agents have advantages over the older agents in this area, and have become the clear first line treatments for first episode psychosis.[8] In particular, newer agents are less likely to cause extrapyramidal side effects than the older agents and are not as likely to elevate plasma prolactin concentrations. The incidence of tardive dyskinesia may also be less, but the evidence awaits longer term use with these agents.

MONITORING SIDE EFFECTS The side effects of antipsychotics are prominent, causing significant morbidity and often limiting treatment. Common side effects include sedation, anticholinergic effects (blurred vision, dry mouth, constipation, urinary hesitancy), weight gain (often to obesity) and sexual dysfunction.

The following side effects are common factors influencing choice of medication or guiding a change of medication:

- obesity, diabetes (type 2), hypertension and dyslipidaemia (all of which increase heart disease) are associated with all antipsychotics. On current evidence, the high risk drugs are olanzapine and clozapine; the moderate risk drugs are risperidone and quetiapine; and the low risk drugs are aripiprazole and ziprasidone. Recent guidelines from both Australia[9] and the US[10] have highlighted the risks and suggested patients with pre-existing risk factors for these conditions avoid the higher risk drugs. Furthermore, monitoring for emergence of these conditions is now recommended— in particular, weight and height (for Body Mass Index), waist circumference, blood pressure, serum glucose and lipid levels;

- hyperprolactinaemia, which can become symptomatic (especially risperidone);
- Electrocardiogram (ECG) QTc interval prolongation, which is associated with life-threatening cardiac events (especially thioridazine, pimozide, ziprasidone and droperidol);
- extrapyramidal side effects, including acute dystonias, Parkinsonism, akathisia and tardive dyskinesia. Anti-Parkinsonian drugs are often required, even prophylactically in high-risk groups with high extrapyramidal side effects medications (see Table 20.4); and
- neuroleptic malignant syndrome (NMS). NMS is a rare but potentially fatal syndrome, consisting of fever, muscle rigidity, autonomic instability and confusion. NMS is a psychiatric emergency, and if suspected, the patient should be referred for urgent review. Rechallenge with any antipsychotic should only be done in a specialist setting, as 30% will redevelop NMS.

MONITORING RELATED HEALTH ISSUES The general health implications of the side effects listed above, in conjunction with the 'lifestyle' illnesses associated with schizophrenia in general (cigarette and marijuana use, poor diet, limited exercise) mean patients with schizophrenia are at risk of many medical problems. GPs are ideally placed to address these problems, especially given that specialist mental health services are more likely to focus on the mental illness rather than the overall health of the patient. Hence the GP should ensure the patient has a thorough assessment prior to beginning medications, and at regular intervals thereafter.

Figure 20.2 highlights some of the key investigations associated with the use of antipsychotic medications.

CEASING ANTIPSYCHOTICS AND CHANGING FROM ONE TO ANOTHER With regard to an acute episode of psychosis, if medications are failing to have any effect on positive symptoms after two weeks of treatment with adequate dose increases, serious consideration should be given to a trial of a different antipsychotic. The rate of improvement varies between patients, with some improving within several hours or days of treatment being initiated. Most of the therapeutic gains are observed within about four weeks, but some gains may continue for up to six months.

Maintenance therapy is necessary in most patients with schizophrenia. Once antipsychotic drugs are withdrawn, relapse is the rule rather than the exception. Within six months of placebo being substituted, about 60% of patients previously responsive to acute treatment with antipsychotic drugs have relapsed. Similarly, when drugs are withdrawn after 2–3 years on medication, relapse rates are the same.

Even with good adherence to medications, many patients experience a relapse. This makes choices about medications very difficult. The clinician never fully knows whether the relapse is related to medication failure or other factors, such as non-compliance, stressors or illicit drug use (especially marijuana). It is easy to fall into the trap of blaming medication failure, and precipitously changing the medication or adding

---

FIGURE 20.2 Antipsychotics and investigations

DIAGNOSTIC INVESTIGATIONS FOR ANY ANTIPSYCHOTIC

- Full blood examination (initiation and 6 monthly)
- Electolytes and urea (initiation and 6 monthly)
- Liver function tests (initiation and 6 monthly)
- Weight and height for Body Mass Index (initiation, monthly for 3 months, then 3 monthly thereafter)
- Waist circumference (initiation and 3 monthly)
- Blood pressure (initiation and 6 monthly)
- Blood glucose (initiation and 3–6 monthly, depending on drug and other risk factors)
- Lipid profile (initiation, 6 months and then annually)

DIAGNOSTIC INVESTIGATIONS FOR SPECIFIC ANTIPSYCHOTICS OR SIDE EFFECTS

- Electrocardiogram for QTc interval if thioridazine, pimozide, ziprasidone or droperidol (initiation and once maintenance dose is reached)
- Prolactin level if symptoms of gynaecomastia, galactorrhoea, amenorrhoea, or sexual dysfunction (dose dependent, mainly risperidone, amisulpiride and olanzapine)
- Clozapine has a mandated range of tests, and the prescriber must be registered as a clozapine prescriber

---

other augmenting medication. This should only be done after careful consideration of the above issues, with a clear long-term pharmacological plan (most patients with chronic schizophrenia try many medications over the years) and in conjunction with specialist services.

CHANGING THE ROUTE OF ADMINISTRATION Non-compliance is common with antipsychotics. It may relate to the disorganisation associated with schizophrenia or to an active decision on the part of the patient to avoid medication (related to a lack of insight regarding their condition). If strategies to improve compliance, such as education and support, fail to improve the situation, depot antipsychotics are often considered. There are depot formulations of both typical and atypical antipsychotics; most require injection on a fortnightly or monthly basis.

ANTI-ANXIETY AND HYPNOTIC AGENTS
HISTORICAL DEVELOPMENT

In the mid-1950s, the Hoffman-LaRoche company, with Leo Sternbach and Lowell Randall heading the effort, began a systematic search for compounds with tranquilising effects. RO 5-0690 was the result of a mistaken synthesis on the part of one of Sternbach's bench chemists. This was the first benzodiazepine, which was initially called methaminodiazepoxide and then chlordiazepoxide (Librium). Subsequently, Hoffman-LaRoche showed that the epoxide moiety on chlordiazepoxide reduced activity. Analysis of the activity of chlordiazepoxide's primary metabolite, demoxepam, led to the introduction of diazepam about four years later. In the 1960s, through to the 1980s, benzodiazepines replaced previously used anxiolytics such as barbiturates and eventually became the largest selling anxiolytics worldwide.

TABLE 20.4 Antipsychotic drugs and usual dose ranges*

DRUG	USUAL DAILY ORAL DOSE RANGE (MG)	SEDATION	POSTURAL HYPOTENSION	ANTI-CHOLINERGIC	EXTRA-PYRAMIDAL	WEIGHT GAIN
ATYPICAL DRUGS						
Amisulpride	400–1000 (acute psychosis) 100–300 (negative symptoms)	+	+	0	++ [NB1]	+
Aripiprazole	10–30	++	+	0	+	+
Clozapine	200–600	+++	+++	+++	+	+++
Olanzapine	5–20	+++	+	++	+	+++
Quetiapine	300–750	+++	++	+	+ [NB1]	++
Risperidone	2–6	++ (initially)	+++(initially)	0	++	++
Ziprasidone	80–160	++	+	+	+	+
TYPICAL DRUGS						
Chlorpromazine	75–500	+++	+++	+++	++	+++
Droperidol	5–10 (IM) [NB2]	++	+	+	+++	+
Fluphenazine	5–20	+	+	+	+++	+++
Haloperidol	1–7.5	+	+	+	+++	++
Pericyazine	15–75	+++	++	+++	+	++
Pimozide	2–12 [NB3]	++	+	+	+++	+
Thioridazine	300–600	+++	+++	+++	+	+++

TABLE 20.4 *continued*

TYPICAL DRUGS *continued*

DRUG	USUAL DAILY ORAL DOSE RANGE (MG)	SEDATION	POSTURAL HYPOTENS ON	ANTI-CHOLINERGIC	EXTRA-PYRAMIDAL	WEIGHT GAIN
Trifluoperazine	5–20	+	++	+	+++	++
Zuclopenthixol acetate	50–150 (IM) [NB4]	+++	+	++	+++	++
Zuclopenthixol dihydrochloride	10–75	+++	+	++	+++	++

Approximate frequencies of adverse effects: 0 (< 2%) = negligible or absent; + (> 2%) infrequent; ++ (> 10%) = moderately frequent; +++ (> 30%) = frequent

NB1: Rarely a problem at usual therapeutic doses.

NB2: Doses > 5 mg should not be given without immediate access to ECG monitoring and resuscitation facilities.

NB3: Use doses > 12 mg only under specialist supervision.

NB4: Single dose, not to be repeated for 2–3 days.

* *Note:* This is the frequency of occurrence of adverse effects, not the intensity with which they occur.

Source: Psychotropic Expert Group; 2003.[4]

EFFICACY OF BENZODIAZEPINES

There is no clinical evidence that one benzodiazepine is superior to another, but some drugs are more likely to be used as anxiolytics and others as hypnotics (sleep inducing). Drugs with longer half-lives—for example, diazepam—are usually chosen for anxiety disorders, while drugs with shorter half-lives are used as hypnotics—for example, temazepam or triazolam. Benzodiazepines usually provide rapid relief of the symptoms of anxiety, but the decision to use medication must be carefully assessed; in particular, organic causes of anxiety must be ruled out.

The efficacy of benzodiazepines in the long-term treatment of anxiety or insomnia is controversial. Evidence for efficacy beyond four months is lacking. Brief interrupted courses of treatment should be proposed from the outset. The drugs should be tapered on withdrawal to avoid a withdrawal syndrome. Medication alone is rarely sufficient to provide complete relief from anxiety, and psychosocial interventions should always be included in the treatment plan.

INDICATIONS

Benzodiazepines have multiple pharmacological actions, with different members of the class showing varying degrees of muscle relaxant, sedative, anxiolytic, anticonvulsant and hypnotic properties.

The primary therapeutic role for benzodiazepines is in the management of generalised anxiety disorder (GAD), panic disorder and insomnia (see Chapter 9). While they are commonly used in other anxiety related disorders, this is more often due to clinical desperation than proven efficacy. Even in GAD and panic disorder, benzodiazepines have fallen from favour in recent years due to problems of dependence and withdrawal syndromes. They have been replaced by antidepressants, usually the SSRIs. Nevertheless, benzodiazepines have a role for the short-term management of anxiety and sleep disorders.

Different agents are recommended for anxiolytic and hypnotic activity (see Table 20.5). While there is some relationship between the elimination half-life of the different members of the class and their use as anxiolytics or hypnotics, elimination half-life is not a good guide to duration of action. Thus flunitrazepam has a half-life of more than 24 hours yet is used as a hypnotic, since plasma levels of the drug are not sustained above the minimum effective dose for more than a few hours.

In recent years, both zopiclone and zolpidem have been introduced for the management of sleep disturbance. Neither drug is a benzodiazepine; however, they do appear to act through similar receptor mechanisms in the brain—that is, the GABA chloride ion channel.

CHOICE OF BENZODIAZEPINE

Many anxiety disorders can be managed by psychotherapeutic means alone or by other psychotropics (such as SSRIs). If a decision is made to use a benzodiazepine, consideration should be given to the proneness of the patient to addiction or abuse of the agents. There is little doubt that these were once prescribed too freely, but if the patient's anxiety is of sufficient severity, short-term access to these drugs should not be denied. The initial choice

TABLE 20.5 Anxiolytic and hypnotic agents

DRUG	USUAL DOSE RANGE	DRUG TRADE NAMES	ELIMINATION HALF LIFE (HOURS)
BENZODIAZEPINES			
Predominantly anxiolytic			
Alprazolam	0.5–4.5 mg/day	Alprax, Kalma, Xanax	9–20
Bromazepam	6–9 mg/day	Lexotan	8–30
Clobazam	10–30 mg/day	Frisium	20–40
Clonazepam	2–6 mg/day	Rivotril, Paxam	19–60
Diazepam	5–40 mg/day	Antenex, Ducene, Valium, Valpam	14–70
Lorazepam	1–10 mg/day	Ativan	8–24
Oxazepam	45–90 mg/day	Alepam, Muelax, Serepax	3–25
Predominantly hypnotic			
Flunitrazepam	1–2 mg/day	Hypnodorm	24 (see page 348)
Nitrazepam	5–10 mg/day	Alodorm, Mogadon	15–48
Temazepam	10–30 mg/day	Euhypnos, Normison, Temaze, Temtabs	3–25
Triazolam	0.125–0.5 mg/day	Halcion	1.5–5
Non-benzodiazepines			
Buspirone	20–30 mg/day	Buspar	1–11
Zopiclone	Up to 7.5 mg/day	Imovane	3–6.5
Zolpidem	5–10 mg/day	Stilnox	1.5–4.5

of drug may be based on previous response or on the convenience of use for the patient (for example, long half-life drugs require once daily dosing). Initially, dose titration may be required, with the bulk of the dose given at night to aid with sleep disturbance.

SPECIAL ISSUES

There are few absolute contraindications for benzodiazepine use, but because of their muscle relaxant properties, the drugs should not be used in patients with myasthenia gravis. In patients with compromised respiratory function, benzodiazepines may aggravate the problems. Benzodiazepine use should be carefully considered in patients who are pregnant or breast-feeding. There are reports of teratogenicity with benzodiazepines, and the drugs pass into breast milk and could affect an infant being breast-fed.

BENZODIAZEPINE DEPENDENCE In the past twenty or so years, doctors have become more aware of tolerance and dependence on benzodiazepines. Tolerance to the sedative effects of the drugs develops rapidly but whether there is tolerance to the anxiolytic effects is more controversial. Some clinical studies have suggested no anxiolytic tolerance even after a year of continuous use.

It is not clear what factors influence the development of withdrawal phenomena in individual patients. Both high and normal dose use has been implicated in the withdrawal syndrome, as has short or long duration of use. In general, higher doses of short-acting drugs are more likely to cause problems than are longer half-life agents. Symptoms of the syndrome (see Figure 20.3) are often pronounced 3–7 days after cessation of medication, with up to four weeks or longer required for the patient to return to normal.

Clinical difficulty can arise in distinguishing between the withdrawal syndrome and the return of the original anxiety symptoms. Often withdrawal is a pattern of symptoms distinct from the original presenting complaints. Clearly it is useful for the doctor to have a list of the original symptoms for comparative purposes.

Withdrawal can usually be managed as an out-patient by using a tapered withdrawal schedule for the drug. Changing to an equivalent dose of diazepam before withdrawal may be useful, as the plasma concentrations of the drug decline more slowly. When psychotic reactions and seizures are present, inpatient care may be necessary for some cases. The tapering schedule should be individualised to the patient's need. It is important to implement some psychological aids—for example, relaxation therapy — with the withdrawal process. There should be close contact with the patient throughout the withdrawal period, and follow-up is mandatory. It is useful to remember that benzodiazepines are cross-tolerant with alcohol, which may be used by patients as a substitute for relief of anxiety.

FIGURE 20.3 Benzodiazepine withdrawal symptoms

- Somatic symptoms of anxiety
- Depressed mood
- Depersonalisation, derealisation
- Tremor, shakiness
- Headache
- Hypersensitivity to touch, pain
- Paranoid reactions
- Muscle aches, twitching
- Sleep disturbance
- Convulsions (rare cases)

ADVERSE EVENTS AND DRUG INTERACTIONS Like all medications, benzodiazepines are associated with a number of unwanted side effects. The most important side effect is excessive sedation. In the elderly, this is frequently associated with falls and hip fractures. Oversedation results in psychomotor impairment, with an increase in the likelihood of accidents (for example, from driving or operating heavy machinery). Fatigue, concentration difficulties, ataxia, dysarthria, confusion and impaired memory may all occur during benzodiazepine use. Disinhibition reactions occur infrequently.

There are few clinically important drug–drug interactions with benzodiazepines. The most important is the potentiation of the sedative effects of other CNS depressants, most notably alcohol. Digoxin plasma levels may be increased by co-prescription with some benzodiazepines. Co-administration with L-DOPA may worsen the symptoms of Parkinson's disease.

BUSPIRONE

Buspirone sits alone as an anxiolytic drug, since it is a member of the azapirone class of drugs, which act as partial agonists of the 5HT1A receptor system. This action is thought to account for its anxiolytic activity. Unlike benzodiazepines, the drug takes longer for a therapeutic effect to become apparent and in this respect is more like an antidepressant. Buspirone is not as sedative as benzodiazepines nor does it have the same potential for psychomotor disturbance, abuse and dependence. In clinical trials buspirone has been shown to be as effective as the benzodiazepines in treating GAD. It does not appear to be effective in panic disorder. The main side effects of treatment are dizziness, drowsiness, nausea, headache, fatigue, nervousness and insomnia. The drug apparently has a benign drug–drug interaction profile, but serotonin syndrome is a possibility when it is co-administered with SSRIs or MAOIs.

MOOD STABILISERS
CASE STUDY: BIPOLAR DISORDER

Louise is 36 years old and has had bipolar disorder for over ten years. During that time she has been depressed on five occasions, each time responding well to tricyclic antidepressants. Louise has also been manic on three occasions, the first two times requiring a brief psychiatric admission due to over-activity, lack of sleep and some high-risk behaviours, such as unprotected casual sex and excessive spending. After the second admission, Louise finally accepted she had bipolar disorder, and elected to go on mood-stabilising medications. She went on lithium after an appropriate work-up four years ago. She ceased after one year, largely because she hated taking daily tablets, but after a minor relapse of mania, went straight back on lithium and has been on it since. There have been no subsequent episodes of mania, and only one period where she was depressed, but this coincided with a significant relationship break-up and only lasted two months.

Louise now presents with tiredness and poor concentration, and looks run down and overweight. She has lost her sex drive and is not socialising much. Her weight seems odd as she denies over-eating, and she has never gained weight on lithium before. She has not been on antidepressants since her last episode of depression.

When questioned about depression, Louise says she feels a little down, but it feels different to the other times she has been depressed.

Physical examination is normal, and so you run basic investigations appropriate to depression and lithium monitoring, including her lithium level, full blood examination, renal function and thyroid tests. All tests are normal except her thyroid, which reveals high TSH and low T4. Given the lithium is working so well, you discuss the option of thyroxine replacement, but Louise would prefer to keep her medications to a minimum, and so you cease lithium in favour of sodium valproate.

You discuss interim thyroxine replacement while waiting the month or two that it usually takes for a return of thyroid function after lithium cessation. Louise feels her symptoms are mild and tolerable, and is reluctant to take extra medications, and so you elect to wait and review the situation fortnightly to ensure her mood, fatigue and concentration return to normal as her thyroid function returns.

HISTORICAL DEVELOPMENT

The mood-stabilising agent with the longest history of use is simple salts of lithium, with lithium carbonate being most widely used. The use of lithium salts in medicine dates back to about 150 years ago, when the salts were used in the treatment of gout. The rationale was that the lithium salt of uric acid is soluble in water, and formation of the salt would remove uric acid from the joints. In the 1950s, lithium salts were widely used as a sodium chloride (table salt) substitute for cardiac patients in the United States. This often led to unintended cases of toxicity and, as a result, the reputation of lithium as a therapeutic agent was tarnished when it was mooted for use in bipolar disorder. An Australian psychiatrist, Dr John Cade, first described the use of lithium for 'states of manic excitement' in 1949.[11] The original publication in the *Medical Journal of Australia* was much ignored, and the cause of lithium as a therapy for bipolar disorder was championed by Danish psychiatrist Dr Mogens Schou. Lithium still remains an important therapeutic agent but alternatives, such as anti-epileptic agents, are now also widely used as mood-stabilising agents.

EFFICACY OF MOOD STABILISERS

Lithium, sodium valproate and carbamazepine are the three main mood stabilisers. They are primarily used in bipolar disorder for prophylaxis against relapse, and acute treatment of mania and depression. Their use has also extended in recent years to other indications, such as augmentation of antidepressants in unipolar depression and augmentation of antipsychotics in schizophrenia (neither of which are well supported by research). There do not appear to be significant clinical differences in efficacy between the three drugs.

In acute mania, the mood stabilisers compete with the antipsychotics for clinical dominance. The antipsychotics have the advantage of being slightly faster in onset, and better for controlling agitation, but the mood stabilisers have the advantage of helping to prevent a swing to depression.

Similarly, in acute bipolar depression, they compete with antidepressants and electroconvulsive therapy (ECT). Antidepressants are probably more effective, but they can precipitate mania, and so mood stabilisers are a safer choice. This risk must be balanced against other risks, such as suicidality, which may make antidepressants or ECT more favourable.

When used for prophylaxis against mania or depression, the mood stabilisers are the clear first choice. Whether to begin mood stabilisers after a single manic episode or after two significant episodes (depression or mania) in a two-year period continues to be a contentious issue. Mood stabilisers reduce the number and severity of relapses in bipolar disorder. It is a moot point whether there are differences in efficacy between the drugs for this indication. Lithium is less likely to be used as a first choice agent, mainly because of the side effects associated with its use (see below), although neither of the two anticonvulsants is without serious adverse events.

PLASMA CONCENTRATION MONITORING

Lithium is one of the few drugs in psychiatric practice that requires careful monitoring of plasma concentrations on a regular basis. There are two reasons for this: lithium has a narrow therapeutic index (the difference between toxic and therapeutic plasma levels) and a therapeutic plasma range has been established empirically over many years of clinical experience. A plasma concentration range of 0.6–1.0 mmol/L is usually accepted as being therapeutic, provided the plasma is sampled 12 hours after the last dose at steady state (the so-called 12-hour steady state level). Above plasma concentrations of 1.5 mmol/L, clinical signs of lithium toxicity may be manifest. Plasma level monitoring is necessary every 5–7 days at the initiation of therapy, and once steady state is established, then monitoring can be less frequent (perhaps every three months or longer if the patient is stable).

Plasma level monitoring has also been advocated for anticonvulsant drugs when used as mood stabilisers. The anti-epileptic plasma concentration range is usually quoted as therapeutic in bipolar disorder. There does not appear to be robust empirical evidence for this contention; nevertheless a therapeutic plasma concentration of 50 mg/l or more may be associated with clinical response for valproate and 4–12 mg/L for carbamazepine. In both cases the trough concentration (that is, 10–15 hours after the last dose) is related to clinical response.

SPECIAL ISSUES

LITHIUM Before prescribing lithium, cardiac, renal and thyroid function should be evaluated. Thereafter these indices should be monitored on a regular basis as lithium not only affects the renal tubules but is also anti-thyroid. If necessary, thyroxine can be used to compensate for decreased thyroid function. Since lithium is only renally cleared, alterations in glomerular filtration rate (GFR) have the potential to alter plasma lithium levels accordingly. Toxic plasma concentrations can occur through interactions with other medications (for example, non-steroidal anti-inflammatory drugs or NSAIDs, diuretics, angiotensin-converting enzyme inhibitors), which may affect renal function.

Lithium toxicity can occur with plasma concentrations >1.5 mmol/L and is characterised by gastrointestinal effects (nausea, vomiting) and effects on the central nervous system (muscle twitching, drowsiness, ataxia, tremor, dysarthria). At higher concentrations, disorientation, seizures and coma may ensue. Haemodialysis may be required in cases of severe toxicity.

VALPROATE Valproate is associated with a number of side effects, including lethargy, confusion, weight gain, hair loss and peripheral oedema. Fulminant liver failure is a rare side effect, as are thrombocytopenia and leucopenia. Polycystic ovary disease in women may also occur. Side effects are dose related and are more likely to occur when plasma levels are > 100 mg/L.

CARBAMAZEPINE Common side effects of carbamazepine include dizziness, drowsiness, ataxia and nausea. Around 3% of patients develop an erythematous rash.

Hyponatraemia has also been reported. Carbamazepine may induce a chronic low white blood cell count. Rarely (about 1 in 20 000 cases), this may develop into an agranulocytosis or aplastic anaemia. Stevens-Johnson syndrome has also been reported with the use of carbamazepine.

USE IN PREGNANCY Mood-stabilising agents should not be used in patients who are pregnant or who are breast-feeding. Lithium has been associated with an increased risk of cardiac malformations, and anticonvulsants with an increased risk of neural tube defects.

DRUG INTERACTIONS As noted above, drug–drug interactions with lithium primarily relate to alterations of lithium renal clearance. Carbamazepine is metabolised by, and is a potent inducer of, the enzyme CYP3A3/4. Plasma concentrations of drugs metabolised by this enzyme are reduced by co-administration of carbamazepine. Valproate is highly protein bound (up to 94%) so it has the potential to interfere with the binding of other highly protein bound drugs. Valproate is hepatically metabolised by, and also inhibits, liver cytochrome enzymes. Thus there is potential for metabolic interactions with drugs that are dependent on these enzymes for their metabolism or that inhibit these enzymes.

DISCLAIMER

This chapter represents the individual views of the authors and does not provide comprehensive drug information, some of which may be particularly important in prescribing for individual patients, such as contraindications and precautions relevant to the various drugs discussed. Responsible use therefore requires that the prescriber is familiar with these matters, and refers to the relevant pharmaceutical literature. This chapter is not a substitute for seeking appropriate advice.

CONFLICT OF INTEREST

Trevor R Norman serves or has served on advisory boards for various companies whose products are mentioned in this article. He provides or has provided educational talks, is in receipt of or has received research funding and travel grants from these companies. In particular he has or has had associations with Alphapharm, Astra-Zeneca, Aventis, Bristol-Myers-Squibb, Eli-Lilly, Glaxo-Smith-Kline, Lundbeck, Organon, Wyeth and Pfizer.

REFERENCES

1. Harrison C, Britt H. The rates and management of psychological problems in Australian general practice. Australian and New Zealand Journal of Psychiatry 2004;38(10):781–8.
2. McManus P, Mant A, Mitchell P, Britt H, Dudley J. Use of antidepressants by general practitioners and psychiatrists in Australia. Australian and New Zealand Journal of Psychiatry 2003; 37(2):184–9.
3. Royal Australian and New Zealand College of Psychiatrists Clinical Practice Guidelines Team for Depression. Australian and New Zealand clinical practice guidelines for the treatment of depression. Australian and New Zealand Journal of Psychiatry 2004;38:389–407.
4. Psychotropic Expert Group. Therapeutic Guidelines: psychotropic. Version 5. Melbourne: Therapeutic Guidelines Limited, 2003.

5. Moses-Kolko EL, Bogen D, Perel J, Bregar A, Uhl K, Levin B, Wisner KL. Neonatal signs after late in utero exposure to serotonin reuptake inhibitors: literature review and implications for clinical applications. Journal of the American Medical Association 2005;293(19):2372–83.

6. Cade J. Mending the Mind: A Short History of Twentieth Century Psychiatry. Melbourne: Sun Books Pty Ltd, 1979.

7. Harrison C, Britt H. Prescriptions for antipsychotics in general practice. Medical Journal of Australia 2003;178(9):468–9.

8. McGorry P, Killackey E, Elkins K, Lambert M, Lambert T. Summary of the Australian and New Zealand clinical practice guideline for the treatment of schizophrenia. Australiasian Psychiatry 2003;11(2):136–47.

9. Lambert TLR, Chapman LH. Diabetes, psychotic disorders and antipsychotic therapy: a consensus statement. Medical Journal of Australia 2004;181(10):544–8.

10. American Diabetes Association, American Psychiatric Association, American Association of Clinical Endocrinologists, North American Association for the Study of Obesity: Consensus development conference on antipsychotic drugs and obesity and diabetes. Diabetes Care 2004;27:596–601.

11. Cade JFJ. Lithium salts in the treatment of psychotic excitement. Medical Journal of Australia 1949;2:349–52.

CHAPTER 21

TOOLS FOR ASSESSMENT AND SELF-MANAGEMENT

M Kyrios and K Hegarty

Quemadmodum gladius neminem occidit, occidentis telum est.

A sword never kills anybody; it is a tool in the killer's hand.

SENECA, *Letters to Lucilius, c. 62 AD*

CASE STUDY 1

Jenny, aged 35, presents to you, a female general practitioner (GP), saying, 'I feel tired all the time.' She has two children, aged 10 and 7, and has been separated from her husband for the last four years. She wonders if there might be something 'physical going on'. She has no other specific physical symptoms and generally feels okay. She does feel that life is 'overwhelming', as she is trying to set up her own jewellery-making business and is currently struggling on the pension to make ends meet. In response to further general questions about what else is happening in her life, she tells you that her son is being bullied at school and this makes her very anxious. You then ask more specific questions that are based on the Primary Care Evaluation of Mental Disorders (PRIME-MD) screening questions[1] (see below). She admits to not enjoying anything at the moment, and feels a bit down and hopeless most of the time. Jenny is having difficulty concentrating, is sleeping poorly, eating a lot of junk food and has felt as if she is being a 'bad mother'. The screening questions and being positive on four of the symptom questions from the PRIME-MD means that she is very likely to have depression (6% false positive rate).

These are questions from the PRIME-MD depression module.

(a) Screening questions:
— Have you been bothered by little interest or pleasure in doing things?
— Have you been feeling down, depressed or hopeless in the last month?

(b) Symptom questions:
- — Sleep disturbance
- — Appetite disturbance
- — Loss of energy
- — Difficulty concentrating
- — Feelings of worthlessness
- — Psychomotor retardation
- — Suicidal thoughts

Score one point for each positive category; the cut-off value is 5.9.

KEY FACTS

- Depression and anxiety are serious psychological disorders that interfere with quality of life and are associated with poorer health outcomes. Patients are more likely to present to primary care settings than anywhere else.

- Depression and anxiety disorders are frequently missed when the focus is on somatic complaints and/or explanations for presenting problems, or when patients are reluctant to discuss psychological distress.

- The use of standardised tools is often a helpful strategy in screening for psychological disorder, in assessing symptoms of psychological dysfunction, and for self-monitoring.

- Screening tools include those for psychological distress, as well as for specific disorders, such as depression and anxiety.

- Screening tools are not a substitute for clinical assessment but can be used to assist with the assessment.

- Assessment tools need to demonstrate a number of properties in order for clinicians to be confident about the accuracy and validity of the information provided.

- Several instruments have been shown to exhibit satisfactory sensitivity and specificity in general practice and other settings.

- Regardless of the quality of the assessment tools clinicians use, standardised measures often miss detailed aspects of a patient's presenting problems, particularly contextual issues.

- Self-monitoring tools can provide contextual and individual details that are useful for developing intervention strategies, including self-monitoring.

INTRODUCTION

Information acquired from interviews with patients regarding their symptoms and difficulties comprises an important feature of the clinical context. This is particularly true of information about mental health as it presents in primary care settings. Furthermore, such information is central to clinicians' decision making and their capacity to make recommendations about patient self-management strategies. It is important, however, for clinicians to consider the accuracy and breadth of the information that patients provide.

Patients can often forget to mention an important aspect of their current difficulties, or their history reporting can be inconsistent and confusing. On the other hand, distracted or busy clinicians can overlook asking about potentially important aspects of patient symptoms or circumstances.

Such concerns relate to the reliability and validity of information collected from clinical interviews. In an attempt to overcome some of the potential pitfalls and limitations of interview based information, clinicians can use:

- standardised measures of psychological and psychiatric phenomena, usually in the form of checklists or questionnaires, based on normative studies; and
- self-monitoring approaches, requiring patients to monitor selected aspects of their symptoms or circumstances while they are in their usual surroundings or in specific situations; these approaches maximise the assessment of the distinctive characteristics of patients or their environments.

A range of assessment options is available to clinicians in order to improve the reliable, valid and efficient collection of patients' reports of psychological and contextual factors as they relate to primary care concerns. One can choose from: measures that allow screening of possible diagnostic categories (for example, depression or anxiety); measures that assess the severity of a particular disorder once diagnosis is clear (for example, obsessive-compulsive disorder); and tools that allow patients to monitor particular aspects of their functioning (for example, anxiety or mood swings over a day). This chapter will outline some of the issues pertaining to the use of such measures, as well as describe some of the more common measures. The chapter will focus on depression and anxiety as these are among the most common presentations in primary care.

CONTEXTUAL ISSUES IN GENERAL PRACTICE

There are many ways in which GPs can use the available tools to measure depression and anxiety in general practice. They can:

- ask all patients a small number of standard questions during the consultation (usually as an initial screening exercise);
- use pen and paper, structured interview or computer based tools to screen for disorder—for example, depression or anxiety in all patients prior to the consultation (usually in the waiting room);
- use pen and paper or computer based tools to assess the severity of a specific disorder and to monitor progress once the diagnosis is made; and
- selectively use tools on patients deemed to be 'high risk' for depression and anxiety on the basis of particular key signs that are assessed during clinical consultation or screening—for example, highly stressful life events, sleep problems, multiple somatic symptoms and scores above a cut-off on a screening measure.

These uses will vary in terms of their sensitivity and the specificity to particular disorders. The suitability of assessment tools also depends on the age, gender, comorbidity, language difficulties and cognitive impairment of the patient in front of you. Some of the scales are available for free, while others require payment of a fee. Which tool to use depends on what you are using it for. While using tools alone is not advisable for making a diagnosis, any measures used need to be valid and reliable, and have high specificity (low false positives) and high sensitivity (low false negatives). For monitoring the progress of treatment, tools need to be reliable over time and also to assess changes in a sensitive enough way to give clinically meaning outcomes. Such tools are compared against a gold standard, usually in the form of a focused, in-depth interview by an experienced mental health professional. The next section will go into further detail about all these issues.

HOW USEFUL IS IT TO USE TOOLS?

Tools are a useful adjunct but not a substitute for the usual clinical skills of history taking, mental state examinations and case formulation. Many practitioners are also reluctant to utilise pen and paper screening tools, rather seeing the consultation as the cornerstone of eliciting emotional health issues in general practice. Despite this, the tools can be useful:

- where the diagnosis is uncertain;
- where the GP is monitoring the progress of treatment;
- where the patient is self-monitoring at home;
- for assessing the severity of the illness;
- for diagnosing comorbidity; and
- for assessing suicide risk.

Only a small number of practitioners screen all patients, and there is currently no evidence that utilising screening tools in general practice will alter health outcomes. Following a review of effectiveness studies, Gilbody et al[2] concluded that the routine administration and feedback of questionnaires measuring depression or quality of life had no impact on the recognition, management or outcomes of depression in non-specialist settings. Detection rates increased only when questionnaires were administered to high-risk patients (that is, those above a diagnostic threshold), and administrative assistants or practice nurses provided feedback. Furthermore, no evidence of follow-on to clinical practice or outcomes was found. Hence, the use of such tools for assessing mental health problems in primary care patients may be advisable or even necessary, but not sufficient to guarantee improved care and positive outcomes.

Where questionnaires and relevant normative data are not readily available, or where questionnaires do not adequately assess features of presentation relevant to a particular individual (for example, specific situations where anxiety is experienced), then it is useful to take time out to develop an individualised self-monitoring measure. The newly developed measure can then be used to structure treatment exercises, and to monitor changes in important issues such as thinking styles during intervention. In such self-monitoring tools, it is useful to include columns for:

- the day and date;
- a description of the problematic situation (who was there, what happened and so on);
- a description of thinking styles and automatic thoughts used in the situation; and
- the associated outcomes, including mood states (for example, depression, anxiety) and severity ratings for specific moods, using a scale of 0 (none) to 10 (most severe).

CASE STUDY 2

Rebecca is a 29-year-old secretary presenting for a check-up on her 'heart'. She has been having episodes of a combination of nausea, difficulty getting her breath and heart racing for the last eighteen months. The first time she experienced this was when she tried some tablets to help her stop smoking: she had a reaction to these and was taken to hospital. Since then she gets the attacks irregularly but they seem to have become more frequent over the last six months, and she is avoiding situations where they are likely to occur. She is worried that she may have a 'heart condition' like her father, who had a heart attack when she was younger. Physical examination suggests no physiological irregularities. Further assessment reveals that the 'heart episodes' are often preceded by stressful events.

A structured diary of 'heart episodes' over a period of a week can be helpful in reaching a differential diagnosis (in Rebecca's case, this is likely to be panic disorder with or without agoraphobia) and in identifying associated cognitive and behavioural factors that underline and then maintain the anxiety disorder. In Rebecca's case, the cognitive factors are likely to relate to her fears about having a heart attack, while the behavioural factors are likely to include avoidance and reassurance seeking. In order to yield useful information, the diary could be structured as shown in Table 21.1.

While self-assessment tools are useful for helping patients monitor their levels of depression, anxiety and related problems, self-management tools can be equally useful as part of a treatment plan in primary care. GPs can consider a self-management approach for patients who prefer a more self-contained or solitary approach to dealing with their problems; however, this should only be done if the GP has made a thorough assessment of risk, and can monitor the patient's progress. There are a variety of websites that provide screening tools and quality evidence based treatment content (for a description and review of Australian depression sites, see Griffiths and Christensen[3]). During psychological treatment, it is often useful to include two additional columns in structured diaries, asking patients to: first, identify alternative thinking; and second, identify alternative outcomes and mood states if the alternative thinking was used. Fuller descriptions of such commonly used column techniques can be found in many self-help books. One of the most widely used measures of depression, the Beck Depression Inventory (BDI[4]), has been published in a widely available self-help book by Burns.[5]

PATIENT BARRIERS TO ASSESSMENT

GPs will often encounter patients who are resistant to the nature of assessment for the following major reasons:

- Patients may not understand the rationale underlying the need for assessment of specific aspects of their presentation. In such cases, it is important for the GP to clearly explain the rationale for monitoring and assessment, and to ask the patient to explain the rationale back to the GP.
- Patients may want to avoid discussing their problems. For patients who are concerned about social judgments by their GP, self-report questionnaires and inventories are particularly useful. For patients who are overwhelmed by the perceived enormity of their problems, a more graded or structured approach to problem identification and

TABLE 21.1 Example of a structured diary

DAY/DATE	DESCRIBE THE SITUATION IN WHICH THE PANIC OCCURRED	WHAT DID YOU DO IN RESPONSE TO THE PANIC ATTACK?	WHAT WERE YOU THINKING AT THE TIME?	HOW DID YOU FEEL AT THE TIME AND AFTERWARDS? (0 = NOT AT ALL; 10 = TOTALLY)
Monday, 16 May	Walking to work. Had an argument with my boss yesterday.	Stopped for a rest. Rang my friend to come and get me and take me to the hospital. Made appointment with my GP.	My heart is beating really fast. Maybe I'm having a heart attack. I could be dying. I should never exercise again. I can't cope by myself.	Initially, I felt extremely anxious (9). Afterwards, I felt like I was a failure (8). I was reassured after going to hospital (7). I then felt relieved after my GP organised some tests (6).

problem solving may be recommended. GPs may need to spend a longer time with such patients, building trust and rapport. With the patient's permission, family and other carers can also be recruited to help with assessment and management.

PROPERTIES OF ASSESSMENT TOOLS

In order to maintain your confidence in their capacity to do what they purport to do, assessment tools are subject to a number of requirements. When choosing an assessment tool, you need to be cognisant of five important properties of instruments: reliability, validity, standardisation, sensitivity and specificity (see Table 21.2 for a summary and definitions). The employment of measures without established reliability, validity and normative data for comparative purposes limits their use in clinical assessment because of the risk of misdiagnosis. Furthermore, when choosing a particular measure, you need to be aware of the likelihood that the measure will be able to identify patients with mental health problems or with a specific disorder of interest—for example, depression. While many measures have been developed for assessing depression and anxiety, not all have been used in primary care settings, nor have norms been established for the primary care population.

Many of the measures also exhibit validity problems. Measures of depression and anxiety contain items assessing somatic symptoms of mental health disorders that might also be due to a physical disorder, especially in a primary care population. Furthermore, even measures demonstrating adequate properties may exhibit limitations with respect to their utility—for example, for developing management strategies. Standardised measures often miss out on detailed aspects of a patient's presentations and difficulties, and on the assessment of an individual's particular circumstances. Self-monitoring can often provide the level of circumstantial and idiosyncratic detail that standardised questionnaires miss, and that is necessary for developing intervention strategies. For instance, in developing cognitive behavioural therapy interventions for panic disorder, it is often essential to gain relevant knowledge through the use of panic diaries that assess the antecedents of panic attacks and the thinking patterns with which they are associated.

TOOLS FOR THE DETECTION AND MANAGEMENT OF DEPRESSION AND ANXIETY

Widely used tools for assessing depression, anxiety and related problems are described in Table 21.3. In general, there are two categories of tools used in general practice:

- screening tools, such as the:
  — General Health Questionnaire (GHQ)[6]
  — Primary Care Evaluation of Mental Disorders (PRIME-MD)[1]
  — Kessler Psychological Distress Scale (K-10)[7]
  — Edinburgh Post-Natal Depression Scale (EPDS)[8]
- tools assessing the severity of specific disorders such as depression and anxiety, such as the:
  — Beck Depression Inventory (BDI)[4]
  — Centre for Epidemiologic Studies Depression Screen (CES-D)[9]

TABLE 21.2 Properties of tools

PROPERTY	DEFINITION	EXAMPLES
Reliability	Degree of consistency in the assessment or diagnostic process	▪ Inter-rater reliability: Do independent observers rate or diagnose the same patient in a similar manner? ▪ Test-retest reliability: Would the same patient consistently rate themselves with similar degrees of severity using the same measure at different assessment points? ▪ Internal consistency: Are all the questions a clinician asks regarding symptoms of depression relevant to an overall severity score for depression?
Validity	Extent to which an assessment tool actually measures what it is supposed to measure	▪ Content validity: Does the measure cover all relevant areas relating to a particular disorder? ▪ Convergent and divergent validity: What is the degree of association between measures of the same or dissimilar disorders, respectively? ▪ Criterion related validity: Do scores on one's chosen measure change in expected ways with changing circumstances? ▪ Face validity: Do recipients of a particular measure feel that the tool is measuring what they have been told it is measuring? ▪ Ecological validity: Does a measure accurately indicate a patient's behaviour in real life situations?
Standardisation	The existence of normative data on which to compare individual data (i.e. norms or cut-off scores on which to compare individuals)	▪ Can one compare a patient's scores on a specific measure against the scores of a cohort of individuals known to have the specified disorder?
Sensitivity	The degree to which a particular measure can accurately indicate that an individual is likely to be experiencing a psychological problem in general	▪ Are individuals scoring beyond a specific cut-off score likely to be diagnosable with any psychological disorder?
Specificity	The degree to which a particular measure can accurately indicate that an individual is likely to have a specific psychological problem	▪ Are individuals scoring beyond a specific cut-off score likely to be diagnosable with a specific condition (e.g. major depression)?

— Beck Anxiety Inventory (BAI)[10]
— Yale-Brown Obsessive-Compulsive Scale (YBOCS)[11]

Some of the severity scales for depression are also used as screening tools, as they provide cut-off scores for probable 'casesness'—for example, BDI, CES-D.

In evaluating the usefulness of tools for identifying depressed patients presenting to primary care, Mulrow et al[12] identified several instruments that exhibited reasonable sensitivity and specificity. Of these, the BDI, GHQ and the depression items from the PRIME-MD exhibited the best sensitivity, although the CES-D exhibited among the best specificity. While the K-10[7] is used very commonly in primary care settings and research, it lacks the specificity of many other scales.

THE BDI

The BDI is a 21-item self-report measure that asks recipients to identify which of four statements per item most closely conveys how they have been feeling over the past week. The BDI comprises cognitive, affective, somatic and vegetative symptoms of depression and dysphoria. A BDI cut-off score of ≥ 14 is usually used to identify 'cases' of major depression.[4] However, research with patients presenting with chronic medical illness—for example, diabetes—has indicated that BDI scores of ≥ 10 are associated with significant risk.[13, 14] An updated version of the BDI, the BDI-II, has been published recently[15] to more closely reflect diagnostic criteria for major depression from the *Diagnostic and Statistical Manual for Mental Disorders*.[16] Shorter versions of the BDIs have also been developed.

THE BAI

Beck and associates have also developed the Beck Anxiety Inventory,[10] a 21-item anxiety symptom checklist that covers core anxiety symptoms commonly experienced by clinically anxious people, particularly those with physiological symptoms of panic.

THE CES-D

The CES-D comprises 20 items that ask recipients to rate the degree of time over the past week that they have experienced a range of depression related symptoms. Scores on the CES-D are used both as a continuous variable and with respect to a standard cut-off score (> 16). The latter is used for definition of probable 'casesness' when used as a screening measure. The CES-D has been found to be a reliable and valid instrument in general community, psychiatric and primary care samples across a range of countries.[17]

THE GHQ

The GHQ was developed as a screening measure to identify individuals likely to present with a psychiatric disorder in primary care settings. Although there are various versions of the GHQ, each differing in length and focus, the 12-item and 28-item versions are commonly encountered in primary care and general population research, and include items assessing depression, anxiety, sleep difficulties and somatic concerns. With threshold scores for the GHQ varying with context, it has been suggested that the GHQ cut-off score is more useful for estimating prevalence in large populations than for screening individual patients.

THE PRIME-MD

The PRIME-MD was designed as a screening tool for primary care attenders. It is a multidimensional questionnaire arranged in several categories, which are used to trigger more detailed questions about specific diagnoses. For instance, the depression module paraphrases DSM-IV criteria for depression. The PRIME-MD depression scale is among the shortest of all measures. However, there is some Australian evidence that the PRIME-MD may overdiagnose depression.

OTHER USEFUL INSTRUMENTS

Some other useful instruments with particular strengths include the Hospital Anxiety and Depression Scale (HADS),[19] the Depression Anxiety Stress Scale (DASS)[20] and the Edinburgh Postnatal Depression Scale (EPDS).[8]

THE HADS The HADS is a 14-item self-report scale, originally developed to identify cases of anxiety disorders and depression in non-psychiatric hospital clinics. It has also been found useful in assessing severity and caseness of anxiety disorders and depression in somatic, psychiatric, primary care and general populations.[21] The HADS exhibits advantages in assessing anxiety and depression in primary care settings where somatic symptoms of anxiety and depression may be of mixed aetiology.

THE DASS Developed in Australia, the DASS is a particularly useful self-report measure that adequately distinguishes features of depression, physical arousal and psychological tension and agitation.[22] The DASS is available in 42-item and 21-item versions, with adequate psychometric properties.

THE EPDS The EPDS is a 10-item self-report scale that screens for post-natal depression in the community. The EPDS has satisfactory sensitivity and specificity, and is sensitive to change in depression severity.

TOOLS FOR ASSESSING ANXIETY AND RELATED PROBLEMS

A range of measures is also available for assessment of specific anxiety related problems. Many of these can be accessed in the *Practitioner's Guide to Empirically-Based Measures of Anxiety*.[23] With respect to the anxiety disorders (see Chapter 9), there is a variety of self-report measures from which to choose for assessing particular aspects of specific disorders. For phobias, one can use the Fear Survey Schedule[24] to assess the degree of anxiety associated with specific situations and the Fear Questionnaire[25] to assess social anxiety and agoraphobia. For panic disorder, it is often useful to assess the degree of mobility and avoidance (Mobility Inventory for Panic and Agoraphobia)[26] or the experience of bodily sensations (Body Sensations Questionnaire).[27] For social phobia, one can use the Liebowitz Social Anxiety Scale[28] to assess severity of social anxiety in particular situations. For post-traumatic stress reactions, one can use the Post-Traumatic Stress Disorder Checklist,[29] which is applicable to any traumatic event and assesses the degree to which particular symptoms bother patients. For generalised anxiety disorder, there is a range of worries measures, including the Penn State Worry Questionnaire[30] and the Worry Domains Questionnaire.[31] For obsessive-compulsive disorder (OCD), relevant severity measures include the Yale-Brown Obsessive-Compulsive Scale (YBOCS)[11] and the Padua Inventory.[32]

The routine use of validated screening instruments to assist with identification of excessive drinking has also been suggested—for example, the CAGE[33] and the Alcohol Use Disorders Identification Test (AUDIT).[34]

The CAGE was developed as a short clinician administered screen for alcoholism or covert problem drinking. The CAGE consists of 4 questions about lifetime alcohol consumption, with a positive response to 2 or more items indicative of problem drinking. While CAGE can detect severe forms of alcohol disorders or dependent drinking, it is less sensitive to hazardous alcohol consumption, defined as drinking over medically recommended limits and that can lead to risk of physical or psychological harm.

The AUDIT, developed by the World Health Organization, is a validated questionnaire consisting of 10 questions (maximum score of 40), and includes items assessing alcohol consumption, problems and dependency (a cut-off score of ≥ 8 is recommended for routine screening of hazardous or harmful use).

TOOLS FOR ASSESSING SUICIDE RISK

Finally, suicide risk has received little attention in primary care research. In a recent review, the US Preventive Services Task Force[35] found only one article assessing an instrument's operating characteristics for identifying suicide risk in primary care. The Symptom-Driven Diagnostic System for Primary Care (SDDS-PC)[36] includes three items ('thoughts of death', 'wishing you were dead', 'feeling suicidal') that assess suicide risk within the past month in adults.[37] Compared with a structured interview for identifying a plan to commit suicide, all three items exhibited adequate sensitivity, specificity and predictive value.

REVISITING CASE STUDY 1

Two months later, Jenny is seeing the same GP again. Although reluctant at first to see her tiredness as being due to psychological reasons, underneath she knows how sad she is feeling. She has been regularly seeing the GP every 1–2 weeks to receive some supportive counselling and cognitive behavioural strategies. She chose this care because she did not want to go on antidepressants, could not afford a psychologist, and was reluctant to see a psychiatrist at this stage. Initially, she borrowed the self-help book *Feeling Good: The New Mood Therapy*[5] and scored herself on the depression scale at the front. This convinced her she was depressed, as she scored in the moderate range. Jenny was unable to concentrate at first on the exercises in the book or on the internet based self-help cognitive behavioural strategies, but she is now feeling a lot better and has been able to do some of this self-help. She has rescored herself and has improved her rating on the scale. Jenny is functioning much better with her work and coping with her child's school issues. She is thinking about accessing a mental health specialist if things get worse again.

CONCLUSION

Many standardised tools are available for the assessment of depression, anxiety and other psychological issues commonly seen in primary care. These tools can be used to

TABLE 21.3 Tools commonly used to assess emotional health in primary care

TOOLS	REFERENCE	NO. OF ITEMS	METHOD	USES	ADVANTAGES/LIMITATIONS
Psychosocial distress					
GHQ	6; 38	12, 28, 30 or 60	Self-report. Costs	Screening tool for primary care settings	Variety of versions with different lengths and foci. Good sensitivity
K-10	7	10	Self-report. No cost	Screening—cut-off for likely 'diagnoses'	Widely used in population studies. Good sensitivity. Poor specificity
Depression					
PRIME-MD depression screen	1	2	Clinician or self-report	Screening tool	Good sensitivity. Poor specificity
PHQ-9 PRIME-MD (depression)	1	9	Clinician and self-rated. No cost	Screening tool for primary care settings	Good sensitivity, but overdiagnoses depression
BDI-I and BDI-II	4; 15	21	Self-rated. Costs	Severity of depression; screening—cut-off for likely 'casesness'	Widely used. More recent version updated for greater consistency with diagnostic criteria. Difficult questions. Good for treatment response
CES-D	9	20	Self-rated. No cost	Severity of depression; cut-off for likely 'casesness'	Consistency with diagnostic criteria; widely used
EPDS	8	10	Self-rated. No cost	To assist in detection of depression in post-natal and antenatal period as eliminates somatic symptoms	Improves detection of post-natal depression. Widely used. Translated into many languages. Easy to complete and score

continued overleaf

TABLE 21.3 *continued*

TOOLS	REFERENCE	NO. OF ITEMS	METHOD	USES	ADVANTAGES/LIMITATIONS
Anxiety					
BAI	10	21	Self-report. Costs	Severity of anxiety	Self-rated. Particularly for somatic symptoms of anxiety and panic
Fear Survey Schedule	24	108	Self-report. No cost	Severity of anxiety in specific situations	Self-rated. Useful screen for phobias
Fear Questionnaire	25	24	Self-report. No cost	Screening for social anxiety and agoraphobia sub-scales	Self-rated. Useful screen for particular anxiety disorders
Mobility Inventory for Panic and Agoraphobia	26	34	Self-report. No cost	Degree of mobility in and avoidance of particular situations when accompanied and when alone, and severity of panic attacks	Self-rated. Useful to assess treatment gains
Body Sensations Questionnaire	27	17	Self-report. No cost	Range and severity of bodily sensations in panic disorder	Self-rated. Useful for assessing treatment gains
Liebowitz Social Anxiety Scale	28	24	Self-report. No cost	Degree of fear in and avoidance of specific situations that trigger social anxiety	Self-rated. Useful for assessing treatment gains
Post-Traumatic Stress Disorder Checklist	29	17	Self-report. No cost. In public domain (www.ncptsd.org/ PILOTS.html)	Degree to which particular PTSD symptoms have bothered respondents	Self-rated. Useful for assessing treatment gains. Applicable to any traumatic event

TABLE 21.3 *continued*

TOOLS	REFERENCE	NO. OF ITEMS	METHOD	USES	ADVANTAGES/LIMITATIONS
Penn State Worry Questionnaire	30	16	Self-report. No cost	Worries associated with generalised anxiety disorder	Self-rated. Useful for assessing treatment gains
Worry Domains Questionnaire	31	30	Self-report. No cost	Worries in generalised anxiety disorder	Self-rated. Useful for assessing levels of worry in specific domains
Obsessive-compulsive disorder					
YBOCS	11	10 main items plus additional questions	Self- and clinician-rated versions. No cost	Severity of OCD	Clinician and self-rated versions. Sensitivity to change with treatment
Padua Inventory	32	60- and 39-item versions	Self-rated. No cost	Distress associated with OCD	Self-rated. Widely used
Mixed symptoms					
HADS	19	14	Self-rated. No cost	Severity of anxiety and depression	As somatic symptoms are selected out, very useful for primary care
DASS	20	42- and 21-item versions. No cost	Self-report. No cost. www.psy.unsw.edu.au/Groups/Dass	Severity of anxiety, depression and stress symptoms	Developed in Australia. Increasing public profile

continued overleaf

TABLE 21.3 *continued*

TOOLS	REFERENCE	NO. OF ITEMS	METHOD	USES	ADVANTAGES/LIMITATIONS
PHQ PRIME-MD	1	26-item (PHQ) self-report screening measure	Self-rated screening measure followed by clinician-rated interview version	Screening tool (PHQ) and diagnostic tool (PRIME-MD Interview) for primary care settings	Good sensitivity. Overdiagnoses depression. Includes alcohol, eating disorders, somatisation and anxiety
Alcohol abuse					
CAGE	33	4	Clinician-rated screen. No cost.	Screens for lifetime alcohol consumption	Detects severe forms of alcohol disorders or dependent drinking, but is less sensitive to hazardous consumption
AUDIT	34	10	Self-rated questionnaire. No cost.	Assesses for alcohol consumption, problems and dependency	Validated, with standardised cut-off score for routine screening of hazardous or harmful use
Suicide					
SDDS-PC: suicide items	36	3	Self-report questionnaire	Screen for suicide risk, especially suicide plan	Adequate sensitivity, specificity and predictive value

screen for disorder, assess the severity of specific disorders and monitor progress. While standardised assessment tools can help overcome many of the limitations of clinical interviews, GPs need to provide a rationale for the use of specific measures, each of which has its own focus and advantages. Furthermore, assessment tools need to exhibit a number of properties in order for GPs to feel confident about the accuracy and validity of the information they provide. Regardless of the quality of the assessment tools that GPs use, standardised measures often miss detailed aspects of a patient's presentations and difficulties, particularly contextual issues. However, individualised and contextual details can be assessed via the use of self-monitoring tools. Structured diaries can include a number of columns so that patients can self-monitor particular aspects of their symptoms and context, yielding information that is often useful in developing tailored interventions. In summary, considered use of tools to assess mental health problems in primary care patients is advisable but not sufficient to guarantee improved care and positive outcomes.

REFERENCES

1. Spitzer RL, Williams JB, Kroenke K, Linzer M, deGruy FV, Hahn SR, Brody D, Johnson JG. Utility of a new procedure for diagnosing mental disorders in primary care. The PRIME-MD 1000 study. Journal of the American Medical Association 1994;272:1749–56.
2. Gilbody SM, Whitty PM, Grimshaw JM, Thomas RE. Improving the detection and management of depression in primary care. Quality and Safety in Health Care 2003;12:149–55.
3. Griffiths KM, Christensen H. The quality and accessibility of Australian depression sites on the World Wide Web. Medical Journal of Australia 2002;176:S97–104.
4. Beck AT, Ward CH, Mendelson M, Mock J, Erbaugh J. An inventory for measuring depression. Archives of General Psychiatry 1961;4:561–71.
5. Burns DD. Feeling Good: The New Mood Therapy. Melbourne: Information Australia Group, 1980.
6. Goldberg DP, Blackwell B. Psychiatric illness in general practice. A detailed study using a new method of case identification. British Medical Journal 1970;2:438–43.
7. Kessler RC, Andrews G, Colpe LJ, Hiripi E, Mroczek DK, Normand ST, Walters EE, Zaslavsky AM. Short screening scales to monitor population prevalences and trends in non-specific psychological distress. Psychological Medicine 2002;32:959–76.
8. Cox JL, Holden JM, Sagovsky R. Detection of postnatal depression. Development of the 10-item Edinburgh Postnatal Depression Scale. British Journal of Psychiatry 1987;150:782–6.
9. Radloff LS. The CES-D Scale: A self-report depression scale for research in the general population. Applied Psychological Measurement 1977;1:385–401.
10. Beck AT, Steer RA. Manual for the Beck Anxiety Inventory. San Antonio, TX: The Psychological Corporation, 1993.
11. Goodman WK, Price LH, Rasmussen SA, Mazure C, Fleischmann RL, Hill CL, Heniger GR, Charney DS. The Yale-Brown Obsessive Compulsive Scale. I. Development, use and reliability. Archives of General Psychiatry 1989;46:1006–11.
12. Mulrow CD, Williams JW Jr, Gerety MB, Ramirez G, Montiel OM, Kerber C. Case-finding instruments for depression in primary care settings. Annals of Internal Medicine 1995;122:913–21.
13. Haire-Joshu D, Heady S, Thomas L, Schechtman K, Fisher EB. Depressive symptomatology and smoking among persons with diabetes. Research in Nursing Health 1994;17:273–82.
14. Leedom L, Meehan WP, Procci W, Zeidler A. Symptoms of depression in patients with type II diabetes mellitus. Psychosomatics 1991;32:280–6.
15. Beck AT, Steer RA, Brown GK. Beck Depression Inventory—Second Edition Manual. San Antonio, TX: The Psychological Corporation, 1996.
16. American Psychiatric Association. Diagnostic and Statistical Manual of Mental Disorders. 4th edn. Washington DC: American Psychiatric Association, 1994.

17. Fleck M, Simon G, Herrman H, Bushnell D, Martin M, Patrick D. Major depression and its correlates in primary care setting in six countries. British Journal of Psychiatry 2005;186:41–7.

18. Goldney R, Hawthorne G, Fisher L. Is the Australian National Health Survey of Mental Health and Wellbeing a reliable guide for health planners? A methodological note on the prevalence of depression. Australian and New Zealand Journal of Psychiatry 2004;38:635–8.

19. Zigmond AS, Snaith RP. The Hospital Anxiety and Depression Scale. Acta Psychiatrica Scandinavica 1983;67:361–70.

20. Lovibond SH, Lovibond PF. Manual for the Depression Anxiety Stress Scales. 2nd edn. Sydney, Australia: Psychology Foundation of Australia, 1995.

21. Bjelland I, Dahl AA, Haug TT, Neckelmann D. The validity of the Hospital Anxiety and Depression Scale: an updated literature review. Journal of Psychosomatic Research 2002;52:69–77.

22. Anthony MM, Beiling PJ, Cox BJ, Enns MW, Swinson RP. Psychometric properties of the 42-item and 21-item versions of the Depression Anxiety Stress Scales in clinical groups and a community sample. Psychological Assessment 1998;10:176–81.

23. Martin MA, Orsillo SM, Roemer L. Practitioner's Guide to Empirically-Based Measures of Anxiety. New York: Kluwer Academic/Plenum, 2001.

24. Wolpe J, Lang PJ. A fear survey schedule for use in behavior therapy. Behaviour Research and Therapy 1964;2:27–30.

25. Marks IM, Mathews AM. Brief standard self-rating for phobic patients. Behaviour Research and Therapy 1979;17:263–7.

26. Chambless DL, Caputo GC, Jasin SE, Gracely E, Williams C. The Mobility Inventory for Agoraphobia. Behaviour Research and Therapy 1985;23:35–44.

27. Chambless DL, Caputo GC, Bright P, Gallagher R. Assessment of fear in agoraphobics: The Body Sensations Questionnaire and the Agoraphobic Cognitions Questionnaire. Journal of Consulting and Clinical Psychology 1984;52:1090–7.

28. Liebowtiz MR. Social phobia. Modern Problems in Pharmacopsychiatry 1987;22:141–73.

29. Weathers FW, Litz BT, Huska JA, Keane TM. PTSD Checklist—Civilian Version. Boston: National Center for PTSD, Behavioural Science Division, 1994.

30. Meyer TJ, Miller ML, Metzger RL, Borkovec TD. Development and validation of the Penn State Worry Questionnaire. Behaviour Research and Therapy 1990;28:487–95.

31. Tallis F, Eysenck MW, Mathews A. A questionnaire for the measurement of nonpathological worry. Personality and Individual Differences 1992;13:161–8.

32. Sanavio E. Obsessions and compulsions: The Padua Inventory. Behaviour Research and Therapy 1988;26:169–77.

33. Mayfield D, McLeod G, Hall P. The CAGE questionnaire: validation of a new alcoholism screening instrument. American Journal of Psychiatry 1974;131:1121–3.

34. Saunders JB, Aasland OG, Babor TF, De La Fuente JR, Grant M. Development of the alcohol use disorders identification test (AUDIT): WHO collaborative project on early detection of persons with harmful alcohol consumption. Addiction 1993;88:791–804.

35. Gaynes BN, West SL, Ford CA, Frame P, Klein J, Lohr KN. U.S. Preventive Services Task Force. Screening for suicide risk in adults: a summary of the evidence for the U.S. Preventive Services Task Force. Annals of Internal Medicine 2004;140:822–35.

36. Broadhead WE, Leon AC, Weissman MM, Barrett JE, Blacklow RS, Gilbert TT, Keller MB, Olfson M, Higgins ES. Development and validation of the SDDS-PC screen for multiple mental disorders in primary care. Archives of Family Medicine 1995;4(3):211–19.

37. Olfson M, Weissman MM, Leon AC, Sheehan DV, Farber L. Suicidal ideation in primary care. Journal of Internal Medicine 1996;11:447–53.

CHAPTER 22
COLLABORATIVE CARE FOR COMMON MENTAL DISORDERS

G Meadows, D Monash and A Cichello

We will surely get to our destination if we join hands.

AUNG SAN SUU KYI, 1945–

CASE STUDY

Caroline is a 41-year-old woman with two teenage children, aged 13 and 17, respectively. She has a background in training as a teacher but works on a part-time freelance basis, doing some industry staff training to add to the income from her husband's job in IT. She recently presented with her third episode of major depressive disorder in the context of some stressful times with the children; she had also not complied with the longer term medication prescribed by a psychiatrist with whom she had never developed a good rapport. She would prefer to see a woman specialist another time. You've prescribed her a selective serotonin reuptake inhibitor (SSRI), choosing one that had seemed to help her in the past, but after some early signs of response, her improvement has not been sustained. An interpersonal therapy (IPT) influenced approach to counselling seems to have helped a bit. But again, improvement has not been maintained; both you and Caroline are feeling rather demoralised.

KEY FACTS

- Successful collaboration requires some investment of time in relationship building and acquiring information about locally available options.

- These options, although influenced by national, state and territory level initiatives, are also very much a local matter.

- In Australia, recent changes in rebate structures for general practitioners (GPs) and specialist mental health practitioners have created some new opportunities for positive collaborations.

continued overleaf

KEY FACTS *continued*

■ Tried and tested models for collaboration include consultation practice, stepped care and co-located practice.

■ The cost of treatment is a common impediment to the provision of care, but there is currently some increase in public funded provisions.

INTRODUCTION
THE AUSTRALIAN CONTEXT

Although this book is primarily targeted at Australian GPs, here is a brief background for those not familiar with the Australian mental health care system. Government funded health care in Australia is supported through two major funding streams:

■ The states and territories in Australia are responsible for providing public hospital systems and associated community services where the focus in practice is oriented towards the multidisciplinary care of people with psychotic and/or severely disabling disorders. They are often open to self-referral although with restrictive entry criteria. Staff in these services are typically salaried and on regular employment contracts.

■ The federal government directly funds private medical care providers and some other clinical inputs on a fee-per-item of service basis through what is effectively a near-universal national health insurance scheme called Medicare. Practitioners billing the government for rebates through Medicare are also permitted to charge a co-payment for their services. Referrals to specialists within this system generally require GP involvement.

GENERAL PATTERNS OF REFERRAL

GPs may refer patients to other sources of mental health care, including private sector psychiatrists, psychologists or other mental health care providers and public sector mental health services. Patients may engage directly with services other than the GP, through various routes, including self-referral, to the public sector mental health services and to a range of other providers of psychology, social work or alternative therapy interventions, or through cross-referral between these groups. Specialists in other mental health sectors may also refer patients to GPs.

These referral relationships vary in terms of the level of collaboration. For example, where the patient has instigated contact with services, there may be no clear mechanism for sharing information between service providers; sometimes patients may even wish to isolate the GP from contact with other health professionals or service providers. As such, referral relationships between providers may or may not shape up to be examples of collaborative care.

A LEGACY OF INEQUITY

Within Australia, there is substantial inequity in mental health care provision, which is affected by geographic, socioeconomic, ethnic and cultural differences. There is a strong historical legacy of geographic and social inequity in the provision of mental health services to the Australian population. The context in which the individual GP practises and the opportunity for successful local service initiatives are both influenced by this broader social and political reality.

The specialist private psychiatry workforce is heavily concentrated in the more affluent suburbs of the major cities. In addition, many services for psychological care provision have until only recently been almost exclusively private sector funded. Consequently, there is a substantial disparity in access to specialist mental health services. GPs working in rural areas and in those parts of major cities characterised by greater socioeconomic disadvantage may be markedly disadvantaged in gaining access to specialist mental health care on behalf of their patients.[1]

People from indigenous backgrounds collectively suffer disadvantage across multiple domains of health care and social welfare, with the health effects compounded by socioeconomic and geographical impediments to accessing services (see Chapter 6). In terms of collaborative care, indigenous populations are often in remote areas and poorer parts of cities where the structural factors of the health service operate strongly against positive collaboration. In parts of the country—such as the Northern Territory, where indigenous populations are greater—primary care may be structured differently from that offered to most of the Australian population—for example, there may be a greater proportion of salaried GPs than in urban areas. Under such circumstances, there may be reduced leverage available from new Medicare funding initiatives that could potentially encourage collaborative care.

Australia's non-indigenous population is characterised by successive waves of migrants, with first generation migrants at any time experiencing particular access and service delivery issues. Generally, these minority groups seem to have poorer access to mental health care,[2] and language barriers will be a significant problem for many (see Chapter 5). Using interpreters for telephone access and for translating both general documentation about service delivery and specific information, such as patient health records, can make a major contribution to care in the transcultural context. Multilingual GPs, including those from specific cultural backgrounds, have the opportunity to make a special contribution to these patients. The problems can be especially severe for migrant groups who are also traumatised by the uncertainty of their status as refugees. Collaborative care in Australian immigrant detention centres has been seriously deficient, as evidenced by recent cases of neglect of the mental health care needs in the refugee population; some of these cases have become notorious.[3]

VARIATIONS IN CONTEXT

Some GPs will have excellent connections and relationships with mental health services, including primary care, specialist counseling and consultative and support services. For many others, the process of establishing communication between the different parties involved in the care of one patient with a mental health problem is more typically a source of recurrent frustration. In these worse case scenarios, GPs often criticise private psychiatrists for lengthy waiting lists and poor communication practices, and are unhappy with public mental health services for having entry criteria that disqualify most of the people they see with mental health problems. In their turn, mental health services also often criticise the appropriateness of referrals from general practice, and the quality and amount of information provided. For one reason or another, limited communication during courses of treatment, little sharing of responsibility for care and, consequently, poorly co-ordinated packages of care seem to be disturbingly common occurrences.

Successful collaborative care in response to the need of an individual presenting patient is generally possible only in the context of substantial prior investment in relationship building, through which common understandings have been developed with mental health care providers. A summary of collaborative care for the practising GP needs to include: first, some information about relevant good practice models in the development of strategies and structures that will support good quality collaborative and shared care; and, second, some comments as to how such collaborative care models can be brought into effective action in support of quality care for an individual patient.

STRUCTURES AND STRATEGIES
A TIME FOR NEW BEGINNINGS

Many GPs will be working in areas where, over recent years, successful collaborative initiatives have been established, and there may now be a local capacity for working together across sector boundaries with scope to build on this work. In addition, relatively recent changes in incentives for GPs and psychiatrists have been introduced, and their full potential has certainly not been exploited yet; there is scope for a new wave of collaborative work if practitioners can find ways to make constructive use of these changes.

STATE AND TERRITORY FUNDED SERVICES

The history of local initiatives has been influenced by national mental health policy, particularly through its effect on the activities of state and territory funded services. Through the 1990s, the focus of the first National Mental Health Plan (1993 to 1998)[4] on deinstitutionalisation and improving the quality of care for those with 'serious mental illness' was dominant within public mental health services. The thrust of developments in mental health shared care was towards care for people with schizophrenia and related disorders. The second and third National Mental Health plans (1998 to 2003 and 2003 to 2008, respectively)[5, 6] have laid out an agenda that suggests a broader focus for the activities of public mental health services, with more emphasis on higher prevalence problems such as affective and anxiety disorders. A range of other initiatives within the public mental health services have followed.

There are many other successful local examples of GP shared care programs throughout Australia. Two of the authors have worked on a model for shared care and collaboration with GPs that has been influential in Australia; it is currently the subject of randomised controlled trials in Canada. The program has a well developed manual available on the internet.[7, 8] Also, in a number of Area Mental Health Services, the Public Mental Health Services provide a GP liaison clinician who oversees GP shared care at the point of discharge and follow-up. Perhaps most significant among more recent changes has been the introduction in Victorian public mental health services of small

Primary Mental Health Teams, who specifically provide a range of services for GPs, including consultancy, training, brief collaborative clinical service delivery and a systems development approach that creates links between sectors.

Whatever exists in terms of specific shared care programs, specialist public mental health services each typically provide an intake service, through which the GP will refer patients into the service as a whole. Upon an intake assessment, the public mental health service then determines the most appropriate care option for the patient—for example, crisis assessment and treatment, community continuing care and inpatient admission. In addition, the intake service may be a source of helpful information for the GP on the types of GP shared care mental health offered within the service and/or within the local area, as well as with other private providers.

COMMONWEALTH FUNDED SYSTEM CHANGES

The Commonwealth government has instigated the Better Outcomes in Mental Health Care (BOiMHC) initiative, and many GPs will be familiar with this. BOiMHC provides some incentives for the training of GPs in specific mental health care issues, with two different levels of accreditation for GPs.

Within the initiative, there is provision for a Division of General Practice based funding pool, from which funds can be drawn to reimburse GPs for short courses on focused psychological strategies, generally although not always, presented by clinical psychologists. These funds are accessed through referral from a Level 1 trained GP but administered according to local agreements. Because the Divisions of General Practice (DGP) receive the funding on a population weighted basis, there are some safeguards in place against the evident inequities that have arisen through the development of private sector psychiatrist services under the incentive of rebates that carry no geographic capping. However, funding for these psychological services is modest compared to the demonstrated need, and rationing of this resource is a developing problem.

BOiMHC has also established a national helpline so GPs can consult with psychiatrists by telephone.

Initiatives such as the BOiMHC have also recently been supplemented by the introduction of a specific item under Medicare, remunerating psychiatrists for providing assessment and management planning on a consultancy basis. As with all new payment items, there is a lag, sometimes a substantial one, between the introduction of new items and their uptake in a way that enables their potential to improve patient care to be realised.

Some of the initiatives have been criticised—most notably by the Australian Medical Association—for being bureaucratically unwieldy and having problems with confidentiality; however, there are also examples of GPs who have substantially redesigned their practices in response to the initiatives and Medicare payment items, and who believe such initiatives are an important factor in their being able to enhance the mental health care of their patients. Uptake of the training offered by the BOiMHC initiative has been higher than anticipated, particularly in rural centres. Adoption and refinement of this initiative, funded by the Commonwealth, continues; however, it is frequently in isolation from state services delivery.

GETTING INVOLVED IN COLLABORATIVE SHARED CARE

GPs can be proactive in seeking out formalised collaborative networks or informal supports for the care of their patients with mental health problems. Ideally, such networks and supports should be developed by clusters of GPs prior to the need for patient referral, so that they can systematically develop an understanding of the specific nature and utility of each service. The ideal is to have a 'continuum of care' available at the local level for GP-sector patients.

DIVISIONS OF GENERAL PRACTICE Local DGP work to improve outcomes for patients in general practice and are an effective conduit for the establishment of formal and informal contacts with relevant specialist Public Mental Health Services, private psychiatrists, clinical psychologists and the broader primary care sector (for example, community health services, local government support programs and Neighbourhood Houses). Many DGP may be members of a local mental health reference group, comprised of senior representatives from the major mental health service sectors and underpinned by a memorandum of understanding. In this way, DGP can assist in developing joint protocols with relevant services and co-location opportunities.

A GP interested in this field would benefit from engaging with local divisional GP mental health special interest groups and DGP facilitated mental health training, including BOiMHC training. Some forms of shared care services, such as those available under BOiMHC and funded by the Commonwealth, may be accessed only by GPs who have completed Level 1 training. Commonwealth and state resources, including the recently funded initiatives for supporting the work of the GP in caring for their patients' mental health needs, are potentially best integrated functionally at the local level.

The DGP and the mental health services may greatly assist the GP in navigating around the often confusing issues of private sector agencies, intake criteria, differing catchment areas for patients among services, GP shared care services, BOiMHC and the new 'Strengthening Medicare' provisions introduced by the government.

DEVELOPMENT OF MODELS OF SHARED CARE

It is rare for successful collaboration to be rapidly and effectively improvised as a first time response to the presenting problem of a particular patient in crisis. Rather it should be developed systematically so that the apparatus is already in place when a specific clinical problem emerges. We will now consider some specific conceptual and practical models.

A joint report between the Royal Australian and New Zealand College of Psychiatrists and the Royal Australian College of General Practitioners[9] grouped shared care models around the themes of: attachment of a mental health professional; employment of a mental health care professional; provision of a shared base model of service; and liaison and consultation liaison.

OVERSEAS MODELS OF SHARED CARE There have been some key contributions to this field from overseas. In the United Kingdom, psychiatrist–GP collaboration has been typified by: shifted outpatients (co-location without collaboration); shared care (identified responsibilities and co-ordinated appointment schedules); and consultation liaison (provision of opinion and support).[10] Counsellors are also common in primary care in the UK, but are often not working in a particularly well integrated way with specialist services.

On an international basis, a group headed up by Professor Wayne Katon in Seattle, in the United States,[11, 12] has done the most substantial and the highest quality research work on collaborative care. Through well conducted randomised controlled trials, the Seattle group has progressively confirmed the advantage of stepped care models for the management of disorders such as depression (see Chapters 1 and 7). Within stepped care models, protocols that provide guidance to GPs to enable them to manage less complicated cases are developed. However, they also give guidance as to when care should be 'stepped up' to involve some level of specialist services. A major contribution of the Seattle group has been to confirm the contribution that can be made by properly trained nursing staff in enhancing adherence by patients to medication regimens and in providing professional support for people with depression.

Canada has some impressive and long-running collaborative initiatives that place both a psychiatrist and a specialist counsellor within the primary care team on a regular basis.[13–15] In the model adopted in Hamilton, Ontario, a GP, a psychiatrist and a counsellor—commonly a social worker—all work in the same building so that they can easily make referrals and discuss cases. The counsellors are directly employed by the GPs and are accountable to the GPs for their work.

COLLABORATIVE CLINICAL CARE
GENERAL PRINCIPLES

To establish and support the collaborative clinical care of patients with mental health problems, the GP should invest some time in establishing local networks; however, this must be referenced against the challenge that the GP faces when dealing with clinical situations. The imperative is quality of patient care, and so there is only one reason to collaborate in the care of a patient and that is to improve the outcome of treatment. In order for this to happen, the collaboration must be underpinned by an appropriate reason, involve people with appropriate skills and have the informed consent of the patient.

There are some general principles from the GP perspective that may be helpful in underscoring day to day clinical practice.

The best treatment outcomes are obtained if the referring GP is clear about the reasons for the referral, and the referral contains this information, along with an appropriate clinical history and social information. Here are the most common reasons why a GP seeks collaboration:

- The disorder fails to respond to the therapy instituted by the GP.
- The patient requires access to therapy that is not provided by the GP.
- The GP seeks advice on how to treat the presenting problem.
- The GP needs to share the burden of a difficult case.

Having decided that assistance is required, the doctor and patient then need to determine the appropriate level of support required. In making this determination, it is important that they consider the resources available in the local area and at the disposal of the patient. This is more important in psychiatry than other disciplines, as multiple visits to the psychiatrist are often necessary, thus increasing the costs of treatment and amplifying any difficulties associated with travelling to and from appointments.

ROLES OF SPECIFIC SPECIALISTS

Psychiatrists can be used for diagnostic assessments, treatment, advice and sharing the load. The service required and the manner in which it is obtained are both determined locally. The greatest difficulty in obtaining such care is often the inability of psychiatrists to see patients quickly or for long periods. Some solutions include the use of the telephone, video-conferencing, email, faxing and the use of specific consultation item numbers for psychiatrists. These items are available for psychiatrists undertaking a diagnostic assessment and providing a management plan for the GP. An advice line for the provision of urgent psychiatric advice is also available.

Psychologists and other allied health professionals are useful for confirming diagnoses and providing courses of therapy, either goal focused short courses of therapy or long-term supportive care. In this way they can share the load of caring for a patient. Frequently, the greatest hurdles with referrals to allied health professionals are the cost of the therapy to the patient and defining the roles of those involved.

ESTABLISHING COLLABORATION

Once a GP has decided to ask for assistance, they must then determine the nature and extent of the collaboration required. It is best if these details are determined prior to the referral in order to minimise confusion and assist in providing seamless collaborative care. If the referring GP is unclear about these details, then a consultative telephone call or case conference may assist in determining the nature of the assistance required as well as what is available.

The options available usually form a continuum, from a one-off consultation that may or may not involve the patient to a complete transfer of care; both extremes of collaboration are rare in practice. The details of GP involvement and responsibility need to be clearly determined by all involved.

Clear directions need to be conveyed at the initial referral and followed by regular communication about the aims, goals and, where appropriate, mechanisms for closure. Collaborative care arrangements become easier when all the practitioners involved in the care of a patient understand the skills of their colleagues and develop secure and simple methods of communication. This understanding, combined with professional respect, makes the process of collaboration a rewarding one for all involved and results in better patient outcomes.

The financial problems of referral often experienced by patients can be circumvented if the GP only refers patients with private insurance, private means or who are funded by compensation payments. Unfortunately, the majority of patients requiring these services do not fall into these categories; this necessitates the use of one of the several government sponsored schemes that subsidise the cost of the therapy. There are three main schemes available:

- the rural based More Allied Health Support programs, where the DGP provide funding for local psychologists or counsellors to treat patients;

- the Access to Allied Psychological Services component of the BOiMHC initiative; and
- the Medicare Plus program that allows a patient up to five therapy sessions per year subsidised by Medicare.

REVISITING THE CASE STUDY

After another consultation with Caroline in which she again complains of sleep disturbance, irritability and pervasive low mood, you decide to telephone the national psychiatry advice line. The duty psychiatrist returns your call within an hour and spends about twenty minutes discussing the case with you. The psychiatrist's advice includes reviewing Caroline's personal and family history for signs of bipolar disorder and switching to another class of antidepressant; seeing that she has not had one before, a serotonic norepinephrine reuptake inhibitor (SNRI) might be most appropriate. Follow-up should be assiduous and every effort should be made to achieve full remission of this episode. As someone who has undergone three episodes of major depression, Caroline is almost certain to suffer further episodes, so it is appropriate for the GP to apply some energy to relapse prevention. Full dose antidepressant prescribing is an important plank of management; also, various psychosocial strategies, including IPT and cognitive behavioural therapy (CBT), may assist in maintaining remission. Development of a relapse signature and relapse drill would be a good idea.

If Caroline's history confirms some suggestion of bipolar disorder, then combination therapy with a mood stabiliser might also help. Regular monitoring with a structured instrument is a good idea in these cases.

Further history taking confirms a close family history of bipolar disorder, and also some low-grade manic episodes in the patient herself. Through the Commonwealth funded allied health program, you gain Caroline access to six sessions of CBT, with a request that the feedback from the sessions should include suggestions about longer term relapse prevention, including what warning signs you and she should be looking for. You should also request some guidance in how you may support her to remain well after she finishes the course of treatment.

Caroline attends the six sessions, and reports both learning a lot from them and feeling somewhat better. She and the psychologist worked on a letter that she wrote to herself, containing guidance about lifestyle, stress management and help-seeking responses to some specific warning signs of returning depression. Caroline gives you a copy of this so you can both use it in support of her management. In parallel with the psychological treatment, you have commenced her on venlafaxine and increased the dose. These combined measures have considerably improved matters, but her Kessler-10 scale scores and the mental state examination still suggest mild depression. Using the recently introduced consultation item template, you refer to a psychiatrist for guidance in managing Caroline. The psychiatrist suggests a careful trial of lithium augmentation, providing advice about dosage and current best practice in regard to therapeutic monitoring.

A year later, you are regularly seeing Caroline every month or so, reviewing possible warning signs, and reinforcing some of her CBT strategies, including event scheduling for mastery and pleasure. She remains on venlafaxine and lithium; reports feeling well; is increasingly confident of keeping free of depressive relapse in the future; and is comfortable with seeing you every 1–2 months as well as seeing a psychiatrist once a year. In addition, because her freelance business is improving, she pays for a private session of psychological treatment about once a month.

CONCLUSION

The ideal format for GP shared care seems to be co-located and interdisciplinary, staffed by relatively senior competent clinicians who have already 'cut their teeth' on the mental health service system; a mixture of formal and informal communication processes; a strong central role for the GP in determining patterns of care in the context of consultation with patient, carer and other professionals involved; and a model of care that is appropriate to the local needs of GP, patient and community. Bureaucratic requirements, such as forms and protocols, need to be GP-friendly, and all processes need to be underpinned by shared understandings of lines of responsibility and accountability.

Although these ideals may be rarely attained in Australian practice, there is a great deal of scope for creating them if some prior investment of time is made, and if some ingenuity is employed in applying available funding schemes. Shared care models can now draw on a substantial accumulated body of practice within Australia. Where there is support and the active involvement of a local DGP and interested private and public sector clinicians, there is some cause for optimism about the development and sustainability of useful collaborative care arrangements.

REFERENCES

1. Meadows G, Singh B, Burgess P, Bobevski I. Psychiatry and the need for mental health care in Australia: findings from the National Survey of Mental Health and Wellbeing. Australian and New Zealand Journal of Psychiatry 2002;36:210–16.
2. Pirkis J, Burgess P, Meadows G, Dunt D. Access to Australian mental health care by people from non-English speaking backgrounds. Australian and New Zealand Journal of Psychiatry 2001; 35(2):174–82.
3. Palmer M. Inquiry into the Circumstances of the Detention of Cornelia Rau. Canberra: Commonwealth of Australia, 2005.
4. Australian health ministers. National Mental Health Plan. Canberra: Mental Health Branch, Commonwealth Department of Health and Family Services, 1992.
5. Australian health ministers. Second National Mental Health Plan. Canberra: Mental Health Branch, Commonwealth Department of Health and Family Services, 1998.
6. Australian health ministers. National Mental Health Plan 2003–2008. Canberra: Australian Government, 2003.
7. http://www.health.vic.gov.au/mentalhealth/publications/clipp/
8. Meadows G, Joubert L, Donoghue J, Keller N, Dobson G, Rippe M, Purtell C. CLIPP Manual. Victoria: Human Services Victoria, 2000.
9. Royal Australian College of General Practitioners and Royal Australian and New Zealand College of Psychiatrists. A Report of the Joint Consultative Committee. Primary Care Psychiatry—The Last Frontier. Canberra: Royal Australian College of General Practitioners and Royal Australian and New Zealand College of Psychiatrists, 1997.
10. Strathdee G. Psychiatrists in primary care: the general practitioner viewpoint. Family Practice 1988;5:111–15.

11. Katon W, Von Korff M, Lin E, Simon G, Walker E, Unutzer J, Bush T, Russo J, Ludman E. Stepped collaborative care for primary care patients with persistent symptoms of depression: a randomized trial. Archives of General Psychiatry 1995;56:1109–15.
12. Katon W, Von Korff M, Lin E, Walker E, Simon GE, Bush T, Robinson P, Russo J. Collaborative management to achieve treatment guidelines: impact on depression in primary care. Journal of the American Medical Association 1995;273:1026–31.
13. Kates N, Craven M, Crustolo AM, Nikolaou L, Allen C. Integrating mental health services within primary care: a Canadian program. General Hospital Psychiatry 1997;19:324–32.
14. Kates N, Craven M, Crustolo AM, Nikolaou L, Allen C, Farrar S. Sharing care: the psychiatrist in the family physician's office. Canadian Journal of Psychiatry 1997;42:960–5.
15. Kates N, Craven M, Bishop JF, Clinton TC, Kraftcheck DC, Leclair KF, Leverette JF, Nash LC, Turner TF. Shared mental health care in Canada. Supplement distributed with the Canadian Journal of Psychiatry 1997;42(8) and the Canadian Family Physician 1997;43.

INDEX